⁹⁹ᵐTc-Sestamibi

Jan Bucerius • Hojjat Ahmadzadehfar
Hans-Jürgen Biersack
Editors

^{99m}Tc-Sestamibi

Clinical Applications

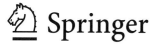

Editors

Priv.-Doz. Dr. med. Jan Bucerius
Department of Nuclear Medicine and
Cardiovascular Research Institute
Maastricht (CARIM)
Maastricht University Medical Center
P. Debyelaan 25
6229 HX Maastricht
The Netherlands
jan.bucerius@mumc.nl

Prof. Dr. med. Hans-Jürgen Biersack
Universitätsklinikum Bonn
Klinik und Poliklinik für Nuklearmedizin
Sigmund-Freud-Str. 25
53127 Bonn
Germany
hans-juergen.biersack@ukb.uni-bonn.de

Dr. med. Hojjat Ahmadzadehfar
Universitätsklinikum Bonn
Klinik und Poliklinik für Nuklearmedizin
Sigmund-Freud-Str. 25
53127 Bonn
Germany
hojjat.ahmadzadehfar@ukb.uni-bonn.de

ISBN 978-3-642-04232-4   e-ISBN 978-3-642-04233-1
DOI 10.1007/978-3-642-04233-1
Springer Heidelberg Dordrecht London New York

Library of Congress Control Number: 2011937232

© Springer-Verlag Berlin Heidelberg 2012

This work is subject to copyright. All rights are reserved, whether the whole or part of the material is concerned, specifically the rights of translation, reprinting, reuse of illustrations, recitation, broadcasting, reproduction on microfilm or in any other way, and storage in data banks. Duplication of this publication or parts thereof is permitted only under the provisions of the German Copyright Law of September 9, 1965, in its current version, and permission for use must always be obtained from Springer. Violations are liable to prosecution under the German Copyright Law.

The use of general descriptive names, registered names, trademarks, etc. in this publication does not imply, even in the absence of a specific statement, that such names are exempt from the relevant protective laws and regulations and therefore free for general use.

Product liability: The publishers cannot guarantee the accuracy of any information about dosage and application contained in this book. In every individual case the user must check such information by consulting the relevant literature.

Cover design: eStudioCalamar, Figueres/Berlin

Printed on acid-free paper

Springer is part of Springer Science+Business Media (www.springer.com)

Foreword

"The owl of Minerva spreads its wings only with the break of dusk"

Georg W.F. Hegel

This volume is uniquely dedicated to the applications of Technetium-99m Sestamibi scintigraphy. It presents an occasion to reflect on the remarkable career of this imaging radiotracer. Belonging to a family of compounds, the isonitriles, it has had a protean evolution.

This family of compounds was first evaluated as a lipophilic compound excreted by the liver into the biliary tract, as a hepatobiliary imaging agent for the evaluation of hepatobiliary excretion and evaluation of gallbladder function and integrity, at a time when that imaging modality was just developing, with the search for compounds with better imaging properties: high affinity, rapid liver transit and excretion. In the course of in vivo experiments, myocardial uptake was noticed. As further experiments revealed flow-dependent myocardial uptake, high affinity and long retention time, its utility as a myocardial perfusion agent became apparent. It would turn out to be of far greater utility, and for its developer, of far greater profit as a myocardial perfusion agent than as a hepatobiliary agent. The rest is history, but it did not have to be that way. Other tracers were promising as cardiac perfusion tracers in animal models, but did not succeed in humans due to inter-species differences in uptake or kinetics. The timing was also fortuitous. At the time, thallium-201 reigned supreme as a myocardial imaging agent. Thallium-201 offered, with one injection, the capability for stress perfusion imaging, the detection of ischemia versus myocardial scarring differentiation due to its redistribution property on delayed imaging, and information of myocardial viability, by virtue of its late redistribution. Its decay scheme produced principally low energy x-ray emissions, limiting image resolution. Its long half-life and decay scheme produced high radiation dosimetry per unit of activity, thus limiting the activity that could be administered with acceptable dosimetry. Thus, thallium-201 images were count-starved and of low resolution, stimulating the search for better tracers.

The development and marketing of Tc-99m sestamibi as a myocardial imaging agent came at a remarkable time, a conjunction of the development and widespread acceptance of SPECT imaging and the application of myocardial perfusion imaging, with thallium-201 paving the way, plus the development of coronary angioplasty, which made the localization of coronary disease important, and the development of non-exercise requiring stress methods, the vasodilator agents dipyridamole and adenosine, dobutamine, and their successors. Without such a conjuction, it is hard to imagine the meteoric success of sestamibi, both in its clinical utilization, and economic volume.

It is said that success breeds success. The success of myocardial perfusion imaging, driven by sestamibi and its competitors, Tc-99m tetrofosmin and thallium, then drove development of SPECT instrumentation and software, in reconstruction, display, and quantification, multiheaded gamma cameras, and more recently, attenuation correction hardware and software, and even hybrid SPECT-CT imaging, combining myocardial perfusion imaging with coronary calcium measurement and coronary angiography. This combination of events, made in heaven, has resulted in myocardial perfusion imaging accounting for some 50% of nuclear medicine imaging.

Early in its myocardial perfusion agent career, sestamibi faced a question of "identity". Was it a "perfusion agent" or a "viability agent"? The first question was easily answered early on in situations of mild to moderate coronary disease severity. In situations of severe myocardial hypoperfusion, sestamibi was shown to underestimate perfusion and viability. This prompted the use of protocols combing stress setamibi person imaging with resting thallium-201 imaging, or combination of F-18 FDG imaging, with SPECT or PET imaging. This question stimulated early research into the mechanisms of sestamibi cell uptake and retention, and the effects of various metabolic and pharmacologic interventions.

Attention turned to MIBI as a perfusion agent of other richly perfused tissues, such a skeletal muscle, in peripheral vascular disease, and uptake in metabolically active tissues, such a thyroid and parathyroid tissues. Pioneering work revealed the affinity to both types of tissue, and the fortuitous differential washout of thyroid and parathyroid tissues, led to sestamibi supplanting thallium-201, for the second time, this time in the detection and localization of parathyroid adenomas, again driven by a conjunction of sestamibi availability, SPECT and later SPECT-CT imaging, and the introduction of minimally-invasive surgery and requirement for pre-op localization.

The story of the evolution of the application of sestamibi was not finished yet. It was demonstrated that sestamibi had affinity not just for normal tissues, but malignant tumors as well. This led to its investigation in breast cancer, lung cancer, and a wide variety of other carcinomas and sarcomas. Limited resolution and the demand for high sensitivity limited an initial success as an adjunct to mammography in breast cancer screening 20 years ago, where the demand for differentiation of even small millimeter-sized tumors outstripped planar or SPECT imaging resolution. The career of sestamibi in lung and other tumors was eclipsed by the success of F-18 fluorodeoxyglucose PET imaging, owing to the remarkable affinity of FDG for tumors of all types, combined with the higher resolution of PET imaging. Sestamibi imaging is making a remarkable come-back with the introduction of dedicated small detectors and solid state technology, that allow the close proximity of the detector to breast tumors, not achievable 20 years ago, that allow the detection of tumors of even a few millimeters, of great value in women with high density breasts, where differentiation of malignant breast tumors from glandular or fibrous tissue is difficult.

The retention of sestamibi in tissue has been found to depend not only on perfusion, uptake and mitochondrial binding, but also on transport of the tracer out of tissue cells. In a number of tumors, the mechanism responsible for transport of sestamibi out the cells is also responsible for the transport of a number of various chemotherapeutic agents, which in turn limits their cytotoxicity, thus limiting their effectiveness, a property that various from individual to individual, that even evolves in the course any particular individual's cancer. Thus, the retention of sestamibi in a particular tumor is an index of its sensitivity to these cytotoxic drugs. This property has not yet found a place in routine clinical treatment of cancer, although its potential in individualized care has been suggested. As this volume shows, applications in other tumors offer intriguing possibilities.

The protean nature of Tc-99m sestamibi and its evolution as a radiotracer of many interesting properties, demonstrates its utility as a valuable tracer with multiple demonstrated and potential applications, whose full utility still remains to be developed, or even to be discovered.

Director, Division of Nuclear Medicine   Josef Machac, MD
The Mount Sinai Medical Center
New York, NY

Preface

Hexakis-2-methoxy-2-methylpropyl-isontrile technetium-99m (^{99m}Tc-Sestamibi) is a single photon emission computed tomography (SPECT-) radiotracer which was firstly introduced to clinical routine in nuclear medicine for myocardial perfusion imaging more than two decades ago. Since that time, several different, non-cardiac applications of ^{99m}Tc-Sestamibi have been reported in the literature although its main application still remains the imaging of myocardial perfusion. It was as early as 1989, that benign and malignant lung tumors were depicted by abnormal uptake of ^{99m}Tc-Sestamibi. Subsequently, further clinical studies have been performed in several oncologic (e.g., brain-, breast-, thyroid cancer) but also in non-oncologic diseases (e.g., thyroid adenoma, parathyroid adenomas). These manifold applications make ^{99m}Tc-Sestamibi an interesting radiotracer in the clinical as well as the out-patient setting even despite the fast-growing diffusion of ^{18}F-fluorodeoxyglucose positron emission tomography (FDG-PET) as an accepted and well-proven imaging technique for several oncologic and non-oncologic diseases.

"^{99m}Tc-Sestamibi - Clinical Applications" aims to provide an overview of almost all oncologic and non-oncologic applications of ^{99m}Tc-Sestamibi including several rather rare indications. It includes not only different disease-related protocols of the tracer but also a comprehensive summary of the pathology and epidemiology of the accordant disease. Thereby, a strong emphasis was set on practical aspects of the use of this widespread SPECT-tracer including instructions for the preparation of several commercially available tracer kits.

Jan Bucerius
Hojjat Ahmadzadehfar
Hans-Jürgen Biersack

Contents

1 Radiochemistry and Radiopharmacy of the SPECT-Tracer Technetium-99m-Hexakis-2-methoxy-2-isobutyl isonitrile (99mTc-Sestamibi) 1
Stefan Guhlke

2 Physics and Radiation Exposure 7
Mark Konijnenberg

3 Preparation of Tc-99m-Sestamibi 25
Hojjat Ahmadzadehfar and Amir Sabet

4 Parathyroid Imaging 31
Hans-Jürgen Biersack and Ursula Heiden

5 Myocardial Perfusion Scintigraphy with 99mTc-MIBI 65
Hojjat Ahmadzadehfar and Amir Sabet

6 99mTc-Sestamibi Scintimammography 87
Jan Bucerius

7 Tc-99m-MIBI for Thyroid Imaging 133
Matthias Schmidt

8 Tc-99m Sestamibi in Miscellaneous Tumors 159
Amir Sabet

9 Oncologic Applications of Sestamibi: *In Vivo* Imaging of Multi-Drug Resistance 175
Ali Gholamrezanezhad

Index 191

Radiochemistry and Radiopharmacy of the SPECT-Tracer Technetium-[99m]-Hexakis-2-methoxy-2-isobutyl isonitrile (^{99m}Tc-Sestamibi)

1

Stefan Guhlke

1.1 Introduction

In modern pharmaceutical development and medicine, radioactivity has increasing impact in the field of diagnostic applications (*in vitro* and *in vivo*) as well as in therapeutic applications [1, 2]. Even though nuclear medicines diagnostic procedures using PET or PET/CT-technology have gained increasing importance over the past decade, still about 70% or even more of all diagnostic scans are performed using technetium-99[m] (^{99m}Tc) labelled radiopharmaceuticals.

Regarding these different forms of applications, radiopharmaceuticals have to be used with respect to their modes of decay. For SPECT, radiopharmaceuticals labelled with isotopes of short (hours to some days) half-life and accompanying gamma emission in the range of 70–250 keV, are most useful. In addition, emission of only one photon per decay is of advantage, but not a must. The gamma emission has to be strong enough to easily penetrate the body barrier and also has to be well detectable by the common SPECT camera systems. Such radionuclides are commonly found among those with the decay mode of electron capture (EC) or internal conversion (IC) and especially Tc-99m fulfils these demands almost ideally.

1.2 [99m]Tc

[99m]Tc decays with a half-life of 6.0 h by isomeric transition to [99g]Tc, thereby emitting a single photon with an energy of 141 keV. This energy almost ideally meets the sensitivity maximum of SPECT camera systems. In addition, the rich complex chemistry of technetium allows incorporation of the radio isotope into a wide variety of ligands stabilising the radionuclide at different oxidation states. Hundreds of

---

S. Guhlke
Department of Nuclear Medicine,
University of Bonn, Bonn, Germany
e-mail: stefan.guhlke@ukb.uni-bonn.de

J. Bucerius et al. (eds.), *[99m]Tc-Sestamibi*,
DOI 10.1007/978-3-642-04233-1_1, © Springer-Verlag Berlin Heidelberg 2012

radiopharmaceuticals labelled with ^{99m}Tc have been developed and some have gained significant market success. However, the main reason for the special role of technetium in SPECT is probably the cost effectiveness and the on-demand availability of the isotope through the ^{99}Mo/^{99m}Tc-generator system [3–5].

The transitional metal technetium (element 43) is located in the seventh group of the periodic chart between the elements manganese and rhenium. All technetium isotopes are radioactive and therefore this element is naturally not present in the earth's crust. It has to be prepared technically by man (this lead to the name 'technetium') and this of course delayed the chemical development of technetium until the respective technology was available. As with manganese and rhenium, oxidation states between +7 and −1 are possible and complexes at all of these oxidation states are known. However, their stability greatly differs and therefore in radiopharmaceuticals the oxidation states + V and + I are dominant.

The basis for all technetium labelled radiopharmaceuticals is the pertechnetate anion ($[^{99m}$Tc]TcO$_4^-$) which is eluted from a commercial ^{99m}Tc-generator. The pertechnetate ion itself (oxidation state (+7)) is quite stable and rather inert to any complex chemistry. In order to form ^{99m}Tc-labelled organic molecules, it is therefore necessary to reduce the pertechnetate anion to a lower oxidation state being reactive towards chelating structures [6–8].

A variety of reducing agents might be used, however stannous(II) ions are used in most cases, especially in commercial kit preparations.

1.3 Development of Tc-99m-Labelled Imaging Agents for the Heart

Among the imaging agents for the heart, for many years the thallium-201 cation has played a dominating role. As surrogate for the potassium cation (K$^+$), it is taken up by the myocard via Na$^+$/K$^+$ ATPase pump system [9]. However, because of the high price of the nuclide and some suboptimal physiological properties, intense research was started with the goal of finding a heart imaging agent on the basis of the highly available Tc-99m.

Earlier studies employing phosphine and arsine complexes of technetium(III) (technetium with the oxidation state +3) had already suggested that cationic species are taken up by the heart to some extent, but unfavourable results in human trials showed that this rather labile oxidation state led to only poor uptake and low retention in the myocard [10]. Thus, a different approach was needed. Tc(I) complexes of the general formula [TcL6]$^+$ were thought to offer high potential as the oxidation state +1 was known to form highly stable technetium complexes and their monocationic form might be recognised by myocardial cells.

Jones et al. [11] studied a variety of isonitrile ligands with various linear and branched alkyl chain moieties and found t-butylisonitrile to be a ligand with rather high heart uptake in animals.

1984 Holman et al. [12] published initial experience in humans using this compound named Tc-99mTBI (Tc-99m-hexakis-t-butylisonitrile) and found it to be a

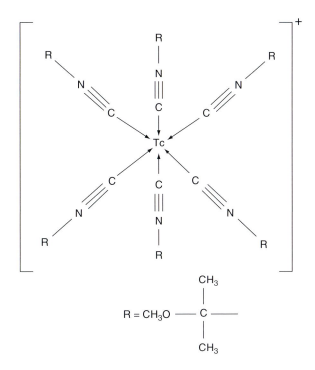

Fig. 1.1 The myocardial perfusion agent ^{99m}Tc-sestamibi as example for a cationic hexameric monoligand complex

promising myocardial imaging agent. However, its high lung and liver uptake and rapid redistribution precluded evaluation of patients during stress. In 1987, again Holman et al. [13] published another progress on using a modified isonitrile ligand bearing an ether group within the isonitrile ligand. The new ligand carboxymethylisopropylisonitrile (CPI) in technetium labelled form named as Tc-99m CPI offered much better results and appeared to have excellent physical and biological properties for use in association with myocardial imaging even with exercise. Further refinement of the isonitrile ligand finally resulted in the development of 2-methoxy-isobutylisonitrile named Tc-99m MIBI (Fig. 1.1) in its radiolabelled form. In 1986, McKusick et al. [14] compared TBI, CPI and MIBI in a preliminary publication for detecting ischaemic heart disease in humans. MIBI showed the highest initial image contrast due to better myocardial uptake and less lung and liver activity. Since then Tc-99m-MIBI was studied intensively in human trials [15] and still remains the Tc-99m heart imaging agent of choice.

Among many other newly developed ^{99m}Tc-agents with useful properties for myocardial imaging (namely, ^{99m}Tc-complexes with teboroxime, Q12-furifosmin, N-NOET) only ^{99m}Tc-tetrofosmin became also a generally accepted radiopharmaceutical for cardiac imaging. It is easy to prepare at room temperature using commercially available Myoview™ labelling kits. Compared to ^{99m}Tc-sestamibi, it may be considered as a 'me-too' radiopharmaceutical with similar or identical indications. Its later introduction in clinical practice might explain its lower popularity. Nevertheless, ^{99m}Tc-tetrofosmin was developed only 3 years later [16] and has some

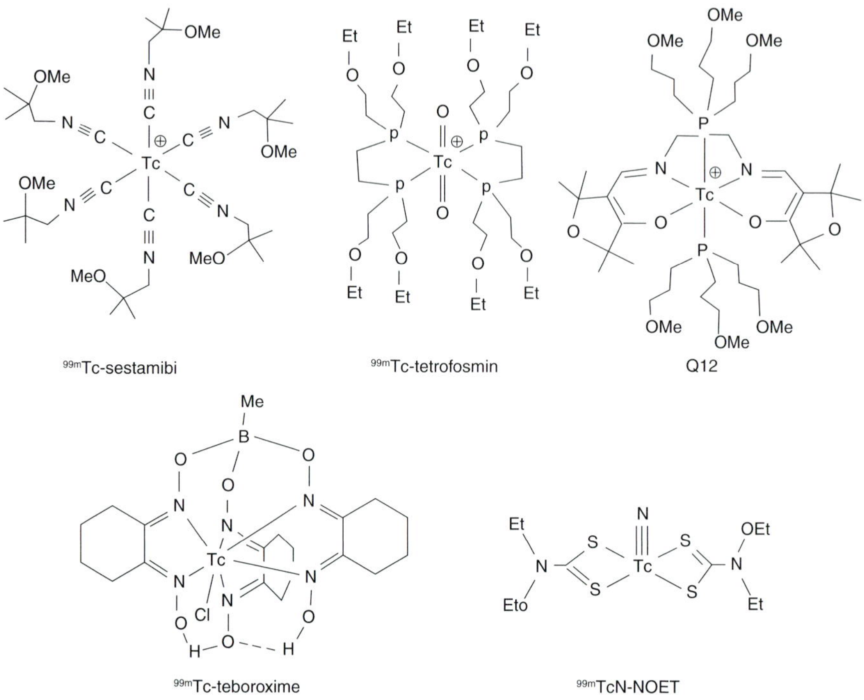

Fig. 1.2 Structures of Tc-99m MIBI and some other selected Tc-99m labelled myocardial imaging agents

more favourable characteristics: a higher myocardial uptake and higher heart-to-liver activity ratio in clinical studies at rest and in addition it can be prepared at room temperature as compared to a required boiling step for ^{99m}Tc-sestamibi. Apparently, nuclear medicine physicians adhere to a radiopharmaceutical that provides them with clinically useful images and information.

1.4 Radiolabelling and Quality Control of Tc-99m-Sestamibi

Monoligands such as isonitriles play an important role especially in more recent attempts to develop Tc-99m-labelled SPECT tracers in the oxidation state +1. The most prominent example among commercially successful tracers is the Tc-99m MIBI complex of which the structure can be seen in Fig. 1.2. The radiopharmaceuticle is used under the trade name Cardiolite™.

Six single isonitrile molecules (as monoligand) bind to one Tc(I) atom. As the isonitrile ligand by itself is volatile and stench, a copper adduct is used as precursor in the commercial labelling kit. Therefore, an exchange labelling with heating is required. The preparation is performed by adding 1–3 mL of TcO_4^- solution (up to 5.5 GBq) to the lyophilised terakis-(2-methoxyisobutylisonitrile)copper

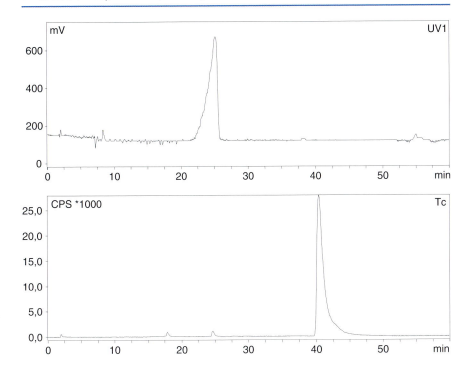

Fig. 1.3 HPLC-chromatogram of Tc-99m-Sestamibi. Chromatography conditions: The column used in the shown chromatogram was a LiChrospher 100 RP-18 EC (250×4 mm) with a particle size of 5 μm (CS-Chromatograpie, Germany). A linear gradient was performed over 60 min starting from 100% aqueous solution (0.1% TFA) to 100% organic solution (acetonitrile): The Tc-99m MIBI complex is eluted at about 40 min. The low intensity UV-peak at approximately 25 min represents the Cu-MIBI precursor

(I)-tetrafluoroborate adduct and stannous chloride used as reducing agent. The mixture is heated at 100°C for 10 min and cooled to be ready for injection.

According to the manufacturer, the quality control is performed by placing a small drop of the QC-sample to the start line of a chromatography strip (Aluminium oxide; Baker-Flex 1B-F) and developed in ethanol. The radiochemical yield is determined by cutting the strip into origin and front halves of which the activity found on the front half represents the Tc-99m MIBI complex. The QC can also be performed by using a radio-HPLC system using reversed phase columns such as C-18 and gradient elution. A sample chromatogram is shown in Fig. 1.3.

References

1. Qaim SM, Coenen HH (2005) Reactors and cyclotrons. Pharmaceutical production of relevant radionuclides. Pharm Unserer Zeit 34(6):460–466

2. Stöcklin G, Qaim SM, Rösch F (1995) The impact of radioactivity on medicine. Radiochim Acta 70/71:249–272
3. Tucker WD, Greene MW, Weiss AJ, Murrenhoff A (1958) Methods of preparation of some carrier-free radioisotopes involving sorption on alumina. Report BNL-3746. Annu. Meet. Am. Nucl. Sot., Los Angeles, Calif. Trans. Am. Nucl. Sot., 1. 160
4. Scadden EM, Ballow NE (1960) The radiochemistry of Molybdenum. Report NAS-NS 3009
5. Molinski VJ (1982) A review of 99mTc generator technology. Znt J Appl Radiat Isot 33:811–819
6. Schwochau K (1994) Technetium radiopharmaceuticals: fundamentals, synthesis, structure and development. Angew Chem Int Ed 33(22):2258–2267
7. Verbruggen AM, De Roo MJK (1992) Renal radiopharmaceuticals. In: Nunn AD (ed) Radio-pharmaceuticals: chemistry and pharmacology. Marcel Dekker, NY, p 365
8. Steigman J, Eckelman WC (1992) The chemistry of technetium in medicine, National Research Council. National Academy Press, Washington, DC
9. Atkins HL, Budinger TF, Lebowitz E, Ansari AN, Greene MW, Fairchild RG, Ellis KJ (1977) Thallium-201 for medical use. Human distribution and physical imaging properties. J Nucl Med 18(2):133–140
10. Deutsch E, Glavan KA, Sodd VJ, Nishiyama H, Ferguson DL, Lukes SJ (1981) Cationic Tc-99m complexes as potential myocardial imaging agents. J Nucl Med 22(10):897–907
11. Jones AG, Abrams MJ, Davison A, Brodack JW, Toothaker AK, Adelstein SJ, Kassis AI (1984) Biological studies of a new class of technetium complexes: the hexakis(alkylisonitrile) technetium(I) cations. Int J Nucl Med Biol 11:225–234
12. Holman BL, Jones AG, Lister-James J, Davison A, Abrams MJ, Kirshenbaum JM, Tumeh SS, English RJ (1984) A new Tc-99m-labeled myocardial imaging agent, hexakis(t-butylisonitrile)-technetium(I) [Tc-99m TBI]: initial experience in the human. J Nucl Med 25(12):1350–1355
13. Holman BL, Sporn V, Jones AG, Sia ST, Perez-Balino N, Davison A, Lister-James J, Kronauge JF, Mitta AE, Camin LL (1987) Myocardial imaging with technetium-99m CPI: initial experience in the human. J Nucl Med 28(1):13–18
14. McKusick KA, Holman LB, Rigo P, Sporn V, Jones AG, Davison A, Dupras G, Taillefer R (1986) Human myocardial imaging with 99mTc-Isonitriles. Circulation 74:296, abstr
15. Taillefer R, Laflamme L, Dupras G, Picard M, Phaneuf DC, Léveillé J (1988) Myocardial perfusion imaging with ^{99m}Tc-methoxy-isobutyl-isonitrile (MIBI); Comparison of short and long time intervals between rest and stress injections. Preliminary results. Eur J Nucl Med 13(10):515–522
16. Higley B, Smith FW, Smith T, Gemmell HG, Das Gupta P, Gvozdanovic DV, Graham D, Hinge D, Davidson J, Lahiri A (1993) Technetium-99m-1,2-bis[bis(2-ethoxyethyl)phosphino]eth-ane: human biodistribution, dosimetry and safety of a new myocardial perfusion imaging agent. J Nucl Med 34(1):30–38

Physics and Radiation Exposure

2

Mark Konijnenberg

2.1 Set-Up Chapter

^{99m}Tc radiation physics, imaging principles, and standard protocol
Traditional dosimetry ^{99m}Tc MIBI, effective dose + dose to gall bladder, etc.
Additional dose by CT in SPECT/CT
Comparison to other myocardial imaging procedures
Consequences of dose and justification of high dose versus benefit
Physical developments, scatter correction, attenuation correction, resolution improvement, smallest lesions, faster acquisition before liver uptake

2.1.1 Radiation Physics ^{99m}Tc-Decay and Imaging Principles

Technetium is an element with only unstable isotopes, although the ground state ^{99}Tc with a decay half-life of 211,100 years can almost be considered to be stable. With the decay of Molybdenum-99 in a ^{99}Mo-^{99m}Tc generator the meta-stable ^{99m}Tc is formed, which is an isomeric state of ^{99}Tc (see the decay chart in Fig. 2.1). This isomeric state decays to its ground state ^{99}Tc with a half-life of 6.015 h. In 89% of all decays, a gamma-ray is released with an energy of 140.5 keV. This gamma-photon is used for imaging of the distribution of the ^{99m}Tc labeled MIBI inside the patient with a gamma camera. In the decay, not only gamma-rays are emitted but also X-rays, low-energy Auger and internal conversion electrons and ^{99}Tc itself decays with the emission of beta-rays. The abundance and energy of each decay

---

M. Konijnenberg
Erasmus MC, Nuclear Medicine Department,
Rotterdam, The Netherlands
e-mail: m.konijnenberg@erasmusmc.nl

J. Bucerius et al. (eds.), ^{99m}Tc-Sestamibi,
DOI 10.1007/978-3-642-04233-1_2, © Springer-Verlag Berlin Heidelberg 2012

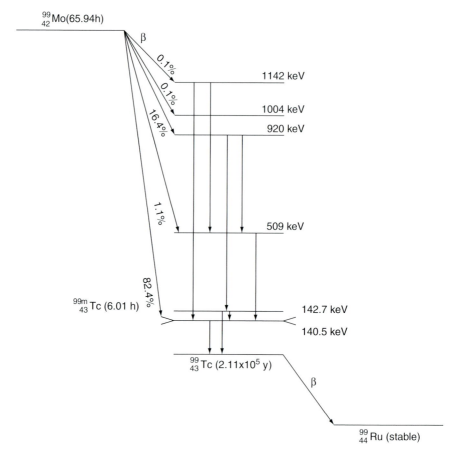

Fig. 2.1 Decay scheme of ^{99}Mo, 82.4% decays to the 142.7 keV level of the metastable ^{99m}Tc which decays to the 140.5 keV level through internal conversion with a half-life of 6.01 h and this level almost immediately decays to the ground state of ^{99}Tc under the emission of 140 keV gamma-rays. By contributions from other levels 89.1% is accumulated in the 142.7 keV ^{99m}Tc level and emits the 140.5 keV gamma-ray

emission is indicated in Table 2.1. The electrons and beta-rays do not interfere with the image quality of the ^{99m}Tc-scan, but do have an influence on the radiation dosimetry of ^{99m}Tc-labeled radiopharmaceuticals.

Imaging of radioactivity uptake patterns in patients after injection of ^{99m}Tc MIBI is performed with the Anger scintillation camera or simply gamma camera, its schematic principle is shown in Fig. 2.2. When the gamma camera is orbited around the patient, 3-dimensional (3-D) tomographic images can be made of the gamma-rays emitted and hence it is called single photon emission gamma camera tomography, or SPECT for short. Several features in radiation transport physics influence the quality and possibilities of the SPECT imaging which are briefly listed here:

2 Physics and Radiation Exposure

Table 2.1 Radiation characteristics of ^{99m}Tc with a half-life of 6.015 h

Radiation	Energy (keV)	Intensity (%/decay)
Conversion electron M	1.6286	74.595
Auger electron L	2.17	10.32
Auger electron K	15.5	2.05
Conversion electron K	119.5	8.84
Conversion electron K	121.6	0.55
Conversion electron L	137.5	1.07
Conversion electron L	139.6	0.172
Conversion electron M	140.0	0.194
Conversion electron NP	140.4	0.0374
Conversion electron M	142.1	0.034
Conversion electron NP	142.6	0.0066
X-ray L	2.42	0.447
X-ray Kα2	18.25	2.14
X-ray Kα1	18.37	4.07
X-ray Kβ3	20.60	0.330
X-ray Kβ1	20.62	0.639
X-ray Kβ2	21.01	0.145
γ-ray	140.511	89.06
γ-ray	142.63	0.0187

2.1.2 Attenuation

Attenuation of the 140 keV gamma-rays in the body distorts the image. Source regions with more or denser tissue in the path to the detector show more attenuation of the gamma-rays than shallower lying source regions. Several methods have been developed for correction of attenuation in the patient's body. The most simple method is by estimating the thickness of tissue d through which the photons travel and correcting the raw image data I(d) with the exponential equation $I(d) = I_0 e^{-\mu d}$. The linear attenuation coefficient μ for 140 keV gamma-rays in water is: 0.15/cm. The attenuation can be simulated by using a phantom with comparable dimensions of the region of interest and various layers of tissue-like material for attenuation. This method applies well for a source within a homogeneous medium.

In reality, however, patient bodies hardly resemble phantoms and especially the heart region with normal density myocardium surrounded by regions with high density as spine, low density lung, and intermediate density breasts, is hardly like the homogeneous phantom. The attenuation correction cannot be expressed by a constant μ factor. Transmission sources can be used to measure the transmission and thus attenuation map along the field of view in the SPECT system. Transmission scans (TCT) and X-ray CT imaging are capable of producing 3-D maps of the attenuation (μ-map) in each voxel of the SPECT image and thus provide patient-specific attenuation correction. SPECT/CT systems are therefore increasingly used. When a low current setting is used for the CT imaging it is possible to obtain a good μ-map at reasonably low patient dose [1].

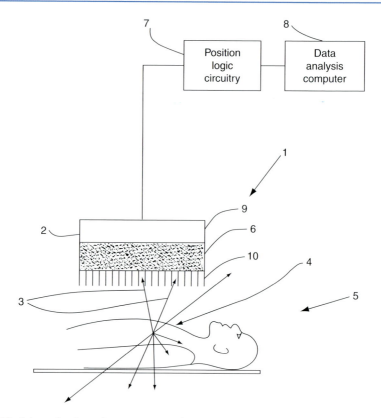

Fig. 2.2 Schematic view of gamma-camera imaging of the gamma-ray emissions (*3*) coming from the myocardiac regions. The gamma-rays that pass through the collimator (*10*), generate light pulses in the scintillation crystal (*6*, usually NaI), which is amplified and transformed into an electronic signal by the photomultiplier tube (*9*), which signal is then used to determine the source position. When the detector is used at different angles around the patient a 3-D image of the emission distribution can be made

2.1.3 Scatter

Scattering of the gamma-rays in the patient not only creates widening of the measured 140 keV energy spectrum, but also scattering from sources neighboring the myocardium, like from the liver, can cause counts within the myocardium region of interest. Apart from scattering in the body, scatter can also occur in the collimator and detector system. Both types of scatter cause deterioration of image resolution. Scatter correction can be solved by using either multiple energy windows on the measured ^{99m}Tc spectrum to determine the scatter component in the signal empirically [2–4]. The other possibility is to use the µ-map and the geometry of the scanner system together with the uncorrected SPECT activity distribution in a Monte Carlo model [5]. This Monte Carlo model can calculate from scatter theory the scatter and photo peak signal contributions in each ROI, as

2 Physics and Radiation Exposure

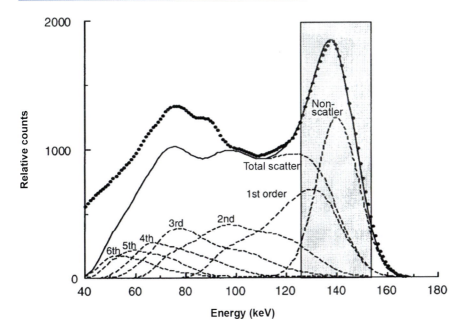

Fig. 2.3 Energy spectrum for the 140 keV ^{99m}Tc line source on the axis of a water-filled cylinder simulated using the Monte Carlo method. The spectrum due to primary and scattered photons (*solid line*) is separated into different contributions (total scattering or different orders of photon scattering). The experimentally measured spectrum is also shown (*dots*)

shown in Fig. 2.3 [6]. It was found that the field of view of the CT scanner should be larger than that of the SPECT camera, as regions outside may cause scatter effects inside its field of view.

2.1.4 Resolution and Partial Volume Effect

The limited spatial resolution of SPECT imaging cameras (for ^{99m}Tc in the order of 4 mm) causes serious blurring of the images. For large organs, in comparison to the spatial resolution, this is not really a problem as the signal measured is formed by equilibrium between gamma-rays scattering in and those scattering out of the central region. At the edges of these large regions and in finite regions, however, this equilibrium will not exist and distortions of the image, as shown in Fig. 2.4, will be the result. Filtering of the signal to control the noise tends to even enhance this partial volume effect. The lower uptake values in the inferior LV wall can be attributed to this liver-heart artifact [7]. Correction of this partial volume effect involves the use of CT anatomical information in a Monte Carlo code to determine the spill in and out, but it is prone to induce false-negative results when a real perfusion defect occurs in the inferior wall [8]. Corrections for attenuation, scatter, and partial volume effects are invaluable when myocardial imaging is not only used for qualitative

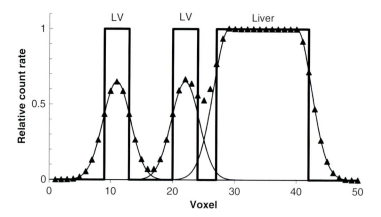

Fig. 2.4 Partial volume effect by small (just three voxels wide) left ventricle (*LV*) region next to liver. The *rectangular blocks* show the theoretical activity distribution over liver and LV myocardium. The *dashed curves* show the spill out from each source region due to scatter and limited resolution. In the four voxel thick LV region, partial coverage of these voxels lowers the detector response

diagnosis of possible perfusion defects, but also to measure the magnitude of myocardial perfusion quantitatively.

2.1.5 Radiation Dosimetry of ^{99m}Tc MIBI

Myocardial perfusion imaging is the medical imaging procedure with the largest radiation dose to the patient, both on individual basis and on patient-population averaged effective dose per person [9]. The reason it is positioned so high on this list is that the majority of the myocardial imaging procedures in the patient group considered was performed with ^{201}Tl, which is known to have a high effective dose of 0.14 mSv/MBq in the adult [21], which leads to a mean dose of 16 mSv at the maximum injected activity of 111 MBq. When all myocardial perfusion imaging would have been performed with ^{99m}Tc MIBI still this procedure would remain in the top contributor segment for annual effective dose together with CT imaging. Theoretically, this high effective dose could cause excess cancer deaths by the radiation, although the individual risk for fatal cancer may be low (approximately 0.02% for a 15 mSv dose given to a 40-year or older patient), when considered over a large patient population the numbers of induced cancers can be substantial [10].

The risk for induction of cancer is assumed to follow a linear relation with the dose given, although it has never been proven below a dose of 100 mSv. This linear no-threshold model for induction of fatal cancer predicts an excess risk of fatal cancer of 0.005% per person per mSv. Still the benefit of the perfusion imaging outweighs the increased risk of cancer induction, as was analyzed by Zanzonico and Stabin for ^{201}Tl [11]. They stated that 24 mSv by ^{201}Tl myocardial perfusion imaging would induce fatal cancer in 11 patients over the US heart patient

2 Physics and Radiation Exposure   13

population, but the procedure would save 109 lives per year by considerably reducing the chance of myocardial infarction during vascular surgery. The net benefit of myocardial perfusion imaging with ^{201}Tl is 98 lives saved per year. When a ^{99m}Tc heart agent would have been used with an effective dose of 15 mSv, the net benefit would rise to 102 lives saved. This clearly makes the high effective dose by myocardial perfusion imaging justifiable, although the ALARA (as low as reasonably achievable) principle in health physics would favor the use of ^{99m}Tc heart perfusion agents instead of ^{201}Tl.

2.2   Biokinitic of ^{99m}Tc MIBI

The biokinetic model is summarized in ICRP 80 and based on papers published by Wackers et al. [12], Leide et al. [13] and Boström et al. [14].

MIBI is accumulated in viable myocardial tissue in proportion to regional blood flow, in a manner similar to thallous chloride. After intravenous injection, the substance is rapidly cleared from the blood and taken up predominantly in muscular tissues (including heart). It is accumulated and excreted by liver and kidneys, with a smaller amount; also, an uptake in the salivary glands and thyroid occurs. Other organs and tissues show a low uptake with a uniform distribution. The principal metabolic pathway for excretion is via the hepatobiliary system to the gastrointestinal tract, with some additional excretion via the kidneys. The major part of injected substance is excreted within 48 h [19].

During the first 60 min after an injection in a resting patient, marked accumulation of Sestamibi is present in the liver and spleen; nevertheless, the heart is as well visualized. In conjunction with a stress test, less uptake in the liver and spleen can be observed with a considerable increase of uptake in heart and skeletal muscles. No redistribution takes place, and there is no evidence of any metabolism of the substance [12, 19]. Substantial excretion in the gallbladder was noted both after exercise and at rest, reaching a maximum at circa 1 h after injection.

2.3   Blood Clearance

Pre- and post-exercise blood decay using clearance curves were measured by Wackers et al. [12].

During rest, at 30 s after injection, blood activity is $22 \pm 18\%$ of injected activity (IA). Maximal activity of $36 \pm 18\%$ of IA was noted at 1 min after injection. Blood activity subsequently decreased to $23 \pm 0.9\%$ of IA at 3 min, $9 \pm 0.6\%$ at 5 min, and $2.5 \pm 0.3\%$ of IA at 10 min after injection. After this time, MIBI blood clearance continues to decrease slowly. At 60 min, $0.8 \pm 0.02\%$ of IA are reached, at 2 h $0.5 \pm 0.03\%$ of IA, at 4 h p.i. At 24 h, blood activity was $0.3 \pm 0.004\%$ of IA. Curve fitting through the data shows that in rest mibi clears bi-exponentially from the blood: $41.9 \pm 0.1\%$ with a clearance half-life of 1.37 ± 0.03 min and $1.28 \pm 0.05\%$

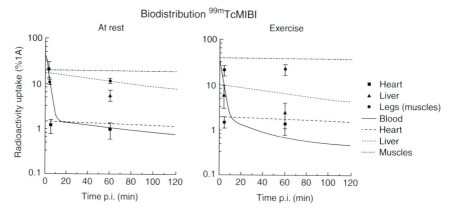

Fig. 2.5 Biodistribution patterns for ^{99m}Tc MIBI injected at rest and injected under peak stress exercise. The data points for heart, liver, and legs were taken from Wackers et al [12]. The blood curves were fitted through the blood data from Wackers. The *curves* for heart, liver, and muscle were taken from ICRP80 [19] and are substantially higher than the data

with a half-life of 88 ± 9 min. These values are different from the curves presented by Wackers. There it was claimed that the fast clearance component proceeds with 2.18 min effective half-life, whereas the curve presented indicated a 19 s half-life (Fig. 2.5).

During exercise, maximal MIBI blood activity (51 ± 28% of IA) was measured at 0.5 min. Blood activity decreased over the following minutes, reaching a level of 11 ± 4% of IA at 4 min, 6.5 ± 2.9% of IA at 5 min, and 2.6 ± 1% of IA at 10 min after injection. Thereafter, blood pool activity continued to decrease slowly: 1.1 ± 0.1% of IA at 30 min, 0.7 ± 0.1% of IA at 1 h, 0.4 ± 0.2% of IA at 4 h, and 0.3 ± 0.3% of IA at 24 h after injection. The blood clearance with exercise proceeds with 3 compartments: 58 ± 36% with a clearance half-life of 1.5 ± 0.5 min, 1.8 ± 0.9% with $T_{1/2} = 22 \pm 16$ min, and 0.44 ± 0.10% with $T_{1/2} = 41$ h. Again, this blood curve differs from the curve originally presented.

2.4 Upper-Body Organ Distribution

Under resting conditions, initially, the highest MIBI concentration was in gallbladder and liver, followed in decreasing order of activity per pixel, by heart, spleen, and lungs. Decay corrected MIBI activity in spleen and lung decreased gradually over time, whereas MIBI activity in the heart remained relatively stable. At 3 h after injection 27 ± 4% of initial activity had cleared from the heart, whereas 67 ± 12%, 76 ± 4%, and 49 ± 4% had, respectively, cleared from spleen, liver, and lungs. Within the first 30–60 min, liver activity decreased with excretion into the biliary system, maximal accumulation in the gallbladder occurred at approximately 60 min p.i. Consequently, since no significant redistribution of MIBI occurs, with regard to laboratory logistics and patient flow, a convenient and practical time for imaging is approximately 1 h after injection. However, with increasing time interval between injection and scan, the relative visualization of the heart will continue to improve.

During exercise, immediately after injection, the highest concentration of MIBI was in the gallbladder, followed by heart, liver, spleen, and lungs. Again, the cardiac, pulmonary, and spleen activity gradually decreased over time. Hepatic activity decreased more rapidly due to excretion in the biliary system. By 3 h after injection, $26 \pm 12\%$ of initial cardiac activity had cleared: at this time, $65 \pm 7\%$ had cleared from the liver, $43 \pm 21\%$ from the spleen, and $39 \pm 10\%$ from the lungs. The count density within the heart was higher than in the immediately adjacent organs. Only the gallbladder had higher count density.

A pharmacokinetic compartment model for ^{99m}Tc MIBI is unfortunately missing. This would support more clearly the additional compartment found in the blood clearance with exercise. Also, the liver uptake kinetics would be better described, thus giving better arguments for doing early myocardial uptake scanning with high speed czt detectors [15]. These experiments indicate that the uptake in the liver proceeds much slower than the myocardial uptake, thus creating an early opportunity for imaging, contrary to the traditional scanning time a half to 1 h after injection.

2.5 Heart-to-Organ Ratios

Wackers et al. (1989) have summarized the heart/liver, heart/lung, and heart/spleen ratios in humans after 5 up to 180 min post injection. For example, the 60 min ratios increased from 0.6 ± 0.1 (rest) to 1.8 ± 0.3 (exercise) for heart and liver, these figures were 2.4 ± 0.1 (rest and exercise) for heart/lung, and 1.3 ± 0.3 (rest) and 2.5 ± 0.3 (exercise) for the heart/spleen ratio.

The data for organ dosimetry were summarized in ICRP 80 and in the paper published by Wackers et al. (1989): in general, organ dosimetry was determined from whole body images by expressing specific organ uptake as percent of injected dose. The 24-h urinary excretion was 29.5% of IA at rest and 24.1% of IA after exercise. The 48-h fecal excretion was 36.9% of IA at rest and 29.1% of ID after exercise.

According to Leide et al. (1992), there is a significant difference in the biodistribution of MIBI between stress and rest for the following tissues: muscle tissue, thyroid, gall bladder, and remaining tissues. The activity content in the small intestine, upper large intestine, and lower large intestine also differs between stress and rest. Since the uptake in the muscle tissue is lower at rest compared to stress, the substance reaches the GI-tract earlier at rest than stress. That is why the content in ULI (upper large intestine) is higher 6 h after injection at rest than stress. It is the same reason why the content in ULI at 24 h is lower at rest. By then the substance has already reached the LLI (lower large intestine).

In conclusion, it can be summarized, that the major metabolic pathway for clearance of Sestamibi is the hepatobiliary system. Activity from the gallbladder appears in the intestine within 1 h of injection (after exercise and at rest). About 27% of the ID is cleared through renal elimination after 24 h and approximately 33% of the ID is cleared through the feces in 48 h.

2.6   Radiation Dosimetry

The effect of radiation exposure in tissue can be expressed by the absorbed dose. Absorbed dose D is defined as the mean absorbed energy $\bar{E}$ in a target region or organ coming from a source region, divided by the mass m of the target organ:

$$D = \frac{dE\left(\text{target} \leftarrow \text{source}\right)}{dm_{\text{target}}}$$

The unit of the dose is J/kg or Gray [Gy], in older literature the unit rad is used for dose with the conversion 1 rad=0.01 Gy. In radionuclide dosimetry the convention to calculate the absorbed dose is by the MIRD-formalism. It makes a division between the kinetics of the radiopharmaceutical distribution and the static part of absorption of the radionuclide's specific energy from source to target combination. The dose rate $\dot{D}(t)$ per activity A, both as function of time t, for a source-to-target combination can be written as:

$$\frac{\dot{D}(t)}{A(t)} = \frac{k\sum_i y_i E_i \varphi_i \left(target \leftarrow source\right)}{m_{target}} = S\left(target \leftarrow source\right)$$

With k a conversion factor from MeV/g to Gy

$$(\text{usually } k=0.16022 \; \frac{mGy}{MBq.s} / \frac{MeV}{g.decay} \; \text{is used}),$$

y_i is the yield per decay of gamma-rays with energy E_i (for ^{99m}Tc see Table 2.1) and ϕ_i is the absorbed fraction of energy in the target organ for a gamma-ray with energy E_i coming from the source organ. The kinetic part of the equation is on the left side, and the static physics part, specific for the radionuclide of interest, is on the right side of the equation. For diagnostically used radionuclides, this physics part, often called S-value or absorbed dose factor, is calculated for reference stylized phantom models, like the MIRD phantoms, with Monte Carlo radiation transport codes. Several dosimetry codes exist that provide S-values for all conventionally used radionuclides and all possible source-to-target organ combinations, like Olinda/EXM [16]. Dosimetry for therapeutic use should be based on patient-specific geometry and not on phantom models.

The kinetic part of the dose rate equation is solved by using the biokinetic distribution of the radiopharmaceutical. The total number of decays that yield an absorbed gamma-ray in the target organ is calculated by integration of the time-activity curve multiplied with the S-value:

$$D = \int_0^\infty A(t)e^{-\lambda t} dt \times S\left(target \leftarrow source\right) = \tilde{A}_{target} \times S\left(target \leftarrow source\right)$$

2 Physics and Radiation Exposure

Table 2.2 Tissue weighting factors w_T for calculating the effective dose, according to ICRP publications 60 [18] and 103 [20]

Tissue	Tissue weighting factor, w_T		
	ICRP26	ICRP60	ICRP103
Bone surfaces	0.03	0.01	0.01
Bladder		0.05	0.04
Brain			0.01
Breast	0.15	0.05	0.12
Colon		0.12	0.12
Gonads	0.25	0.20	0.08
Liver		0.05	0.04
Lungs	0.12	0.12	0.12
Eesophagus		0.05	0.04
Red bone marrow	0.12	0.12	0.12
Salivary glands			0.01
Skin		0.01	0.01
Stomach		0.12	0.12
Thyroid	0.03	0.05	0.04
Remainder	0.3	0.05	0.12
Total	1.0	1.0	1.0

With λ the decay constant of the radionuclide (for ^{99m}Tc: $\lambda = \ln(2)/6.015 = 0.1152/h$), when $A(t)$ is the decay corrected time-activity curve, and $\tilde{A}$ the cumulated activity in a source organ. Often the cumulated activity per injected activity ($\tilde{A}/IA$) is indicated as organ residence time τ. The advantage of this division into kinetic and static part is that the dosimetry can easily be updated with improved calculational models for the static part. The limitations of this model, however, show up when the activity is heterogeneously distributed over the source organ, or when the source and target organ are variable in size, like a rapidly growing tumor.

To enable dose comparisons of different radiation exposures, specifically meant for radiation protection and dose limits for health physics in radiation work situation, the effective dose has been introduced by the ICRP [18]. The effective dose E is a weighted mean organ dose, with weights w_T assigned to each organ expressing its radiosensitivity for induction of fatal cancer or genetic damage:

$$E = \sum_T w_T \sum_R w_R D_{T,R}$$

With w_T the organ or tissue weighting factors, listed in Table 2.2, expressing the relative risk for late radiation effects in these tissues, and w_R the radiation weighting factor, which is 1 for all low LET radiation like gamma-rays and beta-particles, expressing the relative risk associated with high LET radiation. For ^{99m}Tc, therefore, only the first summation over the weighted organ doses D_T is of relevance, as $w_R = 1$ for all LET radiation. The unit for effective dose is the Sievert, or Sv. In older literature rem is used instead of Sv (with 1 rem = 0.01 Sv). Also the definition of effective dose has changed with increasing knowledge of tissue radiosensitivities. With tissue weighting factors according to ICRP26 [17], effective dose equivalents were defined. Although the differences for ^{99m}Tc MIBI are not large, care should be taken in comparing equally defined effective doses.

The radiation dosimetry for ^{99m}Tc MIBI is based on the evaluation in ICRP publication 80 [19]. The biokinetic model is based on the old work by Wackers and by Leide et al. As already shown in the paragraph on biodistribution of MIBI, these reports could be much improved and the dose values given can therefore be taken as approximate values, mere estimates of the dose magnitude. The dose tables indicate dose estimates for each organ and the effective dose according to ICRP60. The effective dose indicates the weighted average organ dose, with weights indicating the susceptibility of each separate organ to radiation-induced cancer. The effective dose is a tool to enable comparisons between different types of radiation exposure, especially in health physics. The newer organ weights from ICRP publication 103 do not alter the effective dose for ^{99m}Tc MIBI significantly [22].

The maximum dose is reached in the gallbladder, both for the rest and the exercise studies (Tables 2.3 & 2.4). Also, the kidneys and colon get higher doses than average. In comparison to the effective dose per activity by ^{201}Tl of 0.14 mSv/MBq, with the highest organ dose in the kidneys (0.48 mGy/MBq), ^{99m}Tc MIBI has a 15-fold lower dose (ICRP publication 106 2008). For that reason ^{201}Tl is used at much lower activities than ^{99m}Tc MIBI: typically 75 MBq for a stress test instead of 1,000 MBq ^{99m}Tc MIBI used. The effective dose from 75 MBq ^{201}Tl is 11 mSv, whereas 1,000 MBq ^{99m}Tc MIBI gives an effective dose of 8 mSv. The doses to each organ for a rest study with 500 MBq ^{99m}Tc MIBI and an exercise study with 1,000 Mbq ^{99m}Tc MIBI (1-day protocol) are given in Tables 2.5 and 2.6.

Although the dose tables suggest that the pediatric doses are known, it is in reality the result of using unchanged adult biokinetics to children in child-size calculational phantoms. No studies were made to confirm that the biodistribution of ^{99m}Tc MIBI in children is equal to the adult situation. Qualitatively, however, no differences have been observed between adult and pediatric myocardial uptake. The recommended activities for ^{99m}Tc MIBI show huge variations in dose reference levels for each country. To make a comparison possible, the maximum activity in clinical practice is taken as example: a 1-day protocol with 500 MBq ^{99m}Tc MIBI at rest and then 1,000 MBq ^{99m}Tc MIBI in an exercise test. These activities are for an adult. The EANM pediatrics committee published recommendations for the dosage of radiopharmaceuticals in children [23]. For ^{99m}Tc MIBI the minimum activity is 80 MBq and the baseline activity for a rest test is 28 MBq and for a stress test it is 84 MBq. These baseline activities must be multiplied with body weight-dependent multiples. The pediatric injected activities in Tables 2.5 and 2.6 were calculated accordingly, using the MIRD phantom body weights of 57, 33, 20, and 10 kg for a 15-, 10-, 5-, and 1-year-old, respectively. The weight of the adult (male) phantom is 74 kg and is conservatively chosen, as the dose is inversely proportional with the weight.

With multimodality imaging, the patients will also receive an additional radiation dose from the other imaging modality, when based on radiation of course. With SPECT/CT imaging low-dose setting of the CT-imaging can be used when the CT image is intended for attenuation correction, then the additional effective dose will be in the order of 0.4–0.9 mSv [1]. When the CT image is to be used for

2 Physics and Radiation Exposure

Table 2.3 Radiation dosimetry table for ^{99m}Tc MIBI in a resting subject from ICRP80 [19]

Dose per activity (mGy/MBq)	Adult	15 years	10 years	5 years	1 year
Adrenals	0.0075	0.0099	0.015	0.022	0.038
Bladder	0.011	0.014	0.019	0.023	0.041
Bone surfaces	0.0082	0.01	0.016	0.021	0.038
Brain	0.0052	0.0071	0.011	0.016	0.027
Breast	0.0038	0.0053	0.0071	0.011	0.02
Gall bladder	0.039	0.045	0.058	0.1	0.32
GI tract					
Stomach	0.0065	0.009	0.015	0.021	0.035
SI	0.015	0.018	0.029	0.045	0.08
Colon	0.024	0.031	0.05	0.079	0.15
Heart	0.0063	0.0082	0.012	0.018	0.03
Kidneys	0.036	0.043	0.059	0.085	0.15
Liver	0.011	0.014	0.021	0.03	0.052
Lungs	0.0046	0.0064	0.0097	0.014	0.025
Muscles	0.0029	0.0037	0.0054	0.0076	0.014
Eesophagus	0.0041	0.0057	0.0086	0.013	0.023
Ovaries	0.0091	0.012	0.018	0.025	0.045
Pancreas	0.0077	0.01	0.016	0.024	0.039
Red marrow	0.0055	0.0071	0.011	0.03	0.044
Salivary glands	0.014	0.017	0.022	0.015	0.026
Skin	0.0031	0.0041	0.0064	0.0098	0.019
Spleen	0.0065	0.0086	0.014	0.02	0.034
Testes	0.0038	0.005	0.0075	0.011	0.021
Thymus	0.0041	0.0057	0.0086	0.013	0.023
Thyroid	0.0053	0.0079	0.012	0.024	0.045
Uterus	0.0078	0.01	0.015	0.022	0.038
Remaining organs	0.0031	0.0039	0.006	0.0088	0.016
Effective dose (mSv/MBq)	0.0090	0.012	0.018	0.028	0.053

The absorbed dose per unit administered activity is given for different age groups, as well as the effective dose [18]

high-resolution CT imaging of the Coronary Arteries (CTCA) effective doses around 15–20 mSv have been reported with high current 64-slice CTCA (A Einstein 2007). Using ECG-controlled current modulation and by adequately adjusting the tube current to the patient's size, high-resolution CTCA can be performed at doses between 5 and 10 mSv. Especially, the effective dose by CT imaging of young children is of great concern [24], but by using appropriate camera setting it is possible to obtain good quality CT scans in children with minimally a 74% reduction in chest doses to around 5 mGy [25].

Combination of 600 MBq ^{99m}Tc MIBI stress test with 185 MBq ^{18}F FDG delivers an effective dose of 8.3 mSv (4.7 mSv from ^{99m}Tc MIBI and 3.5 mSv from ^{18}F FDG [21]) to the adult patient. When combined with CT the total effective dose to this patient will be 13 mSv. Doses from other PET and SPECT radionuclide myocardial perfusion agents are compared in Table 2.7.

Table 2.4 Radiation dosimetry table for ^{99m}Tc MIBI injected at peak stress from ICRP80 [19]

Dose per activity (mGy/MBq)	Adult	15 years	10 years	5 years	1 year
Adrenals	0.0066	0.0087	0.013	0.019	0.033
Bladder	0.0098	0.013	0.017	0.021	0.038
Bone surfaces	0.0078	0.0097	0.014	0.02	0.036
Brain	0.0044	0.006	0.0093	0.014	0.023
Breast	0.0034	0.0047	0.0062	0.0097	0.018
Gall bladder	0.033	0.038	0.049	0.086	0.26
GI tract					
Stomach	0.0059	0.0081	0.013	0.019	0.032
Small intestine	0.012	0.015	0.024	0.037	0.066
Colon	0.019	0.025	0.041	0.064	0.12
Heart	0.0072	0.0094	0.01	0.021	0.035
Kidneys	0.026	0.032	0.044	0.063	0.11
Liver	0.0092	0.012	0.018	0.025	0.044
Lungs	0.0044	0.006	0.0087	0.013	0.023
Muscles	0.0032	0.0041	0.006	0.009	0.017
Esophagus	0.004	0.0055	0.008	0.012	0.023
Ovaries	0.0081	0.011	0.015	0.023	0.04
Pancreas	0.0069	0.0091	0.014	0.021	0.035
Red marrow	0.005	0.0064	0.0095	0.013	0.023
Salivary glands	0.0092	0.011	0.0015	0.002	0.0029
Skin	0.0029	0.0037	0.0058	0.009	0.017
Spleen	0.0058	0.0076	0.012	0.017	0.03
Testes	0.0037	0.0048	0.0071	0.011	0.02
Thymus	0.004	0.0055	0.008	0.012	0.023
Thyroid	0.0044	0.0064	0.0099	0.019	0.035
Uterus	0.0072	0.0093	0.014	0.02	0.035
Remaining organs	0.0033	0.0043	0.0064	0.0098	0.018
Effective dose (mSv/MBq)	0.0079	0.010	0.016	0.023	0.045

The dose per unit administered activity is given for different age groups, as well as the effective dose [18]

2 Physics and Radiation Exposure

Table 2.5 Radiation doses for ^{99m}Tc MIBI procedures in a resting subject

Injected activity (MBq):	500	336	204	136	80
Dose per procedure (mGy):	Adult	15 years	10 years	5 years	1 year
Adrenals	3.8	3.3	3.1	3.0	3.0
Bladder	5.5	4.7	3.9	3.1	3.3
Bone surfaces	4.1	3.4	3.3	2.9	3.0
Brain	2.6	2.4	2.2	2.2	2.2
Breast	1.9	1.8	1.4	1.5	1.6
Gall bladder	20	15	12	14	26
GI tract					
Stomach	3.3	3.0	3.1	2.9	2.8
Small intestine	7.5	6.0	5.9	6.1	6.4
Colon	12	10	10	11	12
Heart	3.2	2.8	2.4	2.4	2.4
Kidneys	18	14	12	12	12
Liver	5.5	4.7	4.3	4.1	4.2
Lungs	2.3	2.2	2.0	1.9	2.0
Muscles	1.5	1.2	1.1	1.0	1.1
Esophagus	2.1	1.9	1.8	1.8	1.8
Ovaries	4.6	4.0	3.7	3.4	3.6
Pancreas	3.9	3.4	3.3	3.3	3.1
Red marrow	2.8	2.4	2.2	4.1	3.5
Salivary glands	7.0	5.7	4.5	2.0	2.1
Skin	1.6	1.4	1.3	1.3	1.5
Spleen	3.3	2.9	2.9	2.7	2.7
Testes	1.9	1.7	1.5	1.5	1.7
Thymus	2.1	1.9	1.8	1.8	1.8
Thyroid	2.7	2.7	2.4	3.3	3.6
Uterus	3.9	3.4	3.1	3.0	3.0
Remaining organs	1.6	1.3	1.2	1.2	1.3
Effective dose (mSv)	4.5	4.0	3.7	3.8	4.2

The absorbed dose and administered activity is given for different age groups, as well as the effective dose [18]

Table 2.6 Radiation doses for ^{99m}Tc MIBI procedures in stress tests

Injected activity (MBq):	1,000	1,000	612	408	228
Dose per procedure (mGy):	Adult	15 years	10 years	5 years	1 year
Adrenals	6.6	8.7	8.0	7.8	7.5
Bladder	9.8	13	10	8.6	8.7
Bone Surfaces	7.8	9.7	8.6	8.2	8.2
Brain	4.4	6.0	5.7	5.7	5.2
Breast	3.4	4.7	3.8	4.0	4.1
Gall bladder	33	38	30	35	59
GI tract					
Stomach	5.9	8.1	8.0	7.8	7.3
Small intestine	12	15	15	15	15
Colon	19	25	25	26	27
Heart	7.2	9.4	6.1	8.6	8.0
Kidneys	26	32	27	26	25
Liver	9.2	12	11	10	10
Lungs	4.4	6.0	5.3	5.3	5.2
Muscles	3.2	4.1	3.7	3.7	3.9
Esophagus	4.0	5.5	4.9	4.9	5.2
Ovaries	8.1	11	9.2	9.4	9.1
Pancreas	6.9	9.1	8.6	8.6	8.0
Red marrow	5.0	6.4	5.8	5.3	5.2
Salivary glands	9.2	11	0.9	0.8	0.7
Skin	2.9	3.7	3.6	3.7	3.9
Spleen	5.8	7.6	7.3	6.9	6.8
Testes	3.7	4.8	4.3	4.5	4.6
Thymus	4.0	5.5	4.9	4.9	5.2
Thyroid	4.4	6.4	6.1	7.8	8.0
Uterus	7.2	9.3	8.6	8.2	8.0
Remaining organs	3.3	4.3	3.9	4.0	4.1
Effective dose (mSv)	7.9	10	9.8	9.4	10

The absorbed dose and administered activity is given for different age groups, as well as the effective dose [18]

Table 2.7 Dose estimates for myocardial perfusion imaging with radiopharmaceuticals

Radiopharmaceutical	IA rest (MBq)	IA stress (MBq)	Effective dose (mSv)
^{99m}Tc MIBI	500	1,000	12.4
^{99m}Tc Tetrofosmin	500	1,000	10.4
^{201}Tl		75	10.5
^{99m}Tc MIBI + ^{201}Tl SDI	500 MBq ^{99m}Tc MIBI	75 MBq ^{201}Tl	14.5
^{82}Rb	1,500	1,500	10.2
^{13}N Ammonia	500	500	2.0
^{15}O Water	1,100	1,100	2.4
^{18}F FDG	275		5.2

2.7 Radiation Exposure from Myocardial Perfusion Agents

The staff in a nuclear medicine department will be inevitably exposed to the radiation coming from the patients. The exposure rates from patients have been worked out by several authors [26, 27]. Per ^{99m}Tc MIBI procedure with an injected activity of 740 MBq at mean dose to the nuclear medicine technician of 1.7 ± 1.0 µSv was measured. With 500 MBq ^{18}F FDG, the dose to the technician is higher 5.9 ± 1.2 µSv. In a PET center handling ^{18}F FDG, ^{13}N Ammonia, and ^{11}C labeled compounds, the average dose to a technologist, handling 831 MBq activity per day, was measured to be 14 µSv.

Reference

1. Preuss R, Weise R, Lindner O, Fricke E, Fricke H, Burchert W (2008) Optimisation of protocol for low dose CT-derived attenuation correction in myocardial perfusion SPECT imaging. Eur J Nucl Med Mol Imaging 35:1133–1141. doi:10.1007/s00259-007-0680-2
2. Narayanan MV, Pretorius PH, Dahlberg ST (2003) Evaluation of scatter compensation strategies and their impact on human detection performance Tc-99m myocardial perfusion imaging. IEEE trans Nucl Sci 50:1522–1527
3. Gur YS, Farncombe TH, Pretorius PH (2002) Comparison of scatter compensation strategies for myocardial perfusion imaging using Tc-99m labeled Sestamibi. IEEE Trans Nucl Sci 49:2309–2314
4. Ogawa K, Harata Y, Ichihara T, Kubo A, Hashimoto S (1991) A practical method for position-dependent Compton-scatter correction in single photon emission CT. IEEE Trans Med Imaging 10:408–412. doi:10.1109/42.97591
5. Xiao J, de Wit TC, Staelens SG, Bezekman FJ (2006) Evaluation of 3D Monte Carlo-based scatter correction for 99mTc cardiac perfusion SPECT. J Nucl Med 47:1662–1669
6. Zaidi H, Koral KF (2004) Scatter modelling and compensation in emission tomography. Eur J Nucl Med Mol Imaging 31:761–782. doi:10.1007/s00259-004-1495-z
7. Nuyts J, Dupont P, Van den Maegdenbergh V, Vleugels S, Suetens P, Mortelmans L (1995) A study of the liver-heart artifact in emission tomography. J Nucl Med 36:133–139
8. Pretorius PH, King MA (2009) Diminishing the impact of the partial volume effect in cardiac SPECT perfusion imaging. Med Phys 36:105–115
9. Fazel R, Krumholz HM, Wang Y, Ross JS, Chen J, Ting HH, et al (2009) Exposure to low-dose ionizing radiation from medical imaging procedures. N Engl J Med 361:849–857. doi:10.1056/NEJMoa0901249
10. Sodickson A, Baeyens PF, Andriole KP, Prevedello LM, Nawfel RD, Hanson R, Khorasani R (2009) Recurrent CT, cumulative radiation exposure, and associated radiation-induced cancer risks from CT of adults. Radiology 251:175–184
11. Zanzonico P, Stabin M (2008) Benefits of medical radiation exposures. Health Phys Soc. Available at: http://hps.org/hpspublications/articles/Benefitsofmedradexposures.html. Accessed on January 1, 2009
12. Wackers FJ, Berman DS, Maddahi J, Watson DD, Beller GA, Strauss HW, et al (1989) Technetium-99m hexakis 2-methoxyisobutyl isonitrile: human biodistribution, dosimetry, safety, and preliminary comparison to thallium-201 for myocardial perfusion imaging. J Nucl Med 30:301–311
13. Leide S, Diemer H, Ahlgren L, et al (1992) In vivo distribution and dosimetry of Tc-99m MIBI in man. In: S-Stelson A, Watson EE (eds) Fifth International Radiopharmaceutical Dosimetry Symposium Conf-910529, Oak Ridge Asoociated Universities, Oak Ridge, TN, pp 483–497

14. Boström P-A, Diemer H, Leide S, Lilja B, Bergqvist D (1993) 99Tcm-Sestamibi uptake in the leg muscles and in the myocardium in patients with intermittent claudication. Angiology 44:971–976
15. Berman DS, Kang X, Tamarappoo B, Wolak A, Hayes SW, Nakazato R, Thomson LE, Kite F, Cohen I, Slomka PJ, Einstein AJ, Friedman JD (2009) Stress thallium-201/rest technetium-99m sequential dual isotope high-speed myocardial perfusion imaging. JACC Cardiovasc Imaging 2:273–282
16. Stabin MG, Sparks RB, Crowe E. (2005) OLINDA/EXM: the second-generation personal computer software for internal dose assessment in nuclear medicine. J Nucl Med 46: 1023–1027
17. ICRP Publication 26 (1977) Recommendations of the ICRP. Ann ICRP 1:3
18. ICRP Publication 60 (1991) The 1990 Recommendations of the International Commission on Radiological Protection, Ann ICRP 21, pp 1–3
19. ICRP Publication 80 (1998) Radiation dose to patients from radiopharmaceuticals (Addendum 2 to ICRP Publication 53). Ann ICRP 28:107–111
20. ICRP Publication 103 (2007) The 2007 Recommendations of the International Commission on Radiological Protection. Ann ICRP 37:2–4
21. ICRP Publication 106 (2008) Radiation dose to patients from radiopharmaceuticals. Addendum 3 to ICRP Publication 53. Ann ICRP 38:159–162
22. Einstein AJ, Moser KW, Thompson RC, Cerqueira MD, Henzlova MJ (2007) Radiation dose to patients from cardiac diagnostic imaging. Circulation 116:1290–1305. doi:10.1161/CIRCULATIONAHA.107.688101
23. Lassmann M, Biassoni L, Monsieurs M, Franzius C, Jacobs F (2007) The new EANM paediatric dosage card. Eur J Nucl Med Mol Imaging 34:796–798. doi:10.1007/s00259-007-0370-0
24. Brenner D, Elliston C, Hall E, Berdon W (2001) Estimated risks of radiation-induced fatal cancer from pediatric CT. AJR Am J Roentgenol 176:289–296
25. Singh S, Kalra MK, Moore MA, Shailam R, Liu B, Toth TL, Grant E, Westra SJ (2009) Dose reduction and compliance with pediatric CT protocols adapted to patient size, clinical indication, and number of prior studies. Radiology 252:200–208. doi:10.1148/radiol.2521081554
26. Chiesa C, De Sanctis V, Crippa F, Schiavini M, Fraigola CE, Bogni A, Pascali C, Decise D, Marchesini R, Bombardieri E (1997) Radiation dose to technicians per nuclear medicine procedure: comparison between technetium-99m, gallium-67, and iodine-131 radiotracers and fluorine-18 fluorodeoxyglucose. Eur J Nucl Med 24:1380–1389
27. Benatar NA, Cronin BF, O'Doherty MJ (2000) Radiation dose rates from patients undergoing PET: implications for technologists and waiting areas. Eur J Nucl Med 27:583–589

Preparation of Tc-99m-Sestamibi

3

Hojjat Ahmadzadehfar and Amir Sabet

3.1 Chemistry and Constituents

Tc-99m-sestamibi or hexakis (2-methoxyisobutyl isonitrile) technetium is a monovalent cation with a central Tc (I) core that is octahedrally surrounded by six identical lipophilic ligands coordinated through the isonitrile carbon. A vial of Tc-99m-sestamibi normally contains a sterile, nonpyrogenic, lyophilized mixture of 1.0 mg Tetrakis (2-methoxyisobutyl isonitrile) Copper (I), Tetrafluoroborate, Stannous Chloride Dihydrate, L-Cysteine Hydrochloride Monohydrate, Sodium citrate, Mannitol Hydrochloric acid, and Sodium hydroxide for pH-adjustment. Sestamibi is available to centers in multidose generator produced vials. The product can be stored at room temperature and has a shelf life of 2 years before preparation and only 10 h after preparation. Preparation includes a boiling step and takes about 15–20 min to complete as described later in this chapter.

3.2 Photon Energy

Tc-99m-sestamibi has a photon energy of 140 keV, which is optimal for scintillation camera imaging. With a standard symmetrical 20% photopeak, most scattered radiation is effectively eliminated.

H. Ahmadzadehfar (✉) • A. Sabet
Klinik und Poliklinik für Nuklearmedizin, Universität Bonn,
Sigmund-Freud- Straße 25, 53127 Bonn, Germany
e-mail: hojjat.ahmadzadehfar@ukb.uni-bonn.de; amir.sabet@ukb.uni-bonn.de

J. Bucerius et al. (eds.), ^{99m}Tc-Sestamibi,
DOI 10.1007/978-3-642-04233-1_3, © Springer-Verlag Berlin Heidelberg 2012

3.3 Organs at Risk for Tc-99m-sestamibi

The organs with the highest absorbed dose per unit administered activity (mGy/MBq) are the gall-bladder and the kidneys. A detailed description of radiation exposure to other organs could be found in package leaflets of Tc-99m-sestamibi.

3.4 Special Warning and Precautions for Use [1]

1. *Women of childbearing potential:* When it is necessary to administer radioactive products to women of childbearing potential, information should be sought about pregnancy. Any woman who has missed a period should be assumed to be pregnant until proven otherwise.
2. *Pregnancy:* Radionuclide procedures carried out on pregnant women also involve radiation dose to the fetus. Only imperative investigations should therefore be carried out during pregnancy, when the likely benefit far exceeds the risk incurred by the mother and fetus. An effective dose to fetus of 1 mSv should not be exceeded, unless clinically justified. However, it should be taken into consideration that any reduction in administered activity must not impact on the likelihood of achieving a diagnostic outcome.
3. *Lactation:* Before administering radiopharmaceutical to a mother who is breast feeding, consideration should be given as to whether the investigation could be reasonably delayed until after the mother has ceased breast feeding and as to whether the most appropriate choice of radiopharmaceuticals has been made, bearing in mind the secretion of activity in breast milk. If the administration is considered necessary, breast feeding should be interrupted for 24 h and the expressed feeds discarded. Close contact with infants should be restricted during this period.
4. Contents of the vial are intended only for use in the preparation of Technetium (99mTc) Sestamibi and are not to be administered directly to the patient without first undergoing the preparative procedure.
5. Because of potential tissue damage extravasal injection has to be strictly avoided.
6. In case of kidney failure, exposure to ionizing radiation can be increased. This must be taken into account when calculating the activity to be administered.
7. In patients with reduced hepatobiliary function, a very careful consideration is required since an increased radiation exposure is possible in these patients.
8. Proper hydration and frequent urination are necessary to reduce bladder irradiation.
9. If hypersensitivity or anaphylactoid reactions occur, the administration must be discontinued immediately and intravenous treatment initiated, if necessary. To enable immediate action in emergencies, the necessary medicinal products and equipment such as endotracheal tube and ventilator must be immediately available.

3 Preparation of Tc-99m-Sestamibi

3.5 Interaction with Other Medicinal Products and Other Forms of Interaction

No drug interactions have been described to date.

3.6 Effects on Ability to Drive and Use Machines

Tc-99m-sestamibi has no influence on the ability to drive and use machines.

3.7 Undesirable Effects [1]

For each patient, exposure to ionizing radiation must be justified on the basis of likely benefit, and the radiation dose should be kept as low as reasonably possible without affecting the intended diagnostic or therapeutic result. As investigations are generally performed with low radiation doses of less than 20 mSv, the adverse events are expected to occur with a very low probability. Higher doses may be justified in some clinical circumstances. Immediately after injection, a metallic or bitter taste, partly in combination with dry mouth and an alteration in the sense of smell may be observed very commonly. Otherwise, the other undesirable effects are very rare including anaphylactic shock (which could be lethal), seizure, dizziness, fatigue, transient headache, syncope, hypotension, dyspnea, flushing, non-itching rash, edema (including larynx edema and angio-edema), pruritus, urticaria (including maculopappular rash), fever, and injection site inflammation.

3.8 Overdosage

In the event of a potential radiation overdose, the absorbed dose to the patient should be reduced by increasing the elimination of the radionuclide from the body by frequent micturation and defecation.

3.9 Technical Aspects

3.9.1 Preparation

Boiling procedure [1]:

Preparation of Tc-99m-sestamibi from the TechneScan Sestamibi Kit is to be performed according to the following aseptic procedure:

1. Waterproof gloves should be worn during the preparation procedure. Remove the flip-off cap from the Technescan Sestamibi Kit vial and swab the top of the vial closure with alcohol to disinfect the surface.

2. Place the vial in a suitable radiation shield appropriately labeled with date, time of preparation, volume, and activity.
3. With a sterile shielded syringe, aseptically obtain additive-free, sterile, non-pyrogenic sodium pertechnetate (99mTc) solution max. 11.1 GBq in approximately 1–3 mL. Not more than 3 mL sodium pertechnetate (99mTc) solution will be used for the maximum activity of 11.1 GBq.
4. Aseptically add the sodium pertechnetate (99mTc) solution to the vial in the lead shield. Without withdrawing the needle, remove an equal volume of headspace to maintain atmospheric pressure within the vial.
5. Shake vigorously, about five to ten quick upward-downward motions.
6. Remove the vial from the lead shield and place upright in an appropriately shielded and contained boiling water bath, such that the vial is suspended above the bottom of the bath, and boil for 10 min. The bath must be shielded. Timing for the 10 min commences as soon as the water begins to boil again. Note: The vial must remain upright during the boiling step. Use a water bath where the stopper will be above the level of the water.
7. Remove the shielded vial from the water bath and allow cooling for 15 min.
8. Inspect visually for the absence of particulate matter and discoloration prior to administration.
9. If needed, a dilution with 0.9% saline solution is possible.
10. Aseptically withdraw material using a sterile shielded syringe. Use within 10 h of preparation.
11. Radiochemical purity should be checked prior to patient administration according to the Radio TLC Method as detailed below.

Note: the potential for cracking and significant contamination exists whenever vials containing radioactive material are heated.

Gagnon et al. [2] and Hung et al. [3] have proposed an alternative method for rapid preparation of Tc-99m-sestamibi using a microwave oven instead of the boiling water bath for labeling Tc-99m-sestamibi which has been shown to be safe and reliable.

The "heating" time was reduced from 10 min with the recommended "standard" method to 13 s with the microwave oven method. The authors have emphasized the need to follow the published specifications, otherwise the user must test the labeling procedure with the user's own microwave oven if the technical specifications differ. These specifications are very important, since the varying power output, microwave frequency, cavity dimensions, and cavity volume may have different impacts on the labeling procedure.

Radiochromatographic quality control methods revealed similar values for both labeling methods mentioned above with a very high labeling efficiency.

3.9.2 Quality Control [1]

The verification of radiochemical purity of Tc-99m-sestamibi is not always required prior to its administration to a patient. However, it is considered to be good radiopharmacy practice to ensure an injection with a radiopharmaceutical of the highest purity, safety, and efficacy. The recommended radiochromatographic procedure for the determination of radiochemical purity of Tc-99m-sestamibi involves the use of an aluminum oxide-coated (Baker-flex) plastic thin-layer chromatography plate with absolute ethanol as developing agent. One drop of ethanol is applied at 1.5 cm from the bottom of a dry plate and two drops of Tc-99m-sestamibi solution are added on top of the ethanol spot. Only the Tc-99m-sestamibi migrates with ethanol to the solvent front. It is not recommended to use Tc-99m-sestamibi if the radiochemical purity is less than 90%.

Similar to the recommended labeling preparation procedure, the recommended quality control is time consuming and needs to be significantly reduced in order to use Tc-99m-sestamibi for emergency purposes. Hung et al. [3] proposed the use of a mini-paper chromatography method. Despite producing similar results, the time for developing mini-paper chromatography strip has been shown to be only 2.3 min compared to 35 min for drying and developing the aluminum oxide-coated thin-layer chromatography plates. Thus, alternative methods could be used to rapidly prepare and perform the quality control of Tc-99m-sestamibi. However, the legal considerations of using these alternative methods should be judged and decided by each individual institution, based on local or federal regulations.

In the following we are describing the Radio-TLC method step by step:

3.10 Radio-TLC Method for the Quantification of Tc-99m-sestamibi

1. Materials
   (a) Baker-Flex-Aluminum Oxide plate, # 1 B-F, pre-cut to 2.5 cm × 7.5 cm.
   (b) Ethanol, >95%.
   (c) Capintec, or equivalent instrument for measuring radioactivity in the 0.74–11.12 GBq (20–300 mCi) range.
   (d) 1 mL syringe with a 22–26 gauge needle.
   (e) Small developing tank with cover (100 mL beaker covered with Parafilm is sufficient).
2. Procedure
   (a) Pour enough ethanol into the developing tank (beaker) to have a depth of 3–4 mm of solvent. Cover the tank (beaker) with Parafilm® and allow it to equilibrate for approximately 10 min.
   (b) Apply one drop of ethanol, using a 1 mL syringe with a 22–26 gauge needle on to the Aluminum Oxide TLC plate, 1.5 cm from the bottom. Do not allow the spot to dry.
   (c) Apply one drop of the kit solution on top of the ethanol spot. Dry the spot. Do not heat!
   (d) Develop the plate a distance of 5.0 cm from the spot.
   (e) Cut the strip 4.0 cm from the bottom, and measure each piece in your dose calibrator.
   (f) Calculate the% Radiochemical purity as:

% Tc-99m-sestamibi = (Activity top portion)/(Activity both pieces) × 100.
% Tc-99m-sestamibi should be >94%; otherwise the preparation should be discarded.

Note: Do not use material if the radiochemical purity is less than 94%.

Tc-99m-sestamibi is to be used within 10 h of reconstitution and the container and any unused contents should be disposed in accordance with local requirements for radioactive materials.

References

1. Le Petten BVMM (ed) Technescan sestamibi, summary of product characteristics, labelling and package leaflet
2. Gagnon A, Taillefer R, Bavaria G, Leveille J (1991) Fast labeling of technetium-99m-sestamibi with microwave oven heating. J Nucl Med Technol 19:90
3. Hung JC, Wilson ME, Brown ML, Gibbons RJ (1991) Rapid preparation and quality control method for technetium-99m-2-methoxy isobutyl isonitrile (technetium-99m-sestamibi). J Nucl Med 32:2162–2168

Parathyroid Imaging

4

Hans-Jürgen Biersack and Ursula Heiden

4.1 Introduction: Parathyroid Glands

The majority of humans have four parathyroid glands, which are located at the upper and lower pole of the thyroid gland. Approximately 3–6% have less than four glands, whereas approximately 5–13% have more than four parathyroids. The parathyroid glands are derived from the third (inferior parathyroid) and fourth (superior parathyroid) branchial pouches. The inferior parathyroid glands migrate caudally with the thymus and are more variable in their location. Ectopic glands are found between the carotid bifurcation and the anterior mediastinum and occur in 15–20% of cases. Parathyroid tissue may be located within the thyroid gland in about 8% of cases.

Parathyroid adenomas may degenerate and form cysts that may be functioning or nonfunctioning. Most of these cysts are located in the lower neck (70–80%) but can also occur in the mediastinum. On CT they may be isodense (high protein content) or reveal low-attenuation values (serous fluid content) with a thin smooth wall. An important diagnostic finding in some patients is the elevation of the parathyroid hormone level in the cyst fluid separating this type of cyst from a thyroid cyst.

Primary hyperparathyroidism (HPT) occurs in 100–200 people per 100,000, with a predilection for women. HPT is caused by a solitary parathyroid adenoma in 80–85% of cases, hyperplasia in 12–15%, multiple adenomas in 2–3%, and parathyroid carcinoma in less than 1% [1, 2]. In the past, chronically elevated calcium levels led to a variety of calcium-related pathologies including bone disease, renal calculi, and systemic symptoms of depression and fatigue. Today however, the

---

H.-J. Biersack (✉)
Klinik und Poliklinik für Nuklearmedizin, Universität Bonn,
Sigmund-Freud-Straße 25, 53127 Bonn, Germany
e-mail: hans-juergen.biersack@ukb.uni-bonn.de

U. Heiden
COVIDIEN Deutschland GmbH, Josef-Dietzgen-Straße 1,
53773 Hennef, Germany
e-mail: ursula.heiden@covidien.com

J. Bucerius et al. (eds.), *99mTc-Sestamibi*,
DOI 10.1007/978-3-642-04233-1_4, © Springer-Verlag Berlin Heidelberg 2012

majority of HPT is detected in asymptomatic patients on routine laboratory screening tests. Parathyroid adenomas range from 0.8 to 1.5 cm in length and between 500 and 1,000 mg in weight (normal weight 35–40 mg). Parathyroid adenomas are encountered most commonly at the superior and inferior poles of the thyroid. Ectopic parathyroid adenomas of the superior gland include a retroesophageal, posterior mediastinal, and intrathyroidal location, whereas ectopic adenomas of the inferior gland include superior mediastinum, thymus, and carotid sheath [2].

As already mentioned, the diagnosis of HPT is usually made on the basis of laboratory tests like (elevated) calcium and parathyroid hormone determination. As in the majority of cases, surgical procedures have to be performed, parathyroid imaging plays an important role in the follow-up of patients with this disease. Imaging procedures comprise ultrasound (US) of the neck, CT, MRI, and parathyroid scintigraphy. This overview deals mainly with parathyroid imaging using radioactive tracers.

4.2 Methods/Image Acquisition (Fig. 4.1)

4.2.1 Parathyroid Imaging: Subtraction and Dual-Tracer Technique

^{99m}Tc-Sestamibi (MIBI) parathyroid scintigraphy is a widely used method for the preoperative localization of hyperfunctional glands in hyperparathyroidic patients for more than 15 years. There are two imaging modalities: (1) subtraction procedure, which is used together with ^{99m}Tc-pertechnetate or ^{123}I, and (2) dual phase imaging procedure.

If the subtraction technique is used, either ^{99m}Tc-pertechnetate or ^{123}I can be given first, followed by ^{99m}Tc-Sestamibi, or ^{99m}Tc-Sestamibi can be given first, followed by ^{99m}Tc-pertechnetate. In case ^{123}I or ^{99m}Tc-pertechnetate is used as the first imaging agent, images are acquired 4 h or 10 min post injection, respectively. Then, Sestamibi is injected and images are obtained 10 min after administration. When ^{99m}Tc-pertechnetate is injected after Sestamibi images are obtained, the patient should be immobilized for 15–30 min after the ^{99m}Tc-pertechnetate injection, and then a 10-min image is acquired. In all cases, both sets of images are normalized to total thyroid counts and computer subtraction of ^{123}I or ^{99m}Tc-pertechnetate images from the Sestamibi images is obtained.

If the dual-phase technique is performed, ^{99m}Tc-Sestamibi is injected and the first images are obtained 10 min later; delayed images are obtained after 1.5–2.5 h p.i. According to the American Guidelines [3], there is no consensus regarding a preference of subtraction imaging versus dual-phase imaging.

Parathyroid scintigraphy was developed in the early 1980s with the introduction of the image subtraction method using ^{201}Thallium and ^{99m}Technetium [4]. One decade later, parathyroid scintigraphy became more common with the introduction of the dual-phase (single-tracer) technique using ^{99m}Tc-Sestamibi [5].

4 Parathyroid Imaging

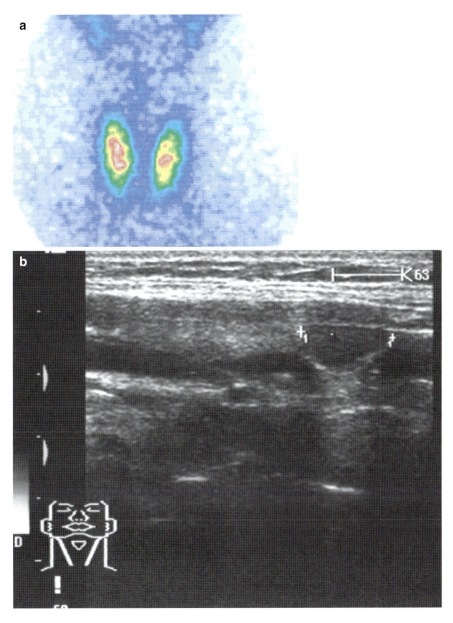

Fig. 4.1 Parathyroid adenoma. (**a**) Thyroid scan with Tc-99m pertechnetate. (**b, c**) Ultrasound with lesion below the right lower pole. (**d**) Delayed MIBI scan with parathyroid adenoma right

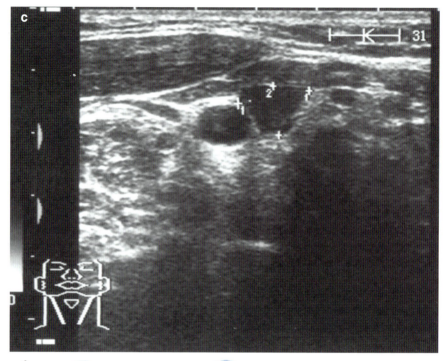

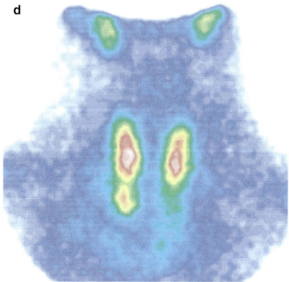

Fig. 4.1 (continued)

4 Parathyroid Imaging

The subtraction technique with Sestamibi was first described by Coakley et al. in 1989 [6] and O'Doherty et al. in 1992 [7]. The protocol was based on the use of ^{123}I as the thyroid agent: first, oral administration of 20 MBq ^{123}I, 4 h later acquisition of a 5-min thyroid scan, and then iv injection of 200 MBq of ^{99m}Tc-Sestamibi followed by a dynamic acquisition. A total of 57 patients have been investigated using this method in the above-mentioned study, and sensitivities of 98% for parathyroid adenoma, and of 55% for hyperplasia were found; no false-positive results due to the presence of nodular goitre were recorded. Although parathyroid scintigraphy is a widely used method in patients with hyperparathyroidism, it has to be taken into account that there are some limitations, in particular because it does not allow the specific evaluation of the thyroid gland [8]. Another criterion of the subtraction technique is that the washout of tracer from adenomas may be variable [8, 9]. The presence of parathyroid adenomas with rapid ^{99m}Tc-Sestamibi wash-out – similar to that of thyroid tissue – can cause false-negative results as reported by some authors [10]; some adenomas will show washout of tracer by 2–2.5 h, and therefore may not be obvious on the delayed images.

Hindie et al. [11] have proposed an improvement of the subtraction technique using ^{123}I as the "thyroid" agent: iv injection of 10 MBq ^{123}I, and 2–4 h later an iv injection of 550 MBq of ^{99m}Tc-Sestamibi, the patient is then positioned under the gamma camera and both tracers are acquired simultaneously [11]. The major advantage of this technique is that by acquiring ^{123}I scan and Sestamibi simultaneously, motion artefacts are avoided. Due to some disadvantages of [123]I (no daily availability, costs, after ^{123}I administration a prolonged time of 2–4 h is required to obtain a constant count rate from the thyroid) a dual-tracer protocol was developed by the Italian task group by Rubello et al. in the early 1990s [12]. By using a modified $^{99m}TcO_4/^{99m}Tc$-Sestamibi-protocol, which includes the oral administration of potassium perchlorate to cause rapid $^{99m}TcO_4$ washout from the thyroid gland and additional neck ultrasound in the same session as scintigraphy, a global sensitivity of 98% in a group of 114 patients with a solitary parathyroid adenoma can be obtained. Moreover, in spite of a coexistence of a nodular goitre in 27% of the patients, all nodular thyroid diseases were correctly diagnosed on the basis of the $^{99m}TcO_4$ and/or US imaging [13].

O'Doherty et al. [7] compared ^{99m}Tc-Sestamibi with ^{201}Tl preoperatively. Out of 40 adenomas, 37 were localized with ^{201}Tl, and 39 with Sestamibi. Although uptake of Thallium was higher in both the parathyroid and thyroid tissue than Sestamibi, the uptake per gram of parathyroid tissue of Sestamibi was higher than the uptake per gram of thyroid tissue. This could not be found with Thallium. This investigation stimulated the use of the Sestamibi-procedure and parathyroid imaging. As already mentioned, the double-phase Sestamibi scintigraphy technique became popular in the late nineties [14]. Nevertheless, the pertechnetate plus perchlorate/ Sestamibi-subtraction scintigraphy proved to be a fast and effective technique [12]. During the last years, the double phase protocol with early (10 min) and delayed (120 min) imaging is now being used at many institutions [15].

This review shows clearly that two technical procedures are recommended for parathyroid imaging: (a) double phase and (b) subtraction ($^{99m}Tc/$ or ^{123}I) technique. This is in accordance with the SNM-guideline [9].

Table 4.1 Sensitivity of SPECT

First author	Year	No/pts	Activity (MBq)	Sensitivity (%)	SPECT
Billotey [16]	1996	43	400–750	Planar 86%	90.5%
Moka [17]	2000	92	740	Planar 87%	95% (preoperative)
Lorberboym [18]	2003	52	740	Planar 79%	96% (preoperative)
Profanter [19]	2004	24	370	CT/MIBI image fusion 93%	50% (preoperative)
Fukumoto [20]	2004	MIBI SPECT			
Schachter [21]	2004	82	740	Planar 78%	96% (preoperative)
Krausz [22]	2006	36	555	SPECT/CT facilitates surgical procedure in 42%	91%

4.2.2 SPECT for Sestamibi Parathyroid Scintigraphy

Since more than 10 years now, SPECT has been added to planar Sestamibi-scintigraphy in HPT. Table 4.1 presents an overview regarding the sensitivity of SPECT [16] obtained Sestamibi scintigrams including SPECT before surgery in 43 patients suffering from HPT. SPECT raised the sensitivity from 86% to 90.5% and from 79.5% to 87% in re-operated patients. Similar findings were published by Moka et al. [17] who could show that SPECT increased the sensitivity from 87% to 95% [17]. Comparable data were published by Lorberboym et al. [18]. Profanter et al. [19] used the CT-Sestamibi image fusion by superimposing the CT on the Sestamibi-SPECT image. Again, a high sensitivity (93%) was found. Fukumoto [20] also proposed Sestamibi for SPECT imaging in this disease. With a view to these excellent results, Sestamibi-SPECT is now proposed as the imaging tool of choice of parathyroid imaging, especially in minimally invasive parathyroidectomy [21, 22].

4.2.3 Recommended Injected Activity and Dosimetry

In Table 4.2, the suggestions for the appropriate amount of activity are given. According to the cited publications [7, 11, 13], an activity of 75–150 MBq ^{99m}Tc-pertechnetate is recommended. The average activity for ^{99m}Tc-Sestamibi ranges from 185 to 740 MBq (in US up to 925 MBq) [3] and reflects the data given in the proposed SmPC.

The resulting organ doses may be adopted from ICRP 80 (resting subject).

4.2.4 General Considerations for Parathyroid Imaging

Although the dual phase protocol has now been accepted as a useful procedure, some authors still advocate the combination with ^{123}I for thyroid tissue imaging [23]. It has been pointed out that this procedure facilitates the differential diagnosis of thyroid nodules and adenomas. However, the application of

Table 4.2 Injected activity

First author	Year	No/pts	Tracer/activity/technique	Sensitivity
O'Doherty	1992	57	Subtraction technique	98% (parathyroid adenoma)
			20 MBq: ^{123}I	55% (hyperplasia)
			4 h later	0 false-positive due to presence of nodular goitre
			200 MBq: MIBI	
Hindié	1998	27	Subtraction technique	93% (parathyroid adenoma)
			10 MBq: ^{123}I	100% in 3/3 with multiglandular disease
			2–4 h later	Only 1 false-negative result due to thyroid nodules
			550 MBq: MIBI	
			Acquisition of both tracers simultaneously	
Casara	2001	143	150 MBq: ^{99m}TcO4 iv	97% (sensitivity of ^{99m}TcO4/MIBI and US/ solitary adenoma)
			20 min later KClO4 400 mg po	
			500 MBq: MIBI iv	
SNM Guideline	2004		75–150 MBq: ^{99m}TcO4 iv	
			185–925 MBq: ^{99m}Tc-MIBI iv	
			7.5–20 MBq: ^{123}I po	
			75–130 MBq: ^{201}Tl	
			Dual-phase and subtraction technique	

^{99m}Tc-pertechnetate before the application of Sestamibi also allows the visualization of thyroid tissue [24, 25].

In a review published by Palestro et al. [26], the different imaging procedures are discussed. It has been stated that not all parathyroid lesions retain Sestamibi and not all thyroid tissue washes out quickly so that subtraction imaging using either ^{99m}Tc–pertechnetate or ^{123}I is helpful. Many Sestamibi-avid thyroid lesions also accumulate ^{99m}Tc-pertechnetate and iodine, and subtraction reduces false positives. The most frequent cause of false positive Sestamibi results is the solid thyroid nodule. It has been found that thyroid nodules can coexist with hyperparathyroidism in up to 30% of cases [8]. This can cause two problems: first, thyroid nodules can be ^{99m}Tc-Sestamibi-avid regardless of whether they are benign or malignant and whether they are hot or cold with ^{99m}TcO$_4$. Such nodules may trap and retain the tracer for a prolonged time, as do parathyroid adenomas, causing false-positive results and thus affecting the accuracy of scintigraphy. Additionally, the discovery of a nodular goitre concomitantly with the hyperparathyroidism can help the surgeon to determine the extension of the required surgical intervention. It will be less extensive in patients with a solitary parathyroid adenoma and a normal thyroid gland, and more extensive in the presence of concomitant thyroid nodules, particularly when the latter is located in the lobe contralateral to the parathyroid adenoma.

Sestamibi scintigraphy is less sensitive for detecting hyperplastic parathyroid glands. In secondary hyperparathyroidism, Sestamibi uptake is more closely related to the cell cycle than to the gland size. Mitochondria-rich oxyphil cells presumably account for Sestamibi uptake in parathyroid lesions. In general, Sestamibi is also less sensitive for detecting multigland disease than solitary gland disease [26].

Stefaniak et al. [27] published a paper on the application of artificial neural network algorithm for the detection of parathyroid adenoma using the ^{99m}Tc-Sestamibi/^{99m}Tc-pertechnetate subtraction scintigraphy combined with ^{99m}Tc-Sestamibi double-phase imaging. They could prove that abnormalities of Sestamibi imaging were depicted more distinctly and visualized more clearly in parametric images received by this network algorithm. The similar procedure had already been published by Blocklet et al. [28] as early as in 1996. A factor analysis of dynamic structures allowed better results of Sestamibi scintigraphy.

Not only data processing procedures have been used to improve Sestamibi scintigraphy. Ho Shon et al. [29] published the paper of the value of oblique pinhole images in preoperative localization with ^{99m}Tc-Sestamibi for primary hyperparathyroidism: oblique pinhole views improved overall sensitivity from 76% to 88% and correctly localized 11 more adenomas than anterior images alone; above that, the confidence of interpretation was improved. Similar results were published by the same group in 86 patients: pinhole images were obtained 15 min and 2–4 h after injection of Sestamibi. The addition of a routine correlative thyroid ^{99m}Tc-pertechnetate scan significantly improved sensitivity so that the pinhole technique is recommended as a procedure of choice for parathyroid imaging.

A lot of papers described some biological factors influencing Sestamibi parathyroid scintigraphy.

Custodio et al. [30] studied patients with secondary hyperparathyroidism and have found that high Sestamibi scores were associated with high estimated gland weight, degree of cell proliferation, and presence of nodular hyperplasia. These factors may explain false negative results of Sestamibi scintigraphy.

Cermik et al. [31] studied the uptake ratios of ^{99m}Tc-Sestamibi and tumor volume, serum biochemical values (i-PTH, Ca, P) and oxyphil cell content. The results may be summarized as follows: there was no significant correlation between Sestamibi uptake ratios and increased gland volume or serum Ca and i-PTH levels. In contrast to Custodio et al. [30], Cermik et al. [31] could not establish a relationship between oxyphil cell content and Sestamibi uptake and retention. However, these authors found an adverse relation between phosphorus and Sestamibi retention so that the phosphorus level is considered prior to Sestamibi imaging.

Pons et al. [32] published a paper on biological factors influencing parathyroid localization. Again, mitochondria-rich oxyphil cells were described to be relevant mechanisms of uptake. They described the relationship between the intensity of focal uptake in the parathyroid glands and the cell cycle phases for patients with secondary hyperparathyroidism. Higher uptake grades correlated with the activity-growing phase, showing that scintigraphy accurately reflects the functional status of the hyperplastic parathyroid glands; in contrast to Cermik et al. [31], serum calcium levels may modify radiotracer kinetics by influencing the membrane

4 Parathyroid Imaging

potential. In addition, P-glycoprotein or multidrug resistance (MDR)-associated protein expression may play an important role in the false-negative results of parathyroid scintigraphy as this protein might be responsible for an early and quick washout of Sestamibi.

Parikshak et al. [33] investigated the impact of hypercalcemia and parathyroid hormone level on the sensitivity of preoperative Sestamibi scanning for primary hyperparathyroidism. They reviewed retrospectively the data of 102 patients with primary hyperparathyroidism and mild hypercalcemia who underwent preoperative Sestamibi. More than 95% of patients with calcium greater than 11.3 mg/dL had a positive scan as compared with 60% of those with lesser values. Similarly, a serum PTH level greater than 160 pg/mL correlated with positive scans in 93% as opposed to 57% in those with lower levels. Lower Ca and PTH levels thus seem to correlate with reduced sensitivity of Sestamibi. These findings were supported by a paper published by Hung et al. [34] who measured intact parathyroid hormone levels in hyperparathyroidism and correlated the data with Sestamibi imaging: visualization of hyperfunctioning parathyroid glands on ^{99m}Tc-parathyroid scintigraphy was more likely with the higher serum i-PTH level in a dose-dependent manner. The same findings have been published by Siegel et al. [35].

Torregrosa et al. [14] investigated the effect of intravenous calcitriol on parathyroid gland activity using double-phase ^{99m}Tc-Sestamibi scintigraphy. After 1 year of treatment with calcitriol, parathormone levels decreased significantly in 95% of the patients. After therapy, Sestamibi-positive areas decreased in 29% of the patients. These authors suggest Sestamibi scintigraphy as a reliable exploratory tool in predicting the response to treatment with intravenous calcitriol in hemodialysis patients with secondary hyperparathyroidism.

Radiochemical purity of Sestamibi may also play an important role in parathyroid imaging: Karam et al. [36] used a procedure to decrease the Technetium to Sestamibi ratio thus improving the radiochemical purity of ^{99m}Tc-Sestamibi. They achieved a higher degree of radiochemical purity (at least 95% bound), which increased the sensitivity from 94% to 84% in patients with disease parathyroid glands.

4.2.5 Sestamibi and Histology in Parathyroid Adenoma

Gupta et al. [37] published data on 35 patients with preoperative Sestamibi localization to optimize a surgical approach. Single-site localization in 21 patients directed a limited unilateral neck exploration with adenomectomy and ipsilateral gland biopsy. Conversion to a bilateral operation was required in one unilateral neck exploration patient because no adenoma was found on one side. The total operative time for the unilateral procedure was significantly shorter than for bilateral neck exploration. All the results were histologically confirmed.

Takebayashi et al. [38] reviewed the Sestamibi scans of 31 patients who underwent parathyroidectomies. The resected glands were investigated histologically. There were 99 resected lesions, including 9 parathyroid adenomas and

61 hyperplastic parathyroids. The sensitivity for localizing the diseased glands in patients with primary HPT (91%) was higher than that in patients with secondary HPT (83%). Significantly greater average parathyroid-to-thyroid count ratios on early and delayed images were observed in the diseased glands. It was pointed out that the uptake of Sestamibi in the hyperfunctional glands is dependent on gland size and the amount of cellular components, chief cells and oxyphil cells.

4.2.6 Parathyroid Imaging in Patients with Concomitant Thyroid Disease

One of the main problems of false-positives in parathyroid imaging is multinodular goitre. It is well known that thyroid nodules – benign or malignant – present with increased Sestamibi uptake and decreased washout so that in dual-phase imaging procedures thyroid nodules look like parathyroid adenomas. As the ultrasound appearance of thyroid nodules and parathyroid adenomas is similar, a higher number of false-positives may be expected. Already in the year 2000, Krausz et al. dealt with this problem [22]. They studied 77 patients with a solitary parathyroid adenoma at surgery, 40 of these patients had concomitant multinodular thyroid disease, whereas 37 patients had no morphologic changes in the thyroid gland on US or at surgery. The combined sensitivity of Sestamibi and ultrasound was 87% in nodular thyroid disease and 89% in patients with no thyroid disease. In patients with no thyroid abnormalities, the PPV of Sestamibi and US was 97%, but it decreased to 91% and 78% in patients with thyroid nodules [39, 40]. Masatsugu et al. [41] published data in patients with and without concomitant thyroid disease. It could be shown that thyroid disease influenced parathyroid localization as well as the indication for minimally invasive parathyroidectomy in a negative way. Lorberboym et al. highly advocated the use of preoperative SPECT imaging of parathyroid adenomas in patients who have multinodular goitres to select those suitable for minimally invasive radioguided surgery [42]. It has been pointed out that in patients with associated thyroid disease, standard neck exploratory surgery has to be recommended, while in patients with normal thyroid gland, minimally invasive procedures may be carried out.

4.2.7 Pitfalls in Parathyroid Imaging

When evaluating parathyroid scans, pitfalls have to be considered. Most common reasons for false-negative results include multiple abnormal glands, ectopic location, and surgical inexperience. Sestamibi is especially suited for detecting ectopic adenomas, for example, in the thorax. Vivian Lee et al. reviewed pitfalls of Sestamibi and MRI and arrived at the conclusion that the absence of definitive findings on both Sestamibi scintigraphy and MRI in patients with high serum parathyroid hormone level should suggest the possibility of multiple small hyperplastic glands [43]. Another reason for reducing the sensitivity of Sestamibi is the application of calcium

4 Parathyroid Imaging

channel blockers. Friedman et al. investigated 235 patients operated for HPT with respect to the potential effect of calcium channel blockers. The odds ratio for a negative study in patients taking this kind of medication was 2.88. Thus, it was concluded that calcium channel blockers reduce the sensitivity of parathyroid Sestamibi-SPECT [44].

In 2004, Kiratli et al. focused on the early phase imaging in hemodialysis patients [45]. It was that Sestamibi-uptake in parathyroid glands was reduced during the early phase imaging in this condition. This paper also discusses the fact that vitamin D supplements can cause diminished uptake of Sestamibi. It is therefore recommended that vitamin D3 metabolites should not be given before parathyroid imaging.

A rare reason for a negative dual-phase scan in parathyroid adenoma is the lack of oxyphil cells within the tumor. In this case, Sestamibi retention is decreased so that false-negative findings may occur [10]; the same holds true also in ectopic parathyroid adenoma [46].

Smith et al. summarized the pitfalls of parathyroid imaging as follows [47]:

- HPT should be confirmed with biochemical testing to minimize false-positive or false-negative study results
- Thyroid cancer may appear as "hot spots"
- Retention of the tracer does not always occur in parathyroid adenomas at dual-phase imaging (lack of oxyphil cells)
- Small parathyroid adenomas may be overlooked, especially when only planar imaging is used
- Ectopic parathyroid adenomas can be overlooked when only a small field of view is used
- Asymmetric activity in the submandibular glands can be mistaken for an ectopic parathyroid adenoma
- Scintigraphy has a lower sensitivity for parathyroid hyperplasia than for parathyroid adenoma
  Above that, medication with calcium channel blockers may lead to a degradation of the images.

4.2.8 Intraoperative Parathyroid Detection

Since more than 10 years now, intraoperative nuclear guidance in benign HPT in parathyroid cancer has been used [48]. Twenty patients undergoing their first operation for HPT, 15 patients undergoing reoperation because of persistent or recurrent HPT, and 2 patients with parathyroid cancer were investigated after the application of Sestamibi. A hand-held gamma detector to identify parathyroid tumors arrived at a sensitivity of 90.5% in first parathyroidectomies, 88.9% in reoperations, and 100% in parathyroid cancer. False-positive results were due to thyroid nodules. This procedure, combined with parathyroid scintigraphy, was used in 36 patients with primary HPT. In 5 of 23 patients, intraoperative gamma probe detection helped to identify the adenoma [49].

Other authors like Casara [13] found a sensitivity of 93.5% for a gamma probe, and 97.7% in a larger series of 70 patients [50]. Rubello et al. [51] extended this series of patients and described a sensitivity of 96.9%. These data were confirmed by Goldstein et al. [52] who claimed a success rate of 98%. The results published during the last 3 years document the high sensitivity of intraoperative procedures, as all of these papers – even in large numbers of patients above 200 – document the high sensitivity [53–61].

It is evident from these data that intraoperative detection of parathyroid adenomas using hand-held probes is a safe and reliable tool, which will also be used in minimally invasive procedures.

4.2.9 Cost-Effectiveness of Sestamibi

One paper has been published on the cost-effectiveness on Sestamibi scanning compared to bilateral neck exploration for the treatment of primary HPT [62]. In the USA, 100,000 cases with primary HPT are diagnosed annually. In approximately 85–90%, this disease is caused by a solitary parathyroid adenoma, amenable to surgical resection. During the last years, unilateral operation procedures have become popular, thus reducing bilateral neck exploration with inspection and identification of all four glands and removal of any abnormal tissue. The unilateral, noninvasive procedures reduce the operation time by the factor of 2 and are combined with a lower rate of complications, and are more comfortable for the patient. Additionally, unilateral procedures are cheaper than bilateral operations. The authors came to the conclusion that a preoperative Sestamibi strategy involving guided minimally invasive radioguided parathyroidectomy and focussed unilateral neck exploration is more cost-effective for the treatment of solitary adenomas than the bilateral approach. These data gave rise to the assumption that Sestamibi should more frequently be used in those patients with primary HPT (before surgery) to reduce costs and reduce morbidity.

4.3 Indications for Parathyroid Imaging

4.3.1 Primary HPT

4.3.1.1 Preoperative Imaging

From 1930 to 1990, bilateral cervical exploration of four glands was considered the gold standard management of HPT [63]. A 95–97% rate of success was reported with this approach, but the operating time was excessive and the hypocalcemia rates remained near 15%. In recent years, the trend toward less invasive surgery in the management of HPT has become popular among physicians.

In 2001, Giordano et al. published a survey on new trends in parathyroid scintigraphy [8]: the authors concluded that parathyroid scintigraphy can be recommended not only in persistent or recurrent hyperparathyroidism, but also in hyperparathyroid patients prior to first surgery. Especially since minimally invasive procedures requiring unilateral exploration of the neck have become popular, a new era of parathyroid scintigraphy has been opened: the preoperative proof of an adenoma can guide the surgeon to reduce operation time and invasiveness of the procedure. As single adenomas of the parathyroid gland are the most frequent cause (approximately 85% of hyperparathyroidism), minimally invasive surgery may become the procedure of choice in the near future. To a lesser extent (up to 15%), multiple adenomas and hyperplastic glands, and in rare cases carcinomas (<1%) are responsible for glandular hyperfunction [64]. Surgical resection is the therapy of choice and offers a cure for nonmalignant disease in more than 95% of all cases [65]. Although the traditional approach for parathyroidectomy (open cervicotomy and bilateral neck exploration) yields very good results in the hands of experienced endocrine surgeon, new procedures such as unilateral open or minimal invasive techniques are getting more common [66]. Udelsman reviewed the outcomes of 656 consecutive parathyroid explorations and compared the results of conventional and minimally invasive parathyroidectomy (MIP) techniques. MIP was associated with reduction of operation time, hospital stay, complication rate, and cost savings. However, these techniques require the preoperative localization of the pathologically altered glands.

The interest in parathyroid surgery is increasing with a paradigm shift in the management of pHPT (primary hyperparathyroidism). This shift arises mainly from the current interest in minimally invasive parathyroid surgery, with special attention to Sestamibi scanning and intraoperative parathyroid hormone (PTH) assay [67].

It is known that the sensitivity of preoperative Sestamibi scintigraphy depends on the cause of HPT, in particular that secondary HPT and multiglandular disease may show sensitivities less than 50%. Contrary to that, due to a single adenoma, primary HPT shows the sensitivity of Sestamibi scintigraphy above 88%. It has to be stated that MIP is predominantly performed in single adenomas, as multiglandular disease requires a complete investigation of the whole neck. The current literature gives evidence for this approach. The respective data are summarized as follows.

Over the past years, several publications have been issued on this topic.

Johnson et al. pointed out that, over the past decade, the surgical treatment of pHPT has changed from predominantly a bilateral approach with four-gland exploration in all cases to unilateral and focused approaches guided by preoperative imaging showing single adenomas [68]. Sonography and ^{99m}Tc-Sestamibi scintigraphy have assumed dominant roles in preoperative location of solitary adenomas, and focused approaches based on concordant findings from both techniques have cure rates equal to that of the traditional approach. Stephen et al. [69] published one of the largest prospective studies, involving 350 patients with pHPT who underwent preoperative Sestamibi subtraction scan and sonography to direct a focal (1-gland) and unilateral (1-sided) parathyroid exploration by using rapid intraoperative PTH determinations. A single gland was predicted by Sestamibi in 83%, by ultrasonography in 85%, and concordance of both in 59%. Unilateral parathyroid exploration would identify single-gland disease in 74% using sonography and 68% for scintigraphy alone, and in 79% when combining both techniques. The addition of intraoperative PTH would increase the success rate to 73% (Sestamibi), 77% (US), and 82% (combination of both) respectively.

A review published by Massaro et al. and Rubello et al. [70, 73] came to the conclusion that in patients with pHPT and solitary adenoma limited or minimally invasive neck exploration including Sestamibi is advisable, given their significant Sestamibi-uptake in the parathyroid adenoma and the absence of coexisting Sestamibi-avid thyroid nodules. Gamma probe guidance increases the accuracy of preoperative Sestamibi scintigraphy. This is also been stated by Ortega et al. [71], Mariani et al. [72] and Rubello et al. [73], who also stressed the necessity of hand-held gamma probes to improve the results of minimally invasive parathyroidectomy.

Murphy et al. [74] used an intraoperative gamma probe to localize an enlarged parathyroid gland in 345 patients with pHPT: therefore, all patients were injected with Sestamibi between 1.5 and 3 h prior to undergoing parathyroidectomy. Patients with a positive Sestamibi scan underwent a minimally invasive radioguided parathyroidectomy and those patients who did not possess a positive Sestamibi scan underwent a standard bilateral neck exploration. A hand-held gamma radiation detecting probe was used during every operation; ex vivo radioactivity was measured in parathyroid and other tissues. Background radioactivity was determined simultaneously within the operative basin after each tissue excision. It was found out that any excised tissue containing more than 20% of background activity in a patient with a positive Sestamibi scan result is a solitary parathyroid adenoma. This technique clearly is a major advance in localizing the parathyroid tissue by a physiologic means rather than by anatomic abnormality and pathologic identification of the enlarged parathyroid gland. If a gland is removed from a patient with pHPT who has a positive Sestamibi scan and it contains more than 20% of the radioactivity that is measurable in the operative basin, that tissue is absolutely a parathyroid adenoma. Frozen-section analysis of that tissue during parathyroid surgery need not be performed, and the intraoperative measurement of parathyroid hormone is unnecessary.

However, Friedman et al. [75] stated in the "Guidelines for Radioguided Parathyroid Surgery" that the ex vivo radioactivity percentages greater than 20% above background clearly can differentiate hyperactive parathyroid tissue from any other tissue, but no definitive conclusions can be made to differentiate single-gland disease from multigland disease (parathyroid hyperplasia or multiple adenoma). It was concluded that as radioactivity percentages are proportional to specimen size, the use of the ex vivo background radioactivity percentages for confirmation of the presence of parathyroid adenoma should incorporate the size of the specimen.

A paper published by Chung-Yau Lo [76] summarized 100 consecutive HPT-patients being candidates for minimally invasive parathyroidectomy. Ultrasound (US) and Sestamibi findings were correlated with intraoperative findings and postoperative outcome. The final pathology included 98 patients with solitary adenoma and 2 patients with multiglandular disease. The sensitivities, accuracies, and positive predictive values found for the different two different options, that is, US and Sestamibi, were as follows:

	US (%)	Sestamibi (%)
Sensitivities	57	89
Accuracies	56	85
Positive predictive values	97	94

4 Parathyroid Imaging

From these data it was concluded that Sestamibi is preferred over ultrasound in pHPT patients being scheduled for minimally invasive procedures.

A recent paper published by Nichols et al. [77] focused on preoperative parathyroid scintigraphic lesion localization and investigated the accuracy of various types of readings (early pinhole images, late pinhole images, subtraction images, SPECT images, all planar images, and all images including SPECT). A total of 534 parathyroid lesions were excised. Of the 462 patients, 409 had one lesion, whereas 53 had multiple lesions. Per-lesion sensitivity for reading all images was significantly higher for single-gland disease than for multigland disease (90% vs 66%). Since more than 10 years now, SPECT has been added to planar Sestamibi scintigraphy in HPT. Civelek et al. [78] prospectively analyzed delayed Sestamibi SPECT scans in 338 patients with biochemically confirmed pHPT. Two hundred and eighty-seven unexplored and 51 re-explored patients participated. The abnormal parathyroid glands included 88% single adenomas, 7% double adenomas, and 4% multigland hyperplasia. Sestamibi SPECT correctly lateralized abnormal parathyroid glands with an overall sensitivity of 87% (sensitivity for solitary adenomas 96%, 83% for double adenomas, and 45% for multiglandular hyperplasia), an accuracy of 94%, and a PPV of 86%. It was concluded that delayed Sestamibi SPECT imaging is a promising procedure in the preoperative detection and localization of parathyroid adenomas in both unexplored and re-explored patients. The sensitivity of Sestamibi is limited in multiglandular disease.

Another paper published by Miccoli et al. [79] compared endoscopic bilateral neck exploration versus quick intraoperative parathormone assay (qPTHa: as a standard procedure for patients with pHPT) during endoscopic parathyroidectomy in forty (40) patients with primary HPT and Sestamibi-positive for a single parathyroid adenoma. With respect to mean operative time and outcome of the surgical procedure it was concluded that bilateral neck exploration can be performed endoscopically avoiding both the time necessary for qPTHa and the related healthcare cost.

The following two publications give undoubtedly evidence of the clinical usefulness of Sestamibi in preoperative situations:

In 2005, the American Association of Clinical Endocrinologists and the American Association of Endocrine Surgeons (AACE/AAES) position statement on the diagnosis of PHPT "convened a meeting of the AACE/AAES Task Force on primary hyperparathyroidism [80]." It was concluded that *parathyroid imaging has no role in the diagnosis of PHPT, but ultrasonography or sestamibi scanning (or both) of the parathyroid glands should be used for operative planning. Specifically, if preoperative ultrasonography or sestamibi scanning localizes an adenoma, this information facilitates a focused or minimally invasive surgical approach.*" Sestamibi scanning can be helpful in localizing an ectopic parathyroid gland. Here, it has also proposed to use hand-held intraoperative gamma probe and Sestamibi to facilitate localization of abnormal parathyroid glands. In the paragraph of "Surgical Strategies," it is recommended that "...preoperative localization by ^{99m}Tc-sestamibi scanning with use of single-photon-emission computed tomography" ...should be used in the respective patients.

The second important publication is the "Summary Statement from a Workshop in Asymptomatic Primary Hyperparathyroidism: A Perspective for the 21st Century", published by Bilezikian et al. [81]. Here, it is stated that *a variety of minimally invasive procedures have been introduced. One of the most promising techniques, minimally invasive parathyroidectomy, is performed with preoperative localization using ^{99m}Tc-labeled Sestamibi-SPECT."*

Further on it is recommended that *"The ^{99m}Tc-labeled Sestamibi scan should be the first procedure with SPECT whenever possible."*

In addition to surgical adjuncts, such as the use of rapid intraoperative PTH assays, intraoperative ^{99m}Tc-labeled Sestamibi with γ-detection probes and intraoperative ultrasound have been found to be helpful in some centers.

A survey of the members of the International Association of Endocrine Surgeons [82] indicated that already in the year 2000 ^{99m}Tc-Sestamibi-based MIP had been adopted by >50% of the surgeons worldwide (59% from America, 56% from Australia, and 49% from Europe and the Middle East).

These last three publications make clear that nowadays preoperative Sestamibi scintigraphy is a clinically significant procedure especially for patients being considered as candidates for minimally invasive parathyroidectomy. This is true especially for primary HPT.

From this literature overview, it can be concluded that the use of nuclear imaging, in combination with improved ultrasound imaging and the availability of rapid intraoperative parathyroid hormone assays has changed the strategy of surgical treatment of primary HPT [83, 84]. Previously, the standard treatment for all patients with primary HPT was the bilateral neck exploration with the goal of identifying and evaluating four parathyroid glands. Visual inspection of the glands, sometimes used in conjunction with intraoperative pathological frozen section assessment, allowed experienced surgeons to identify the pathologic glands and remove them with a success rate in excess of 90% [83]. The ability to preoperatively localize pathologic parathyroid glands has enabled a more focused surgical approach. Most centers now use preoperative imaging and intraoperative rapid parathyroid hormone testing with either a unilateral neck exploration or, increasingly, a minimally invasive single gland exploration for the treatment of patients with primary HPT. These focused surgical approaches are only possible when preoperative nuclear imaging suggests the presence of a localized parathyroid adenoma.

In conclusion, it can be stated that the Sestamibi scintigraphy provides a clear benefit for patients being potential candidates for minimally invasive parathyroidectomy.

4.3.2 Secondary HPT

A large number of uremic patients develop secondary HPT [85]. In a minority of patients, parathyroid overfunction persists, progressively escapes medical control, and eventually becomes extremely severe, requiring surgical correction. Lomonte et al. [85] have used dual-phase ^{99m}Tc-Sestamibi scintigraphy in uremic patients undergoing a first parathyroidectomy after performing Sestamibi scintigraphy.

4 Parathyroid Imaging

Sestamibi scintigraphy showed focal areas of increased uptake in at least one gland, which was the case in 25 out of 35 patients (71.4%). In total, only 42 of 121 glands removed were positive (sensitivity 34.7%, specificity 100%). It was concluded that Sestamibi scintigraphy did not show high sensitivity in identifying hyperplastic glands. The results were somewhat better in nodular disease, compared to diffuse disease. Similar findings were described by Nishida et al. [86], who described a sensitivity of 78.6% in the nodular type and 26.6% in the diffuse type. It was proposed that Sestamibi or Tetrofosmin scintigraphy may be used clinically to distinguish the nodular from the diffuse type parathyroid gland hyperplasia.

Owda et al. [87] investigated 16 chronic hemodialysis patients who received calcitriol for 3 years or longer, and who had a Sestamibi scan at the beginning of therapy or within the first 6 months of therapy. A positive uptake was observed in 9/16 cases. Interestingly, all patients with negative uptake responded to calcitriol while the majority of patients 8/9 (89%) of the positive uptake group did not respond, giving rise to the assumption that nodular types of secondary HPT may be therapy refractory.

4.3.2.1 Recurrent or Persistent HPT

Approximately 90% of patients with primary HPT are cured by parathyroidectomy at the initial neck exploration [88]. Those not cured either remain hypercalcemic in the immediate postoperative period or develop hypercalcemia after a long period of normocalcemia. Recurrent or persistent HPT is caused either by an overlooked parathyroid adenoma or an incomplete resection of hyperplastic parathyroid tissue. A successful neck exploration is primarily dependent on the experience of the operating surgeon, the anatomic location of the parathyroid glands, or normal or ectopic sites, in the presence of a single enlarged parathyroid gland. In cases where an enlarged parathyroid gland is not identified at operation, noninvasive imaging procedures like Sestamibi have to be used. This technique identifies an enlarged parathyroid gland in 65–80% of cases. SPECT may increase the sensitivity up to 85%. However, Sestamibi-SPECT or planar scintigraphy is less reliable in patients with multiglandular disease. Again, ultrasound and CT are also less sensitive. Re-operations, although being associated with higher complication rates, lead to a success in 90% of cases. The success rate of the re-operation depends primarily on the results of the localization procedure and whether the patient has a single enlarged parathyroid gland or multiglandular disease. Sestamibi helps to detect these enlarged glands in recurrent or persistent HPT [88].

The success rate in patients undergoing repeat cervical exploration after an initial failed surgery in HPT may be as low as 60% [89]. This explains that preoperative localization studies before reoperation are often used in patients with recurrent or persistent HPT. The preoperative investigations usually include ultrasonography, CT, MRI, selective venous sampling, selective arteriography, and more recently, ^{99m}Tc-Sestamibi scintigraphy. Use of preoperative imaging provides a directed surgical approach, the success rate of subsequent surgery is improved, and surgical morbidity is decreased when such techniques are used. Preoperative imaging studies have been compared in several investigations [89] and "tailored approaches for preoperative imaging have been suggested." Although MRI imaging has been shown to be useful in the preoperative assessment of recurrent or persistent HPT, Sestamibi scintigraphy has been found to have a high sensitivity and specificity for the detection of abnormal glands in patients with primary and/or recurrent or persistent HPT. The sensitivity and predictive value for the detection of abnormal parathyroid tissue on a per-gland basis increased to 94% and 98%, respectively, when MRI or Sestamibi were required to be positive [89]. These data confirm the excellent results of Sestamibi scintigraphy in the evaluation of recurrent or persistent HPT.

4.4 Sensitivity and Specificity of ^{99m}Tc-Sestamibi in Patients with HPT

The accuracy of Sestamibi scintigraphy in HPT has been described in several papers (Table 4.3) including a literature review on 20,225 patients by Ruda et al. [100]. This review described a sensitivity of 88.4% in adenoma and of only 44.5% in multiglandular disease. The data derived from the other papers cited here show an increase in sensitivity from 80.2% up to 96 and 100% in singular adenoma. The positive predictive value ranges from 86.4% to 100%. In general, it is evident that parathyroid imaging is extremely successful in detecting singular adenomas while in polyglandular disease, sensitivity goes down to 44.5% till 39%.

Table 4.3 Sensitivity and specificity of ^{99m}Tc-Sestamibi patients with hyperparathyroidism

Author	Pts	Sensitivity	Specificity	PPV	NPV
Martin et al. [90]	63	82%[a] 31%[b]			
Castellani et al. [91]	97	84.4%[a]	95.5%[a]	86.4%	95.3%
Sprouse et al. [92]	50	89.3%		91.5%	
Zettinig et al. [93]	35	100%[a]		100%	
Panzironi et al. [94]	77	96.1%			
Clark et al. [95]	125	89%[a]			
Prager et al. [96]	150	86%		89%	
Khaliq et al. [97]	23	91%[a]			
Gotthardt et al. [98]	178 (+ literature review)	45% pr. HPT 39% sec. HPT 50–91%	94% pr. HPT 40% sec. HPT		
Mortier et al. [99]	454	63–95% depending on localization			
Ruda et al. [100]	20,225 (literature review)	88.4%[a] 44.5%[b] 33% carcin.			
Carneiro-Pla et al. [101]	519	80% pr. HPT 80w%[a] 14%[b]			

[a]Adenomas
[b]Multiglandular disease

4 Parathyroid Imaging

A significant number of papers (Table 4.4) documented the additional value of SPECT, especially concerning sensitivity. SPECT imaging, in conjunction with planar imaging, provides increased sensitivity and more precise anatomical localization (SNM guideline [3]). This is particularly true in detecting both primary and recurrent HPT resulting from ectopic adenomas (SNM-guideline).

4.5 Comparison of ^{99m}Tc-Sestamibi and Other Diagnostic Imaging Modality Results in Patients with HPT

Table 4.4 presents an overview on the correlative imaging using Sestamibi scintigraphy mainly in comparison to ultrasound. Here, it has to be mentioned that the first imaging procedure will routinely be ultrasound of the neck. However, this procedure fails to visualize ectopic adenomas, for example, in the thorax. CT is hampered by relatively high radiation exposure to the patient. Above that there are far less studies dealing with Sestamibi, ultrasound, and CT. Another procedure being suited for the diagnosis of HPT is MRI. The disadvantage of ultrasound is that this procedure can identify lesions, but is not able to allow the differential diagnosis between lymph nodes and adenoma. On the contrary, the positive Sestamibi scan is indicative of a parathyroid adenoma, with the exception of thyroid nodules.

In the majority of papers, Sestamibi turned out to be superior to ultrasound. Especially in single adenomas, Sestamibi showed an approximately 10% advantage over ultrasound, while sensitivity of CT is acceptable in those studies where no correlation with Sestamibi has been found. Papers comparing CT and Sestamibi come to the conclusion that Sestamibi is superior to CT. Papers comparing Sestamibi and MRI arrive at a similar conclusion: this literature review makes it evident that Sestamibi is a reliable tool and imaging procedure of choice – together with ultrasound – to detect especially singular adenoma. All procedures described here have similar problems when multiglandular disease is present.

4.6 Radiation Exposure for Different Radiopharmaceuticals

In Table 4.5 dosimetry is given for different radiopharmaceuticals like ^{201}Tl, ^{99m}Tc-Pertechnetate, and ^{99m}Tc-Sestamibi: Sestamibi shows the lowest radiation exposure (largest dose and effective dose) [3].

4.7 Summary and Conclusion

4.7.1 Preoperative Parathyroid Imaging

The management of primary HPT has dramatically changed in the last 5 years. Many more patients now undergo focused, limited or minimally invasive parathyroidectomy instead of traditional bilateral neck exploration [122]. This change has taken place because of the improved accuracy of preoperative localizing studies in

Table 4.4 Comparison of 99mTc-sestamibi (MIBI) and other diagnostic imaging modalities results in patients with hyperparathyroidism

Author	Year	No/pts	Indication	Sensitivity (%)			Specificity (%)			PPV (%)			NPV (%)	
				MIBI	US/CT/MRI	MIBI/US concordant	MIBI	US	MIBI/US	MIBI	US	MIBI/US	MIBI	US
Kairys et al. [102]	2006	65	Preoperative localization with pr HPT, US/ MIBI	63.3% single aden / 35.4% multigland disease	83.3% single aden / 46.2% multigland disease		95.6% single aden / 95% multigland disease	95.6% s a / 100% m d		82.6% s a / 94.4%m d	86.2% s a / 100% m d		88.7% s a / 38% m d	94.5% s a / 41.7% m d
Gawande et al. [103]	2006	569	pr HPT, preoperative MIBI/US	69	63	56	92	90	60	89	89	99		
Fuster et al. [104]	2006	48	sek HPT, preoperative MIBI/US	72%	55%		95%	67%		80%	28%		97%	87%
Solorzano et al. [105]	2005	180	pr HPT; preoperative SUS and MIBI; localization of abnormal parathyroid glands	80%	83%	Sens US+MIBI 93%								
Ruda et al. [100]	2005	20,225	Literature review, diagnosis, and treatment of pr HPT from 1995 to 2003	88.4% aden / 44.46% multi d / 33% carcinoma	78.55% aden / 34.86% multi d / 100% carcinoma									
Mekel et al. [63]	2005	146	Preoperative localization for minimal invasive surgery	74/18.8/38.1% (aden/pr hyperplasia/ sek hyperplasia)	61/6.3/19% (aden/pr hyperplasia/ sek hyperplasia)	Sens US+MIBI 83% aden 25%pr hyperplasia 43% sek hyperplasia								

Seehofer et al. [106]	2004	21	Persistent or recurrent HPT, comparison SVS and MIBI	69% MIBI 71% SUV	50%	MR 54% CT 45%			6/8 (75%)	5/16 (31%)
Clark et al. [107]	2004	8	Recurrent parathyroid carcinoma; preoperative	67% carcinoma	CT 53%					
Ruf et al. [1]	2004	17	Preoperative localization	86% aden (12/17) 33% hyperpl (1/3)	MR 71% aden (10/17) 33% hyperpl (1/3)	MIBI-SPECT fused with MRI Diagnostic improvement 54% (7/13) In 38% patients improved topographic assignment of scintigraphic foci In 15% help to differentiate hyperactive parathyroid tissue from lymph nodes				
Saint Marc et al. [108]	2004	149	Selecting patients with pr HPT for UNE	73.8%	60.4%	US+MIBI 44.1%	US+MIBI 55.6%	US+MIBI 91.1%	US+ MIBI 8.8%	

(continued)

Table 4.4 (continued)

Author	Year	No/pts	Indication	Sensitivity (%)			Specificity (%)			PPV (%)			NPV (%)	
				MIBI	US/CT/MRI	MIBI/US concordant	MIBI	US	MIBI/US	MIBI	US	MIBI/US	MIBI	US
Gross and Wax [109]	2004	22	Preoperative localization with persistent HPT; diagnostic utility of CT		CT 86% localization of abnormal parathyroid glands 76% aden 24% hyperplasia 71% (5/7 pat) detection of aberrant or ectopic parathyroid glands									
Kebapci et al. [110]	2004	52	High-resolution ultrasonography and MIBI (dual-phase) in the preoperative evaluation of parathyroid lesions with concomitant thyroid disease	With thyroid d 70% Without 75%	With thyroid d 78% Without 90%	Combined with 89% Without 93%				With 90% Without 100%	With 88% Without 96%	Combin with 92% Without 100%		
Miura et al. [111]	2002	115	Intraoperative parathyroid hormone assay and MIBI	83% aden	71%	Combined 95%								

Wakamatsu et al. [112]	2001	28	Tetrofosmin compared with MIBI, Tl, MRI, and US	Single gland: Tetro 63.2% MIBI 68.4% Tl 57.9% MR 55.6% US 63.2%	Multigland: Tetro 41.7% MIBI 41.7% Tl 37.5% MR 58.3% US 54.2%	Weight < 200 mg → Sens between 20% and 40% for all modalities; weight > 200 mg 69.2–78.6%						
Gotway et al. [89]	2001	98	Recurrent or persistent HPT	85%	MR 82%	Combination MR + MIBI 94%				89%	MR 89%	Combination 98%
Weber et al. [2]	2000		Review article	70–100%	70–80% US	80–85% MR 90% accuracy ectopic adenoma	90–96%					
De Feo et al. [113]	2000	49	MIBI, US, and CT in parathyroid glands; retrospective study	57%	27% US 17% MR 13% CT	Combined US + MIBI 96%	85%	65% US 65% MR 39% CT	Combin US + MIBI 83%		Combin US + MIBI 88%	Combin US + MIBI 94%
Wada et al. [114]	1999	24	Sek HPT; MR and MIBI	Small glands (<0.5 mL) 40.7% (>0.5 mL parathy. volume) 90%	Small glands (<0.5 mL) 74% MR (>0.5 mL parathy. volume) 95% MR							

(continued)

Table 4.4 (continued)

Author	Year	No/pts	Indication	Sensitivity (%)			Specificity (%)			PPV (%)			NPV (%)	
				MIBI	US/CT/MRI	MIBI/US concordant	MIBI	US	MIBI/US	MIBI	US	MIBI/US	MIBI	US
Pattou et al. [115]	1998	175	Blood sampling; MIBI or Tetrofosmin (TTF)	63% MIBI 71% TTF 49% PTH			98% M 98% T 90% P			96% M 96% T 85% P			82% 87% 61%	
Ishibashi et al. [116]	1998	20	Comparison MIBI, TTF, US, and MR	Sens overall:	Sens overall:		Overall	Overall						
				83% MIBI	78% US		83% M	40% U						
				87% TTF	80% MR		83% T	60% M						
				Sens aden ($n=9$)	Sens aden		Aden	Aden						
				100% MIBI	78% US		100%M	67% U						
				100% TTF	100% MR		100%T	100%M						
				Hyperpl ($n=37$)	Hyperpl		Hyperpl	Hyperpl						
				78% MIBI	78% US		75% M	43%U						
				84% TTF	73% MR		75% T	60%M						
Peeler et al. [117]	1997	25	Recurrent persistent HPT	74% MIBI 50% Tl-Tc	45% US 57% MR 68% CT									

Mazzeo et al. [118]	1996	73	Comparison high-resolution US, double-tracer subtraction scint (Tl-Tc), double-phase scint (MIBI), pr HPT preoperative	Sens overall 82% MIBI Without thyroid disease 87% With thyroid disease 80%	85% 90% 77%	201Tl-^{99m}Tc 62% 59% 67%			
Lee et al. [119]	1996	25	MRI and double-phase MIBI for preoperative localization	79% overall 89% aden 68% hyperplas	MR 84% overall 94% aden 74% hyperpl		94%	MR 75%	

MEN multiple endocrine neoplasia type 1, *UNE* unilateral neck exploration, *MGD* multiglandular disease, *SVS* selective venous sampling

Table 4.5 Radiation dosimetry: adults

Radiopharmaceuticals	Administered activity MBq (mCi)	Organ receiving the largest radiation dose[a] mGy/MBq (rad/mCi)	Effective dose[a] mSv/mBq (rem/mCi)
^{201}Tl-chloride	75–130 iv (2.0–3.5)	0.54 Kidney (2.0)	0.23 (0.85)
^{99m}Tc-perchlorate No blocking agent	75–150 iv (2–4)	0.062 Upper large intestine (0.23)	0.013 (0.048)
^{99m}Tc-sestamibi	158–925 iv (5–25)	0.039 Gallbladder (0.14)	0.0085 (0.031)
^{123}I 15% uptake	7.5–20 po (0.2–0.5)	1.9 Thyroid (7.0)	0.075 (0.28)

[a]International Commission on Radiological Protection [120]; International Commission on Radiological Protection [121]

selecting patients who have single-gland parathyroid disease (single adenoma) and can therefore have a minimally invasive parathyroidectomy.

While in earlier days, Sestamibi has predominantly been used in persistent or recurrent HPT, the development over the last 10 years clearly shows that the spectrum for Sestamibi scintigraphy has been widened: with the introduction of less invasive surgical procedures like unilateral neck exploration, Sestamibi has been extremely useful to guide the surgeon when a bilateral procedure should be avoided. Thus, nowadays Sestamibi is effectively used in the presurgical follow-up of patients being candidates for unilateral surgical procedures. Above that, the high sensitivity for the detection of singular adenomas has also lead to a frequent use of Sestamibi before surgery. Sestamibi facilitates surgery by reducing the operation duration. However, all the procedures mentioned here are by far less effective in detecting multiglandular disease.

In general, a combination of ultrasound with Sestamibi is advocated when enlarged glands have to be detected. CT and MRI will mainly be used when both procedures are negative or equivocal.

4.8 Conclusion

The benefits of preoperative imaging can be summarized as follows:
- Unilateral surgical exploration if adenoma is identified
- Recognition of ectopic adenoma
- Detection of other masses (up to 40–48% of patients have incidental thyroidal abnormalities) [123]
- Decrease of surgical complications (recurrent laryngeal nerve damage, hypoparathyroidism), and
- Reduction in operating room time and increased operative success rate [105, 124, 125]

As minimally invasive approaches to parathyroid surgery have gained in popularity, preoperative imaging of patients with primary hyperparathyroidism has played an important role [102]; based on the sensitivity and cost of the techniques, ultrasound and Sestamibi scanning have become the primary techniques for preoperative localization in patients with primary HPT [102, 103, 105, 111].

4.8.1 Persistent or Recurrent HPT

The main indication for a Sestamibi study in earlier years had been patients with persistent or recurrent HPT after primary surgery. This indication continues to play a major role in diagnosing patients with this disease. As these patients already had bilateral neck operations, it is not easy for the surgeon to detect possible adenomas, which have been newly developed or were overlooked during the first surgical procedure. Especially in these cases, parathyroid imaging allows detecting pathological parathyroid glands and thus can guide the surgeon.

To conclude, it has been shown that Sestamibi should not be used as a screening method but is a great adjunct in the preoperative assessment of patients scheduled for surgery in the different kinds of HPT, be it before limited neck exploration or in recurrent and persistent HPT. It has to be concluded that the diagnostic spectrum should be widened in so far that "pre-operative" imaging has to be added to the hitherto approved indication "recurrent or persistent HPT."

So we would like to propose the following indication statement for parathyroid imaging using Sestamibi in the proposed SmPC:

^{99m}Tc-Sestamibi may be used as… diagnostic aid to detect and localize parathyroid tissue in patients with recurrent and persistent HPT, and in patients who are scheduled to undergo surgery of the parathyroid glands.

References

1. Ruf J, Lopez Hanninen E et al (2004) Preoperative localization of parathyroid glands. Use of MRI, scintigraphy, and image fusion. Nuklearmedizin 43(3):85–90
2. Weber AL, Randolph G et al (2000) The thyroid and parathyroid glands. CT and MR imaging and correlation with pathology and clinical findings. Radiol Clin North Am 38(5):1105–1129
3. Greenspan B, Brown ML, et al (2004) The society of nuclear medicine procedure guideline for parathyroid scintigraphy, version 3.0
4. Ferlin G, Borsato N et al (1983) New perspectives in localizing enlarged parathyroids by technetium-thallium subtraction scan. J Nucl Med 24(5):438–441
5. Taillefer R, Boucher Y et al (1992) Detection and localization of parathyroid adenomas in patients with hyperparathyroidism using a single radionuclide imaging procedure with technetium-99m-sestamibi (double-phase study). J Nucl Med 33(10):1801–1807
6. Coakley AJ, Kettle AG et al (1989) 99Tcm sestamibi – a new agent for parathyroid imaging. Nucl Med Commun 10(11):791–794
7. O'Doherty MJ, Kettle AG et al (1992) Parathyroid imaging with technetium-99m-sestamibi: preoperative localization and tissue uptake studies. J Nucl Med 33(3):313–318

8. Giordano A, Rubello D et al (2001) New trends in parathyroid scintigraphy. Eur J Nucl Med 28(9):1409–1420
9. Greenspan BS, Brown ML et al (1998) Procedure guideline for parathyroid scintigraphy. Society of Nuclear Medicine. J Nucl Med 39(6):1111–1114
10. Benard F, Lefebvre B et al (1995) Rapid washout of technetium-99m-MIBI from a large parathyroid adenoma. J Nucl Med 36(2):241–243
11. Hindie E, Melliere D et al (1998) Parathyroid imaging using simultaneous double-window recording of technetium-99m-sestamibi and iodine-123. J Nucl Med 39(6):1100–1105
12. Rubello D, Saladini G et al (2000) Parathyroid imaging with pertechnetate plus perchlorate/MIBI subtraction scintigraphy: a fast and effective technique. Clin Nucl Med 25(7):527–531
13. Casara D, Rubello D et al (2001) Clinical role of 99mTcO4/MIBI scan, ultrasound and intraoperative gamma probe in the performance of unilateral and minimally invasive surgery in primary hyperparathyroidism. Eur J Nucl Med 28(9):1351–1359
14. Torregrosa JV, Palomar MR et al (1998) Has double-phase MIBI scintigraphy usefulness in the diagnosis of hyperparathyroidism? Nephrol Dial Transplant 13(Suppl 3):37–40
15. Fujii H, Kubo A (2000) Parathyroid imaging with technetium-99m sestamibi. Biomed Pharmacother 54(Suppl 1):12s–16s
16. Billotey C, Sarfati E et al (1996) Advantages of SPECT in technetium-99m-sestamibi parathyroid scintigraphy. J Nucl Med 37(11):1773–1778
17. Moka D, Voth E et al (2000) Technetium 99m-MIBI-SPECT: a highly sensitive diagnostic tool for localization of parathyroid adenomas. Surgery 128(1):29–35
18. Lorberboym M, Minski I et al (2003) Incremental diagnostic value of preoperative 99mTc-MIBI SPECT in patients with a parathyroid adenoma. J Nucl Med 44(6):904–908
19. Profanter C, Wetscher GJ et al (2004) CT-MIBI image fusion: a new preoperative localization technique for primary, recurrent, and persistent hyperparathyroidism. Surgery 135(2):157–162
20. Fukumoto M (2004) Single-photon agents for tumor imaging: 201Tl, 99mTc-MIBI, and 99mTc-tetrofosmin. Ann Nucl Med 18(2):79–95
21. Schachter PP, Issa N et al (2004) Early, postinjection MIBI-SPECT as the only preoperative localizing study for minimally invasive parathyroidectomy. Arch Surg 139(4):433–437
22. Krausz Y, Bettman L et al (2006) Technetium-99m-MIBI SPECT/CT in primary hyperparathyroidism. World J Surg 30(1):76–83
23. Hindie E, de LV, et al (2002) Parathyroid gland radionuclide scanning—methods and indications. Joint Bone Spine 69(1):28–36
24. Bergson EJ, Sznyter LA et al (2004) Sestamibi scans and intraoperative parathyroid hormone measurement in the treatment of primary hyperparathyroidism. Arch Otolaryngol Head Neck Surg 130(1):87–91
25. Mullan BP (2004) Nuclear medicine imaging of the parathyroid. Otolaryngol Clin North Am 37(4):909–939, xi–xii
26. Palestro CJ, Tomas MB et al (2005) Radionuclide imaging of the parathyroid glands. Semin Nucl Med 35(4):266–276
27. Stefaniak B, Cholewinski W et al (2003) Application of artificial neural network algorithm to detection of parathyroid adenoma. Nucl Med Rev Cent East Eur 6(2):111–117
28. Blocklet D, Martin P et al (1997) Presurgical localization of abnormal parathyroid glands using a single injection of technetium-99m methoxyisobutylisonitrile: comparison of different techniques including factor analysis of dynamic structures. Eur J Nucl Med 24(1):46–51
29. Shon IH, Roach PJ et al (2001) Superimposed double parathyroid adenoma on Tc-99m MIBI imaging: the value of oblique images. Clin Nucl Med 26(10):876–877, x
30. Custodio MR, Montenegro F et al (2005) MIBI scintigraphy, indicators of cell proliferation and histology of parathyroid glands in uraemic patients. Nephrol Dial Transplant 20(9):1898–1903
31. Cermik TF, Puyan FO et al (2005) Relation between Tc-99m sestamibi uptake and biological factors in hyperparathyroidism. Ann Nucl Med 19(5):387–392
32. Pons F, Torregrosa JV et al (2003) Biological factors influencing parathyroid localization. Nucl Med Commun 24(2):121–124

33. Parikshak M, Castillo ED et al (2003) Impact of hypercalcemia and parathyroid hormone level on the sensitivity of preoperative sestamibi scanning for primary hyperparathyroidism. Am Surg 69(5):393–398; discussion 399
34. Hung GU, Wang SJ et al (2003) Tc-99m MIBI parathyroid scintigraphy and intact parathyroid hormone levels in hyperparathyroidism. Clin Nucl Med 28(3):180–185
35. Siegel A, Alvarado M et al (2006) Parameters in the prediction of the sensitivity of parathyroid scanning. Clin Nucl Med 31(11):679–682
36. Karam M, Dansereau RN et al (2005) Increasing the radiochemical purity of 99mTc sestamibi commercial preparations results in improved sensitivity of dual-phase planar parathyroid scintigraphy. Nucl Med Commun 26(12):1093–1098
37. Gupta VK, Yeh KA et al (1998) 99m-Technetium sestamibi localized solitary parathyroid adenoma as an indication for limited unilateral surgical exploration. Am J Surg 176(5):409–412
38. Takebayashi S, Hidai H et al (1999) Hyperfunctional parathyroid glands with 99mTc-MIBI scan: semiquantitative analysis correlated with histologic findings. J Nucl Med 40(11):1792–1797
39. Krausz Y, Lebensart PD et al (2000) Preoperative localization of parathyroid adenoma in patients with concomitant thyroid nodular disease. World J Surg 24(12):1573–1578
40. Krausz Y, Shiloni E et al (2001) Diagnostic dilemmas in parathyroid scintigraphy. Clin Nucl Med 26(12):997–1001
41. Masatsugu T, Yamashita H et al (2005) Significant clinical differences in primary hyperparathyroidism between patients with and those without concomitant thyroid disease. Surg Today 35(5):351–356
42. Lorberboym M, Ezri T et al (2005) Preoperative technetium Tc 99m sestamibi SPECT imaging in the management of primary hyperparathyroidism in patients with concomitant multinodular goiter. Arch Surg 140(7):656–660
43. Lee VS, Spritzer CE (1998) MR imaging of abnormal parathyroid glands. AJR Am J Roentgenol 170(4):1097–1103
44. Friedman K, Somervell H et al (2004) Effect of calcium channel blockers on the sensitivity of preoperative 99mTc-MIBI SPECT for hyperparathyroidism. Surgery 136(6):1199–1204
45. Kiratli PO, Ceylan E et al (2004) Impaired Tc-99m MIBI uptake in the thyroid and parathyroid glands during early phase imaging in hemodialysis patients. Rev Esp Med Nucl 23(5):347–351
46. Khan MS, Khan S et al (2006) Ectopic parathyroid adenoma with Tc-99m MIBI washout: role of SPECT. Clin Nucl Med 31(11):713–715
47. Smith JR, Oates ME (2004) Radionuclide imaging of the parathyroid glands: patterns, pearls, and pitfalls. Radiographics 24(4):1101–1115
48. Bonjer HJ, Bruining HA et al (1997) Intraoperative nuclear guidance in benign hyperparathyroidism and parathyroid cancer. Eur J Nucl Med 24(3):246–251
49. Dackiw AP, Sussman JJ et al (2000) Relative contributions of technetium Tc 99m sestamibi scintigraphy, intraoperative gamma probe detection, and the rapid parathyroid hormone assay to the surgical management of hyperparathyroidism. Arch Surg 135(5):550–555; discussion 555–557
50. Casara D, Rubello D et al (2002) 99mTc-MIBI radio-guided minimally invasive parathyroidectomy: experience with patients with normal thyroids and nodular goiters. Thyroid 12(1):53–61
51. Rubello D, Fig LM et al (2006) Radioguided surgery of parathyroid adenomas and recurrent thyroid cancer using the "low sestamibi dose" protocol. Cancer Biother Radiopharm 21(3):194–205
52. Goldstein RE, Billheimer D et al (2003) Sestamibi scanning and minimally invasive radioguided parathyroidectomy without intraoperative parathyroid hormone measurement. Ann Surg 237(5):722–730; discussion 730–721
53. Bekis R, Aydin A et al (2004) The role of gamma probe activity counts in minimally invasive parathyroidectomy. Preliminary results. Nuklearmedizin 43(6):190–194
54. Bozkurt MF, Ugur O et al (2003) Optimization of the gamma probe-guided parathyroidectomy. Am Surg 69(8):720–725
55. Farley DR (2004) Technetium-99m 2-methoxyisobutyl isonitrile-scintigraphy: preoperative and intraoperative guidance for primary hyperparathyroidism. World J Surg 28(12):1207–1211

56. Rubello D, Casara D et al (2003) Importance of radio-guided minimally invasive parathyroidectomy using hand-held gamma probe and low (99m)Tc-MIBI dose. Technical considerations and long-term clinical results. Q J Nucl Med 47(2):129–138
57. Rubello D, Casara D et al (2003) Optimization of peroperative procedures. Nucl Med Commun 24(2):133–140
58. Rubello D, Mariani G et al (2006) Minimally invasive radio-guided parathyroidectomy: long-term results with the 'low 99mTc-sestamibi protocol'. Nucl Med Commun 27(9):709–713
59. Rubello D, Pelizzo MR et al (2005) Radioguided surgery of primary hyperparathyroidism using the low-dose 99mTc-sestamibi protocol: multiinstitutional experience from the Italian Study Group on Radioguided Surgery and Immunoscintigraphy (GISCRIS). J Nucl Med 46(2):220–226
60. Takeyama H, Shioya H et al (2004) Usefulness of radio-guided surgery using technetium-99m methoxyisobutylisonitrile for primary and secondary hyperparathyroidism. World J Surg 28(6):576–582
61. Ugur O, Bozkurt MF et al (2004) Clinicopathologic and radiopharmacokinetic factors affecting gamma probe-guided parathyroidectomy. Arch Surg 139(11):1175–1179
62. Ruda J, Stack BC Jr et al (2004) The cost-effectiveness of sestamibi scanning compared to bilateral neck exploration for the treatment of primary hyperparathyroidism. Otolaryngol Clin North Am 37(4):855–870, x–xi
63. Mekel M, Mahajna A et al (2005) Minimally invasive surgery for treatment of hyperparathyroidism. Isr Med Assoc J 7(5):323–327
64. Marx UC, Adermann K et al (2000) Solution structures of human parathyroid hormone fragments hPTH(1–34) and hPTH(1–39) and bovine parathyroid hormone fragment bPTH(1–37). Biochem Biophys Res Commun 267(1):213–220
65. Perrier ND, Ituarte PH et al (2002) Parathyroid surgery: separating promise from reality. J Clin Endocrinol Metab 87(3):1024–1029
66. Udelsman R (2002) Surgery in primary hyperparathyroidism: the patient without previous neck surgery. J Bone Miner Res 17(Suppl 2):N126–N132
67. Shaha AR (2004) Parathyroid re-exploration. Otolaryngol Clin North Am 37(4):833–843, x
68. Johnson NA, Tublin ME et al (2007) Parathyroid imaging: technique and role in the preoperative evaluation of primary hyperparathyroidism. AJR Am J Roentgenol 188(6): 1706–1715
69. Stephen AE, Chen KT et al (2004) The coming of age of radiation-induced hyperparathyroidism: evolving patterns of thyroid and parathyroid disease after head and neck irradiation. Surgery 136(6):1143–1153
70. Massaro A, Cittadin S et al (2007) Accurate planning of minimally invasive surgery of parathyroid adenomas by means of [(99m)Tc]MIBI SPECT. Minerva Endocrinol 32(1):9–16
71. Ortega A, Perez de Prada MT et al (2007) Effect of parathyroid-hormone-related protein on human platelet activation. Clin Sci Lond 113(7):319–327
72. Mariani G, Gulec SA et al (2003) Preoperative localization and radioguided parathyroid surgery. J Nucl Med 44(9):1443–1458
73. Rubello D, Mariani G (2007) Hand-held gamma probe or hand-held miniature gamma camera for minimally invasive parathyroidectomy: Competition, evolution or synergy? Eur J Nucl Med Mol Imaging 34(2):162–164
74. Murphy C, Norman J (1999) The 20% rule: a simple, instantaneous radioactivity measurement defines cure and allows elimination of frozen sections and hormone assays during parathyroidectomy. Surgery 126(6):1023–1028, discussion 1028–1029
75. Friedman M, Gurpinar B et al (2007) Guidelines for radioguided parathyroid surgery. Arch Otolaryngol Head Neck Surg 133(12):1235–1239
76. Lo CY, Lang BH et al (2007) A prospective evaluation of preoperative localization by technetium-99m sestamibi scintigraphy and ultrasonography in primary hyperparathyroidism. Am J Surg 193(2):155–159
77. Nichols KJ, Tomas MB et al (2008) Preoperative parathyroid scintigraphic lesion localization: accuracy of various types of readings. Radiology 248(1):221–232

4 Parathyroid Imaging

78. Civelek AC, Ozalp E et al (2002) Prospective evaluation of delayed technetium-99m sestamibi SPECT scintigraphy for preoperative localization of primary hyperparathyroidism. Surgery 131(2):149–157
79. Miccoli P, Ambrosini CE et al (2007) New technologies in thyroid surgery. Endoscopic thyroid surgery. Minerva Chir 62(5):335–349
80. Kukora JS, Zeiger M (2005) The American Association of Clinical Endocrinologists and the American Association of Endocrine Surgeons position statement on the diagnosis and management of primary hyperparathyroidism. Endocr Pract 11(1):49–54
81. Bilezikian JP, Potts JT Jr et al (2002) Summary statement from a workshop on asymptomatic primary hyperparathyroidism: a perspective for the 21st century. J Clin Endocrinol Metab 87(12):5353–5361
82. Sackett WR, Barraclough B et al (2002) Worldwide trends in the surgical treatment of primary hyperparathyroidism in the era of minimally invasive parathyroidectomy. Arch Surg 137(9):1055–1059
83. McHenry CR (2002) What's new in general surgery: endocrine surgery. J Am Coll Surg 195(3):364–371
84. Pasieka JL (2004) What's new in general surgery: endocrine surgery. J Am Coll Surg 199(3):437–445
85. Lomonte C, Buonvino N et al (2006) Sestamibi scintigraphy, topography, and histopathology of parathyroid glands in secondary hyperparathyroidism. Am J Kidney Dis 48(4):638–644
86. Nishida H, Ishibashi M et al (2005) Comparison of histological findings and parathyroid scintigraphy in hemodialysis patients with secondary hyperparathyroid glands. Endocr J 52(2):223–228
87. Owda AK, Mousa D et al (2002) Long-term intravenous calcitriol in secondary hyperparathyroidism: the role of technetium-99m-MIBI scintigraphy in predicting the response to treatment. Ren Fail 24(2):165–173
88. Wells SA Jr, Debenedetti MK et al (2002) Recurrent or persistent hyperparathyroidism. J Bone Miner Res 17(Suppl 2):N158–N162
89. Gotway MB, Reddy GP et al (2001) Comparison between MR imaging and 99mTc MIBI scintigraphy in the evaluation of recurrent of persistent hyperparathyroidism. Radiology 218(3):783–790
90. Martin D, Rosen IB et al (1996) Evaluation of single isotope technetium 99M-sestamibi in localization efficiency for hyperparathyroidism. Am J Surg 172(6):633–636
91. Castellani M, Reschini E et al (2001) Role of Tc-99m sestamibi scintigraphy in the diagnosis and surgical decision-making process in primary hyperparathyroid disease. Clin Nucl Med 26(2):139–144
92. Sprouse LR 2nd, Roe SM et al (2001) Minimally invasive parathyroidectomy without intraoperative localization. Am Surg 67(11):1022–1029
93. Zettinig G, Prager G et al (2002) Value of a structured report for the interpretation of parathyroid scintigraphy in primary essential hyperthyroidism. Acta Med Austriaca 29(2):68–71
94. Panzironi G, Falvo L et al (2002) Preoperative evaluation of primary hyperparathyroidism: role of diagnostic imaging. Chir Ital 54(5):629–634
95. Clark PB, Case D et al (2003) Enhanced scintigraphic protocol required for optimal preoperative localization before targeted minimally invasive parathyroidectomy. Clin Nucl Med 28(12):955–960
96. Prager G, Czerny C et al (2003) Impact of localization studies on feasibility of minimally invasive parathyroidectomy in an endemic goiter region. J Am Coll Surg 196(4):541–548
97. Khaliq T, Khawar A et al (2003) Unilateral exploration for primary hyperparathyroidism. J Coll Physicians Surg Pak 13(10):588–591
98. Gotthardt M, Lohmann B et al (2004) Clinical value of parathyroid scintigraphy with technetium-99m methoxyisobutylisonitrile: discrepancies in clinical data and a systematic metaanalysis of the literature. World J Surg 28(1):100–107
99. Mortier PE, Mozzon MM et al (2004) Unilateral surgery for hyperparathyroidism: indications, limits, and late results—New philosophy or expensive selection without improvement of surgical results? World J Surg 28(12):1298–1304

100. Ruda JM, Hollenbeak CS et al (2005) A systematic review of the diagnosis and treatment of primary hyperparathyroidism from 1995 to 2003. Otolaryngol Head Neck Surg 132(3):359–372
101. Carneiro-Pla DM, Solorzano CC et al (2006) Consequences of targeted parathyroidectomy guided by localization studies without intraoperative parathyroid hormone monitoring. J Am Coll Surg 202(5):715–722
102. Kairys JC, Daskalakis C et al (2006) Surgeon-performed ultrasound for preoperative localization of abnormal parathyroid glands in patients with primary hyperparathyroidism. World J Surg 30(9):1658–1663; discussion 1664
103. Gawande AA, Monchik JM et al (2006) Reassessment of parathyroid hormone monitoring during parathyroidectomy for primary hyperparathyroidism after 2 preoperative localization studies. Arch Surg 141(4):381–384; discussion 384
104. Fuster D, Ybarra J et al (2006) Role of pre-operative imaging using 99mTc-MIBI and neck ultrasound in patients with secondary hyperparathyroidism who are candidates for subtotal parathyroidectomy. Eur J Nucl Med Mol Imaging 33(4):467–473
105. Solorzano CC, Carneiro-Pla D et al (2005) Surgical management of primary hyperparathyroidism: the case for giving up quick intraoperative PTH assay in favor of routine measurement the morning after. Ann Surg 242(6):904, author reply 904–905
106. Seehofer D, Steinmuller T et al (2004) Parathyroid hormone venous sampling before reoperative surgery in renal hyperparathyroidism: comparison with noninvasive localization procedures and review of the literature. Arch Surg 139(12):1331–1338
107. Clark P, Wooldridge T et al (2004) Providing optimal preoperative localization for recurrent parathyroid carcinoma: a combined parathyroid scintigraphy and computed tomography approach. Clin Nucl Med 29(11):681–684
108. Saint Marc O, Cogliandolo A et al (2004) Prospective evaluation of ultrasonography plus MIBI scintigraphy in selecting patients with primary hyperparathyroidism for unilateral neck exploration under local anaesthesia. Am J Surg 187(3):388–393
109. Gross ND, Wax MK (2004) Unilateral and bilateral surgery for parathyroid disease. Otolaryngol Clin North Am 37(4):799–817, ix–x
110. Kebapci M, Entok E et al (2004) Preoperative evaluation of parathyroid lesions in patients with concomitant thyroid disease: role of high resolution ultrasonography and dual phase technetium 99 m sestamibi scintigraphy. J Endocrinol Invest 27(1):24–30
111. Miura D, Wada N et al (2002) Does intraoperative quick parathyroid hormone assay improve the results of parathyroidectomy? World J Surg 26(8):926–930
112. Wakamatsu H, Noguchi S et al (2001) Technetium-99m tetrofosmin for parathyroid scintigraphy: a direct comparison with (99m)Tc-MIBI, (201)Tl, MRI and US. Eur J Nucl Med 28(12):1817–1827
113. De Feo ML, Colagrande S et al (2000) Parathyroid glands: combination of (99m)Tc MIBI scintigraphy and US for demonstration of parathyroid glands and nodules. Radiology 214(2): 393–402
114. Wada A, Sugihara M et al (1999) Magnetic resonance imaging (MRI) and technetium-99m-methoxyisonitrile (MIBI) scintigraphy to evaluate the abnormal parathyroid gland and PEIT efficacy for secondary hyperparathyroidism. Radiat Med 17(4):275–282
115. Pattou F, Oudar C et al (1998) Localization of abnormal parathyroid glands with jugular sampling for parathyroid hormone, and subtraction scanning with sestamibi or tetrofosmine. Aust N Z J Surg 68(2):108–111
116. Ishibashi M, Nishida H et al (1998) Comparison of technetium-99m-MIBI, technetium-99m-tetrofosmin, ultrasound and MRI for localization of abnormal parathyroid glands. J Nucl Med 39(2):320–324
117. Peeler BB, Martin WH et al (1997) Sestamibi parathyroid scanning and preoperative localization studies for patients with recurrent/persistent hyperparathyroidism or significant comorbid conditions: development of an optimal localization strategy. Am Surg 63(1):37–46
118. Mazzeo S, Caramella D et al (1996) Comparison among sonography, double-tracer subtraction scintigraphy, and double-phase scintigraphy in the detection of parathyroid lesions. AJR Am J Roentgenol 166(6):1465–1470

119. Lee VS, Spritzer CE et al (1996) The complementary roles of fast spin-echo MR imaging and double-phase 99m Tc-sestamibi scintigraphy for localization of hyperfunctioning parathyroid glands. AJR Am J Roentgenol 167(6):1555–1562
120. International Commission on Radiological Protection (1988) Radiation dose to patients from radiopharmaceuticals. IRRP publication 53. ICRP, London p 199,264,373
121. International Commission on Radiological Protection (1993) Radiation protection in biomedical research. ICRP publication 62. Pergamon Press, New York, p 23
122. Uruno T, Kebebew E (2006) How to localize parathyroid tumors in primary hyperparathyroidism? J Endocrinol Invest 29(9):840–847
123. Funari M, Campos Z et al (1992) MRI and ultrasound detection of asymptomatic thyroid nodules in hyperparathyroidism. J Comput Assist Tomogr 16(4):615–619
124. Petti GH Jr, Chonkich GD et al (1993) Unilateral parathyroidectomy: the value of the localizing scan. J Otolaryngol 22(4):307–310
125. Yousem DM (1996) Parathyroid and thyroid imaging. Neuroimaging Clin N Am 6(2):435–459

Myocardial Perfusion Scintigraphy with 99mTc-MIBI

5

Hojjat Ahmadzadehfar and Amir Sabet

5.1 Kinetics and Scientific Basis of Myocardial Perfusion Imaging with Tc-MIBI

5.1.1 Photon Energy

Tc-MIBI has photon energy of 140 keV, which is optimal for scintillation camera imaging. With a standard, symmetrical 20% photopeak, most scattered radiation is effectively eliminated.

5.1.2 Physical and Biological Half-Life

Tc-MIBI's physical half-life is 6 h. The myocardial biological T½ in normal myocardium is approximately 11 h [1]. The much shorter physical half-life of Tc-99m (6 h vs 73 h for Tl-201) and the biodistribution characteristics of Tc-MIBI permit the administration of a 10-times higher dose compound than Tl-201. This yields better image quality in a shorter acquisition time in a shorter time period [2]. Studies of organ dosimetry showed that a 30 mCi dose (1,100 MBq) of Tc-MIBI can be administered safely [3]. Higher doses are often used in obese patients. The activities should be modified for children according to the recommendations of nuclear medicine guidelines [4, 5].

H. Ahmadzadehfar (✉) • A. Sabet
Klinik und Poliklinik für Nuklearmedizin, Universität Bonn,
Sigmund-Freud-Straße 25, 53127 Bonn, Germany
e-mail: hojjat.ahmadzahdefar@ukb.uni-bonn.de

J. Bucerius et al. (eds.), *99mTc-Sestamibi*,
DOI 10.1007/978-3-642-04233-1_5, © Springer-Verlag Berlin Heidelberg 2012

5.1.3 Radiation Exposure Levels to the Patients, Hospital Staff, and to Relatives of Patients and a Comparison Between Tc-99m-Labeled Tracers and Tl-201

In general, radiation exposure to relatives is limited and no special precautions are needed for studies with either ^{99m}Tc-labeled tracers or ^{201}Tl chloride. However, performing one-day protocols for patients who take care of infants should be avoided. Radiation exposure to the environment is lower with ^{201}Tl chloride than with ^{99m}Tc-labeled tracers. In the contrary, the absorbed dose to the patients with ^{99m}Tc-labeled tracers such as Tc-MIBI is much lower than that of ^{201}Tl. While, the effective dose of Tl-201 is about 18 mSv, the effective dose of Tc-MIBI in a 1 day and 2 days protocols is about 8 and 5–7 mSv, respectively. Using the new camera systems like D-SPECT (Spectrum-Dynamics) or the so-called smartzoom collimators (IQ.SPECT; Siemens) the radiation exposure to the patients could be reduced even further.

5.1.4 Initial Myocardial Uptake of Tc-MIBI

Sestamibi is lipophilic and enters myocardial cells via passive transport driven by the negative membrane potential of the intact cell. Once within the myocardium it is localized mostly inside mitochondria [6, 7]. Cardiac uptake of sestamibi is therefore dependent on normal mitochondrial function. Uptake is depressed and washout increased when there is cellular hypoxia secondary to severe myocardial ischemia and cells are close to death [8]. Studies have confirmed that myocardial uptake of Tc-MIBI, as with Tl-201, is proportional to regional myocardial blood flow over the physiologic flow rates with decreased extraction at hyperemic flows and increased extraction at low flows [9]. Overall, there is a positive, linear relationship between myocardial tissue distribution of Tc-Sestamibi and coronary flow. However, there is an evidence of diffusion limitation at flow levels above 1.5–2 mL/min/g. The proportion of injected activity taken up by the myocardium is $1.5 \pm 0.4\%$ of injected dose at stress and $1.2 \pm 0.4\%$ of injected dose at rest.

5.1.5 Myocardial Redistribution

In contrast to Tl-201, Tc-MIBI shows a very slow myocardial clearance after its initial myocardial uptake. The Tc-MIBI only undergoes minimal (10–15%) redistribution over a period of 4 h.

5.1.6 Blood Clearance

The blood clearance of sestamibi is very rapid and biexponential. There is an initial fast clearance phase (T½ less than 3 min at stress and rest) followed by a slow clearance phase [10]. At 5 min after injection only less than 10% of the injected dose remains in circulation [3].

5.1.7 Biodistribution at Rest and Stress

The major metabolic pathways of clearance are the hepatobiliary system (48 h fecal excretion: 37% of injected dose at rest and 29% at stress) and kidneys (24 h urinary excretion of 30% of injected dose at rest and 24% of injected dose after exercise).

After an injection at rest, the highest Tc-MIBI concentration is initially found in the gallbladder and liver, followed by heart, spleen, and lungs. Within the first hour, liver activity decreases with excretion into the biliary system, while maximal accumulation in the gallbladder occurs at 60 min. Tc-MIBI activity in the heart remains relatively stable over the time, whereas splenic and lung activity gradually decreases. At 110 min after injection, the count density in the heart is higher than in the adjacent organs (only the gallbladder shows a higher activity).

After stress injection, the highest initial tracer concentration, in descending order, is seen in the gallbladder, heart, liver, and spleen. Pulmonary activity is negligible. At all times after a stress injection, cardiac activity is higher than that in the immediately adjacent organs. Hepatic activity decreases more rapidly than activity in any other organ during the first hour [11].

5.2 Tc-MIBI as an Agent for Myocardial Perfusion Imaging

Myocardial perfusion scintigraphy (MPS) is an established imaging technique that is already an integral part of the management of coronary heart disease (CHD) and is included in a number of professional guidelines. Its most important applications are the diagnosis of CHD, prognostication, selection for revascularization, and assessment of acute coronary syndromes [12]. MPS is the only widely available method of assessing myocardial perfusion directly. An inducible perfusion abnormality indicates impaired perfusion reserve, which in turn usually corresponds to epicardial coronary obstruction. The site, depth, and extent of the abnormality provide diagnostic and management information that cannot be determined reliably from other tests such as the ECG. Conversely, normal stress MPS indicates the absence of coronary obstruction and hence of clinically significant disease [13]. It is important to note that normal perfusion does not exclude nonobstructive coronary disease, but such disease is unlikely to be related to symptoms and is not prognostically important.

In 1990, the Food and Drug Administration approved the use of Tc-MIBI for myocardial perfusion imaging. Compared with thallium-201, Tc-MIBI emits higher energy photons, and the shorter half-life of Tc-99m allows the administration of a higher dosage. As a result of higher count rates as well as better tissue penetration, attributable to the 140 keV emission energy, imaging with Tc-MIBI results in sharper images [14]. Uptake of Tc-MIBI and thallium-201 has been shown to be comparable in different myocardial zones and defect magnitude. Sestamibi activity 1 h after rest injection has been found to parallel redistribution thallium-201 activity. Sestamibi can accurately quantify myocardial scarring and is a good indicator of myocardial viability determined with microscopy, although the uptake may underestimate myocardial viability in comparison with FDG-PET in segments with moderately reduced Tc-MIBI activity [14, 15].

5.3 Exercise and Pharmacologic Stress Testing

Myocardial perfusion SPECT images are routinely obtained in two sets of images, one at rest and the other after either exercise or pharmacological stress.

Dynamic exercise is usually performed with a treadmill or bicycle ergometer with continuous patient monitoring and it is the preferred stress modality in patients who can have exercise to an adequate workload.

However, it should not be performed in patients who cannot achieve an adequate hemodynamic response because of noncardiac physical limitations such as pulmonary, peripheral vascular, or musculoskeletal abnormalities or because of poor motivation. These patients, as well as those who are unable to exercise at all for noncardiac reasons (e.g. arthritis, amputation, or neurological disease), should undergo pharmacological stress perfusion imaging, a very good alternative to dynamic exercise [5]. The pharmacological stress can be performed using vasodilator agents such as dipyridamole, adenosine, and regadenoson or dobutamine as a sympathomimetic agent. Since the introduction of dipyridamole-induced coronary vasodilation as an adjunct to Tl-201 MPI [16–18], pharmacologic interventions have become an important tool in noninvasive diagnosis of coronary artery disease (CAD) [19–21]. Dipyridamole SPECT imaging with Tl-201 or Tc-MIBI appears to be as accurate as is exercise SPECT, and its accuracy in detecting multivessel disease is similar for men and women [22]. Results of MPI during adenosine infusion are similar to those obtained with dipyridamole and exercise imaging (Tables 5.2 and 5.3) [19].

There are large variations in the recommendations from country to country considering the dose of Tc-MIBI, with injected activities ranging from 250 to 1,100 MBq subject to exercise protocol (1 day or 2 days).

Concerning the stress techniques, image acquisition methods and doses have been described in detail in the guidelines of American Society of Nuclear Cardiology (http://www.asnc.org) and also in the guideline of European association of Nuclear Medicine (http://www.eanm.org).

5.4 Stress-Only Myocardial Perfusion SPECT with Tc-MIBI

A stress-only imaging strategy approach may be more accurately termed a selective stress-only imaging strategy, in which stress images are obtained and then a decision is made by the interpreting physician about whether to proceed with resting images. If the stress study is completely normal, resting images would not be obtained. A rest study would be obtained if there is any questionable abnormality on the stress study. It may be appropriate at times to consider some nonimaging factors such as a high clinical risk profile or an abnormal ECG response to low-level stress in deciding whether or not to proceed with rest imaging, because of missing important subtle abnormalities such as transient ischemic dilatation.

Patients who cannot exercise are generally at higher risk for cardiac events even after a normal SPECT study. Therefore, a stress-only imaging strategy maybe best applied to patients who can exercise [23]. A stress-only imaging strategy may have less attenuation problems if a high dose of technetium were utilized for the stress images, with rest images if needed performed on a second day. However, a low-dose stress-only strategy allows a 1 day testing strategy [24].

Utilization of attenuation correction and prone imaging may help to reduce the number of patients that need to return for rest images by reducing attenuation artifacts on the stress images.

The best use of a stress-only imaging strategy is likely to be in the selected low or low-intermediate risk population, in whom it is anticipated that the stress study will be normal.

5.5 Sensitivity and Specificity of Myocardial Perfusion Tc-MIBI-SPECT for Detecting CAD

In patients with suspected or known chronic stable coronary disease, the largest accumulated experience in MPI has been with the tracer Tl-201, but available evidence suggests that the Tc-MIBI yield similar diagnostic accuracy [3, 25–29]. The sensitivity and specificity of myocardial perfusion Tc-MIBI-SPECT for the detection of angiographically significant (more than 50% stenosis) CAD is presented in Tables 5.1–5.3.

A meta-analysis of diagnostic test performance has summarized evidence documenting that the sensitivity of exercise electrocardiography is significantly lower than that of myocardial perfusion SPECT [13].

5.6 Tc-MIBI in Assessment of Myocardial Viability

In patients with chronic coronary disease and LV dysfunction, there exists an important subpopulation in which revascularization may significantly improve regional or global LV function as well as symptoms and potentially natural fate. Therefore it is very important to distinguish between stunning, hibernation and necrosis. *Stunning* is characterized by a reduced function, after a period of transient ischemia, in the presence of normal perfusion and preserved metabolic activity; myocardial functional reserve is also preserved. This condition spontaneously recovers after days or weeks. *Hibernating*, viable myocardium, is characterized by a functional impairment, due to a chronic reduction in perfusion, with a persistent blood flow reduction, in the presence of a preserved metabolic activity and a preserved contractile reserve. This condition recovers after coronary revascularization, in

Table 5.1 Sensitivity and specificity of exercise myocardial perfusion Tc-MIBI-SPECT for detecting CAD (≥50% stenosis)

First author	Year	Number of patients	Sensitivity (%)	Specificity (%)
Kiat [30]	1990	61	94	80
Pozzoli [31]	1991	75	84	88
Berman [32]*	1993	63	96	82
Solot [33]	1993	128	96	74
Minoves [34]*	1993	64	90	92
Van Train [35]	1993	160	97	67
Sylven [36]	1994	160	72	50
Van Train [37]	1994	161	89	36
Palmas [38]	1995	70	91	75
Rubello [39]	1995	120	93	61
Hambye [40]	1996	128	82	76
Yao [41]	1997	51	94	93
Heiba [42]	1997	72	93	50
Candell-Riera [43]	1997	235	93	94
Taillefer [44]	1997	85	72	81
Budoff [45]	1998	33	75	71
Santana-Boado [46]	1998	702	91	90
Acampa [47]	1998	32	92	71
San Roman [48]	1998	102	87	70
Olszowska [49]	2003	44	93	84

*MIBI and Tl

Table 5.2 Sensitivity and specificity of vasodilator stress myocardial perfusion Tc-MIBI-scintigraphy for detecting CAD (≥50% stenosis)

First author	Year	Vasodilator	N of Patients	Sensitivity (%)	Specificity (%)
Marwick [50]	1993	Adenosine	97	86	71
Amanullah [51]	1996	Adenosine	201[a]	93	78
Miller [52]	1997	Dipyridamole	244	91	28
Schillaci [53][b]	1997	Dipyridamole	40	95	72
Soman [54]	1997	Dipyridamole	27	90	66
Amanullah [55]	1997	Adenosine	222	93	73
Ogilby [56]	1998	Dipyridamole	26	90	100
Jamil [57]	1999	Adenosin	32	75	73
Smart [58]	2000	Dipyridamole	183	80	73
Onbasili [59]	2004	Dipyridamole	20	85	92
Fan [60]	2006	Adenosine	79	88	66

[a]Only female
[b]>70% stenosis

weeks or months. *Necrotic,* nonviable tissue is characterized by a reduced-absent function, in the absence or severely reduced metabolic activity, and no functional response to inotropic stimuli. This condition is not modified after

Table 5.3 Sensitivity and specificity of dobutamine myocardial perfusion Tc-MIBI-scintigraphy for detecting CAD (≥50% stenosis)

First author	Year	Number of patients	Sensitivity (%)	Specificity (%)
Gunalp [61]	1993	27	94	89
Forster [62]	1993	21	83	89
Marwick [50]	1993	97	80	74
Marwick [63]	1993	217	76	67
Mairesse [64]	1994	129	76	65
Marwick [65]	1994	82	65	68
Senior [66]	1994	61	95	71
Di Bello [67]	1996	45	87	86
Iftikhar [68]	1996	38	79	90
Kisacik [69]	1996	69	96	64
Slavich [70]	1996	46	82	83
San Roman [48]	1998	92	87	70
Elhendy [71]	1998	70	64	72

Table 5.4 Comparison of PET, sestamibi, and echocardiography for detection of hibernating myocardium [80]

Methods	PPV (%)	NPV (%)
NH3-PET	45	95
FDG-PET	75	100
MIBI	50	96
Echocardiography	100	87

coronary revascularization [72]. Because various radionuclide tracers identify preserved cell membrane integrity and aspects of metabolic activity, radionuclide techniques play an important role in the assessment of myocardial viability and, thus, the potential identification of patients with LV dysfunction and CAD who may benefit significantly from revascularization. Many investigators believe that Tc-MIBI is an effective viability tracer [73–79].

In a study comparing the diagnostic accuracy of Tc-MIBI, NH3/FDG-PET and echocardiography to detection of hibernating myocardium, the nuclear technique was found to have high negative predictive values (NPV) of ≥95% but lower positive predictive values (PPV) of 45–75% as compared with echocardiography, which had an NPV of 87% and a PPV of 100%. PET was the most powerful predictor of hibernation, however combination of a technique with a high PPV (echocardiography) and a high NPV (PET or sestamibi) may represent the optimal clinical choice (Table 5.4) [80].

Intravenous/sublingual administration of nitrates prior/during Tc-MIBI injection has been proven to improve the accuracy in detection of viable myocardium and prediction of functional recovery [81, 82]. Nitrates are thought to increase blood flow to severely hypoperfused regions, thereby increasing tracer delivery and uptake in these severely hypoperfused but viable regions. Besides nitrate-enhanced imaging, the development of ECG gated SPECT, enabling the simultaneous assessment of perfusion and function [83, 84], has further improved the accuracy to assess viability.

5.7 Tc-MIBI for Risk Stratification in Patients with Known or Suspected CAD

Nuclear medicines procedures are best applied for risk stratification in patients with a clinically intermediate risk of a subsequent cardiac event. For prognostic testing, patients known to be at high risk or low risk would not be appropriate patients for cost-effective risk stratification, because they are already risk stratified sufficiently for clinical decision making [85]. In general, low risk has been defined as a less than 1% cardiac mortality rate per year, high risk as a more than 3% cardiac mortality rate per year. Intermediate risk refers to the 1–3% cardiac mortality rate per year range [86]. In chronic CAD, it has been suggested that a more than 3% per year mortality rate can be used to identify patients with minimal symptoms whose mortality rate can be improved by coronary artery bypass grafting (CABG) [87] and can be considered high risk. Because the mortality risk for patients undergoing either CABG or angioplasty is at least 1% [88], mildly symptomatic patients with a less than 1% mortality rate would not generally be candidates for revascularization to improve survival. These are, however, general thresholds and may vary according to the age of the patient and comorbidities. For example, in the very elderly, both the low- and high-risk levels would be higher (in the range of 2–5% for annual cardiac death), reflecting the higher rate of yearly cardiac death in elderly patients undergoing revascularization.

Many of the major determinants of prognosis in CAD can be assessed by measurements of stress-induced perfusion and function changes with Tc-MIBI. These include the amount of infracted myocardium, the amount of jeopardized myocardium (supplied by vessels with hemodynamically significant stenosis) and the degree or severity of ischemia (tightness of the individual coronary stenosis). Of additional importance in prognostic assessment is the stability (or instability) of the CAD process, a factor that may explain an apparent paradox.

Studies including large patient samples have demonstrated that factors estimating the extent of LV dysfunction (LVEF, the extent of infarcted myocardium, transient ischemic dilation [TID] of the LV, and increased lung uptake of Tl-201/Tc-MIBI) [89] are excellent predictors of cardiac mortality. In contrast, markers of provocative ischemia (exertional symptoms, electrocardiographic changes, the extent of reversible perfusion defects, and stress-induced ventricular dyssynergy) are better predictors of the subsequent development of acute ischemic syndromes [90]. Other reports have indicated that stress myocardial perfusion SPECT yields incremental prognostic value over clinical and exercise data with respect to cardiac death as an isolated endpoint [91, 92].

To maximally extract the information regarding prognostic determinants in CAD, it is necessary to consider the full extent and severity of abnormalities, either quantitatively [93, 94] or semiquantitatively [32], rather than simply determining that the nuclear study is normal or abnormal. The evaluation of prognosis can be facilitated by assessing global perfusion abnormalities by using a composite variable incorporating the extent and severity of hypoperfusion during stress.

5 Myocardial Perfusion Scintigraphy with 99mTc-MIBI

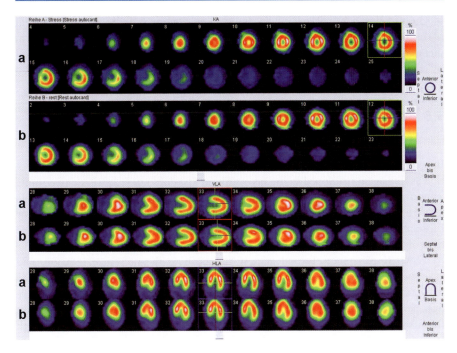

Fig. 5.1 Normal SPECT study in a 55 year-old woman referred because of dyspnea

Quantitative analysis of myocardial perfusion SPECT has been developed by using a variety of approaches [35, 37, 93–98] and, in general, has similar sensitivities and specificities compared with those of expert visual analysis. Quantitative analysis has also been shown to be equal to expert visual interpretation in the assessment of prognosis [99]. These quantitative approaches decrease inter- and intraobserver variability and facilitate serial assessment of myocardial perfusion and function.

In summary, quantitative data necessary for prognostication are:
1. Extent and Severity of perfusion and functional abnormalities
2. Amount of LV ejection fraction changes during stress
3. LV volumes (at rest and after stress)
4. Transient ventricular dysfunction (TID and lung uptake)
   TID: threshold of TID index = 1.14 for a same-day post-exercise stress/rest Tc-MIBI protocol [100] and 1.19 by use of 2-day protocol [101]
   High lung uptake: preliminary data for Tc-MIBI lung-to-heart ratio suggests an upper limit of 0.44 [102]).

A normal scan (Fig. 5.1) is associated with a very low cardiac event rate and the annualized hard cardiac events rate is below 1% [103–111].

Even in the presence of an angiographic CAD, the cardiac event rate remains very low if stress nuclear MPI is normal. A review of 14 trials including over 12,000 patients with stable chest pain confirmed that normal Tc-MIBI SPECT is associated with a hard cardiac event rate of 0.6% per year [112].

On the other hand, according to new studies, abnormal findings on myocardial perfusion imaging labeled false positive based on coronary angiography may predict a higher prevalence of coronary and peripheral vascular events than suggested by a normal coronary angiogram [113, 114].

5.8 Tc-MIBI in Diagnosis and Follow-up of Acute Coronary Syndrome

In contrast to Tl-201, there is no need for immediate imaging after Tc-MIBI injection as this agent is trapped in the myocardium and does not redistribute over time. Thus, tracer injection may be performed in the emergency department, and patients may be transferred to the nuclear medicine or nuclear cardiology laboratory for subsequent imaging as these late images reflect myocardial blood flow (MBF) at the time of injection.

Tc-MIBI can precisely and acutely demonstrate the presence, location, and severity of the perfusion defect causing the infarct, even in the absence of ECG evidence of infarction. It provides a quantitative measure of the zone at risk. In addition, perfusion information can be obtained serially to document improvement with thrombolysis or percutaneous transluminal coronary angioplasty. However, although it detects occlusions, it cannot distinguish old from new ones.

In acute myocardial infarction, heralded by severe chest pain, Tc-MIBI is particularly useful in confirming the diagnosis when the electrocardiogram and enzyme assays are not definitive, that is, left bundle branch block, ventricular pacing, or nontransmural myocardial infarction.

In patients with chest pain receiving resting perfusion imaging, sensitivity and specificity has been shown to be better than clinical factors and the resting ECG [115–117]. Accuracy is the highest when patients are injected while they have chest pain.

The diagnostic accuracy of sestamibi SPECT has also been compared with that of cardiac troponin I (cTnI) [118] TnI as well as Serum troponin-T. They have been found to be as specific as sestamibi SPECT for AMI but have a low sensitivity at presentation with serial determinations being necessary to achieve a high sensitivity.

Furthermore, data acquisition in a gated mode for additional wall motion information results in a significant increase of specificity while the overall sensitivity remains unchanged. Therefore, especially after an acute adverse cardiac event has been ruled out, exercise testing in the form of myocardial perfusion imaging is part of many triage strategies in dedicated chest pain centers or emergency departments [119–122].

Compared to coronary angiography in assessing the presence of myocardial infarction, the overall sensitivity of Tc-MIBI imaging is about 90%.

Tc-MIBI perfusion defect size is closely correlated with values for ejection fraction, regional wall motion score, and creatine kinase release. It also predicts patient outcomes in patients with myocardial infarction [123, 124] and could be a reliable measure of relative infarct size reduction during early reperfusion [125].

5 Myocardial Perfusion Scintigraphy with 99mTc-MIBI

A large number of studies have used Tc-MIBI to predict recovery of regional contractile function after revascularization, showing a sensitivity of about 80% with a specificity of 66%. For most of these studies, segments were classified as viable if activity exceeded a certain threshold, frequently 50–60% [126].

Despite this well-validated body of experimental and clinical knowledge for diagnosis, assessment of myocardium at risk, and management of AMI, the availability of alternative methods and the logistics and time demands of performing MPI in the setting of AMI has limited its widespread clinical application. This technique has value in clinical trials for treatment of acute infarction as it can sometimes reduce the number of patients required to obtain significant results between treatment groups.

5.9 First Pass Technique for Determination of Ejection Fraction and/or Regional Wall Motion

First-pass radionuclide ventriculography (FPRNV) utilizes rapidly acquired images on a high count rate gamma camera with high temporal resolution to track a tracer bolus through the venous system into the right atrium (RA), right ventricle (RV), pulmonary arteries (PA), lungs, left atrium (LA), left ventricle (LV), and finally, the aorta. Several cardiac cycles are sampled continuously. The change in radiotracer content over time is used to calculate functional information, such as ejection fraction, cardiac output, and transit times, as well as to assess regional wall motion by comparison of end-diastolic (ED) and end-systolic (ES) images. The first-pass approach is uniquely suited for the detection of intracardiac left to right shunting, by mathematical analysis of time-activity curves generated by a region of interest placed over the lung. The first-pass approach can be applied to patients both at rest and during exercise stress [127].

Tc-99m diethylamine triamine pentaacetic acid (DTPA) is the radionuclide of choice for standard first pass radionuclide angiography (FPRNA) because of its renal excretion, minimizing patient radiation exposure. Tc-99m pertechnetate or other technetium-based compounds, such as the technetium sestamibi may also be used. Different studies have documented similar accuracy of measurements of right and left ventricular function using Tc-MIBI in comparison to other radiopharmaceuticals [128].

5.10 ECG-Gated SPECT with Tc-MIBI

Tc-MIBI offers the opportunity to obtain, simultaneously, LV myocardial perfusion and function with gated SPECT (Fig. 5.2) [129, 130] or to perform FPRNV [131, 132]. The latter allows the determination of RV and LV function at peak stress and at rest, in contrast to gated SPECT in which functional information is generally restricted to the left ventricle and based on rest data, due to the delayed imaging procedure [90±30 min postinjection (p.i.)] and the long acquisition time (15–30 min). LV function at peak exercise or pharmacological stress, however, has

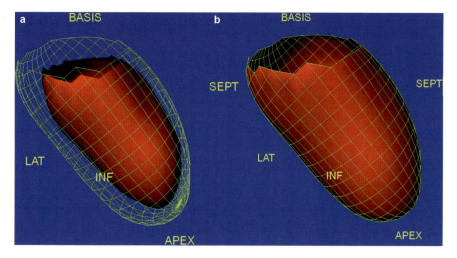

Fig. 5.2 Three-dimensional rendering of left ventricular (LV) function. The end systolic (**a**) and diastolic (**b**) volume shown in poststress show a normal wall motion

been shown to be of great diagnostic and prognostic value in patients with coronary artery disease, greater than many other noninvasively or invasively derived variables [38, 133, 134].

Observing myocardial contraction in segments with apparent fixed perfusion defects permits the nuclear test reader to discern attenuation artifacts from true perfusion abnormalities. Although this phenomenon is difficult to verify and quantify, it is reasonable to expect that it would also result in a reduction in the number of "equivocal" scans reported [84].

The ability of gated SPECT to provide measurement of LVEF, segmental wall motion, and LV absolute volumes also adds to the prognostic information that can be derived from a SPECT perfusion study. A large study including [135] 1,680 patients demonstrated that both poststress LVEF and endsystolic volume provides significant information regarding the extent and severity of perfusion defect as measured by the sum stress score (SSS) in prediction of cardiac death. It could be shown that LV end-systolic volume provides additional information over poststress LVEF in prediction of cardiac death. In a subsequent study of patients undergoing stress Tc-MIBI myocardial perfusion SPECT, it has been [90] demonstrated that poststress EF and the extent of stress-induced ischemia, as assessed by the summed difference score (SDS), provide complementary information in the prediction of risk of cardiac death. EF was the strongest predictor of mortality, whereas the SDS was the strongest predictor of MI. The combined variables were more effective in risk stratification of patients than were the stress variables or poststress EF alone.

In a large study population, a good agreement was observed in the evaluation of LV ejection fraction between gated SPECT and radionuclide angiocardiography.

5 Myocardial Perfusion Scintigraphy with 99mTc-MIBI

However, in patients with perfusion abnormalities, a slight underestimation in poststress LV ejection fraction was observed using gated SPECT as compared to equilibrium radionuclide angiocardiography [136].

Thus, gated myocardial perfusion SPECT may enhance the prognostic and diagnostic content of Tc-MIBI MPI, combining the poststress and/or rest LV function with rest and/or stress perfusion measurements.

Studies revealed no significant differences between Tl-201 and Tc-MIBI gated-SPECT series with respect to test sensitivity, but specificity tends to be greater with Tc-MIBI [137].

With gated SPECT, it is important to distinguish the poststress LVEF from the resting EF because, in patients with severe CAD, stress-induced stunning can result in prolonged depression of LVEF [138–140].

Furthermore, a recent study has shown the impact of complementary information provided by gated SPECT Tc-MIBI, determining functional importance of morphological malformations, in clinical decision making in children and adolescents with severe CHD as well as in children with myocarditis [141, 142].

References

1. Munch G, Neverve J, Matsunari I, Schroter G, Schwaiger M (1997) Myocardial technetium-99m-tetrofosmin and technetium-99m-sestamibi kinetics in normal subjects and patients with coronary artery disease. J Nucl Med 38(3):428–432
2. Beller GA, Watson DD (1991) Physiological basis of myocardial perfusion imaging with the technetium 99m agents. Semin Nucl Med 21(3):173–181
3. Wackers FJ, Berman DS, Maddahi J et al (1989) Technetium-99m hexakis 2-methoxyisobutyl isonitrile: human biodistribution, dosimetry, safety, and preliminary comparison to thallium-201 for myocardial perfusion imaging. J Nucl Med 30(3):301–311
4. Piepsz A, Hahn K, Roca I et al (1990) A radiopharmaceuticals schedule for imaging in paediatrics. Paediatric Task Group European Association Nuclear Medicine. Eur J Nucl Med 17(3–4):127–129
5. Hesse B, Tagil K, Cuocolo A et al (2005) EANM/ESC procedural guidelines for myocardial perfusion imaging in nuclear cardiology. Eur J Nucl Med Mol Imaging 32(7):855–897
6. Piwnica-Worms D, Kronauge JF, Delmon L, Holman BL, Marsh JD, Jones AG (1990) Effect of metabolic inhibition on technetium-99m-MIBI kinetics in cultured chick myocardial cells. J Nucl Med 31(4):464–472
7. Carvalho PA, Chiu ML, Kronauge JF et al (1992) Subcellular distribution and analysis of technetium-99m-MIBI in isolated perfused rat hearts. J Nucl Med 33(8):1516–1522
8. Piwnica-Worms D, Chiu ML, Kronauge JF (1992) Divergent kinetics of 201Tl and 99mTc-SESTAMIBI in cultured chick ventricular myocytes during ATP depletion. Circulation 85(4):1531–1541
9. Canby RC, Silber S, Pohost GM (1990) Relations of the myocardial imaging agents 99mTc-MIBI and 201 Tl to myocardial blood flow in a canine model of myocardial ischemic insult. Circulation 81(1):289–296
10. Glover DK, Okada RD (1990) Myocardial kinetics of Tc-MIBI in canine myocardium after dipyridamole. Circulation 81(2):628–637

11. Taillefer R (2003) Kinetics of myocardial perfusion imaging radiotracers. In: Iskandrian AE, Verani MS (eds) Nuclear cardiac imaging principles and applications, 3rd edn. Oxford University Press, Oxford, pp 57–58
12. Underwood SR, Anagnostopoulos C, Cerqueira M et al (2004) Myocardial perfusion scintigraphy: the evidence. Eur J Nucl Med Mol Imaging 31(2):261–291
13. Fleischmann KE, Hunink MG, Kuntz KM, Douglas PS (1998) Exercise echocardiography or exercise SPECT imaging? A meta-analysis of diagnostic test performance. JAMA 280(10):913–920
14. Travin MI, Bergmann SR (2005) Assessment of myocardial viability. Semin Nucl Med 35(1): 2–16
15. Kailasnath P, Sinusas AJ (2001) Comparison of Tl-201 with Tc-99m-labeled myocardial perfusion agents: technical, physiologic, and clinical issues. J Nucl Cardiol 8(4):482–498
16. Gould KL (1978) Noninvasive assessment of coronary stenoses by myocardial perfusion imaging during pharmacologic coronary vasodilatation. I. Physiologic basis and experimental validation. Am J Cardiol 41(2):267–278
17. Gould KL, Westcott RJ, Albro PC, Hamilton GW (1978) Noninvasive assessment of coronary stenoses by myocardial imaging during pharmacologic coronary vasodilatation. II. Clinical methodology and feasibility. Am J Cardiol 41(2):279–287
18. Albro PC, Gould KL, Westcott RJ, Hamilton GW, Ritchie JL, Williams DL (1978) Noninvasive assessment of coronary stenoses by myocardial imaging during pharmacologic coronary vasodilatation. III. Clinical trial. Am J Cardiol 42(5):751–760
19. Ogilby JD, Iskandrian AS, Untereker WJ, Heo JY, Nguyen TN, Mercuro J (1992) Effect of intravenous adenosine infusion on myocardial perfusion and function - hemodynamic angiographic and scintigraphic study. Circulation 86(3):887–895
20. Verani MS (1993) Pharmacologic stress myocardial perfusion imaging. Curr Probl Cardiol 18(8):481–525
21. Parodi O, Marcassa C, Casucci R et al (1991) Accuracy and safety of technetium-99m hexakis 2-methoxy-2-isobutyl isonitrile (Sestamibi) myocardial scintigraphy with high dose dipyridamole test in patients with effort angina pectoris: a multicenter study. Italian Group of Nuclear Cardiology. J Am Coll Cardiol 18(6):1439–1444
22. Travin MI, Katz MS, Moulton AW, Miele NJ, Sharaf BL, Johnson LL (2000) Accuracy of dipyridamole SPECT imaging in identifying individual coronary stenoses and multivessel disease in women versus men. J Nucl Cardiology 7(3):213–220
23. Navare SM, Mather JF, Shaw LJ, Fowler MS, Heller GV (2004) Comparison of risk stratification with pharmacologic and exercise stress myocardial perfusion imaging: a meta-analysis. J Nucl Cardiol 11(5):551–561
24. Cheetham AM, Naylor V, McGhie J, Ghiotto F, Al-Housni MB, Kelion AD (2006) Is stress-only imaging practical when a 1-day stress-rest 99mTc-tetrofosmin protocol is used? Nucl Med Commun 27(2):113–117
25. Taillefer R, Laflamme L, Dupras G, Picard M, Phaneuf DC, Leveille J (1988) Myocardial perfusion imaging with 99mTc-methoxy-isobutyl-isonitrile (MIBI): comparison of short and long time intervals between rest and stress injections. Preliminary results. Eur J Nucl Med 13(10):515–522
26. Maddahi J, Kiat H, Van Train KF et al (1990) Myocardial perfusion imaging with technetium-99m sestamibi SPECT in the evaluation of coronary artery disease. Am J Cardiol 66(13):55E–62E
27. Kahn JK, McGhie I, Akers MS et al (1989) Quantitative rotational tomography with 201Tl and 99mTc 2-methoxy-isobutyl-isonitrile. A direct comparison in normal individuals and patients with coronary artery disease. Circulation 79(6):1282–1293
28. Maisey MN, Mistry R, Sowton E (1990) Planar imaging techniques used with technetium-99m sestamibi to evaluate chronic myocardial ischemia. Am J Cardiol 66(13):47E–54E
29. Reyes E, Loong CY, Harbinson M et al (2006) A comparison of Tl-201, Tc-99m sestamibi, and Tc-99m tetrofosmin myocardial perfusion scintigraphy in patients with mild to moderate coronary stenosis. J Nucl Cardiol 13(4):488–494

30. Kiat H, Van Train KF, Maddahi J et al (1990) Development and prospective application of quantitative 2-day stress-rest Tc-99m methoxy isobutyl isonitrile SPECT for the diagnosis of coronary artery disease. Am Heart J 120(6 Pt 1):1255–1266
31. Pozzoli MM, Fioretti PM, Salustri A, Reijs AE, Roelandt JR (1991) Exercise echocardiography and technetium-99m MIBI single-photon emission computed tomography in the detection of coronary artery disease. Am J Cardiol 67(5):350–355
32. Berman DS, Kiat H, Friedman JD et al (1993) Separate acquisition rest thallium-201/stress technetium-99m sestamibi dual-isotope myocardial perfusion single-photon emission computed tomography: a clinical validation study. J Am Coll Cardiol 22(5):1455–1464
33. Solot G, Hermans J, Merlo P et al (1993) Correlation of 99Tcm-sestamibi SPECT with coronary angiography in general hospital practice. Nucl Med Commun 14(1):23–29
34. Minoves M, Garcia A, Magrina J, Pavia J, Herranz R, Setoain J (1993) Evaluation of myocardial perfusion defects by means of "bull's eye" images. Clin Cardiol 16(1):16–22
35. Van Train KF, Areeda J, Garcia EV et al (1993) Quantitative same-day rest-stress technetium-99m-sestamibi SPECT: definition and validation of stress normal limits and criteria for abnormality. J Nucl Med 34(9):1494–1502
36. Sylven C, Hagerman I, Ylen M, Nyquist O, Nowak J (1994) Variance ECG detection of coronary artery disease–a comparison with exercise stress test and myocardial scintigraphy. Clin Cardiol 17(3):132–140
37. Van Train KF, Garcia EV, Maddahi J et al (1994) Multicenter trial validation for quantitative analysis of same-day rest-stress technetium-99m-sestamibi myocardial tomograms. J Nucl Med 35(4):609–618
38. Palmas W, Friedman JD, Diamond GA, Silber H, Kiat H, Berman DS (1995) Incremental value of simultaneous assessment of myocardial function and perfusion with technetium-99m sestamibi for prediction of extent of coronary artery disease. J Am Coll Cardiol 25(5):1024–1031
39. Rubello D, Zanco P, Candelpergher G et al (1995) Usefulness of 99mTc-MIBI stress myocardial SPECT bull's-eye quantification in coronary artery disease. Q J Nucl Med 39(2):111–115
40. Hambye AS, Van Den Branden F, Vandevivere J (1996) Diagnostic value of Tc-99m sestamibi gated SPECT to assess viability in a patient after acute myocardial infarction. Clin Nucl Med 21(1):19–23
41. Yao Z, Liu XJ, Shi R et al (1997) A comparison of 99mTc-MIBI myocardial SPET with electron beam computed tomography in the assessment of coronary artery disease. Eur J Nucl Med 24(9):1115–1120
42. Heiba SI, Hayat NJ, Salman HS et al (1997) Technetium-99m-MIBI myocardial SPECT: supine versus right lateral imaging and comparison with coronary arteriography. J Nucl Med 38(10):1510–1514
43. Candell-Riera J, Santana-Boado C, Castell-Conesa J et al (1997) Simultaneous dipyridamole/maximal subjective exercise with 99mTc-MIBI SPECT: improved diagnostic yield in coronary artery disease. J Am Coll Cardiol 29(3):531–536
44. Taillefer R, DePuey EG, Udelson JE, Beller GA, Latour Y, Reeves F (1997) Comparative diagnostic accuracy of Tl-201 and Tc-99m sestamibi SPECT imaging (perfusion and ECG-gated SPECT) in detecting coronary artery disease in women. J Am Coll Cardiol 29(1):69–77
45. Budoff MJ, Gillespie R, Georgiou D et al (1998) Comparison of exercise electron beam computed tomography and sestamibi in the evaluation of coronary artery disease. Am J Cardiol 81(6):682–687
46. Santana-Boado C, Candell-Riera J, Castell-Conesa J et al (1998) Diagnostic accuracy of technetium-99m-MIBI myocardial SPECT in women and men. J Nucl Med 39(5):751–755
47. Acampa W, Cuocolo A, Sullo P et al (1998) Direct comparison of technetium 99m-sestamibi and technetium 99m-tetrofosmin cardiac single photon emission computed tomography in patients with coronary artery disease. J Nucl Cardiol 5(3):265–274
48. San Roman JA, Vilacosta I, Castillo JA et al (1998) Selection of the optimal stress test for the diagnosis of coronary artery disease. Heart 80(4):370–376

49. Olszowska M, Kostkiewicz M, Tracz W, Przewlocki T (2003) Assessment of myocardial perfusion in patients with coronary artery disease. Comparison of myocardial contrast echocardiography and 99mTc MIBI single photon emission computed tomography. Int J Cardiol 90(1):49–55
50. Marwick T, Willemart B, D'Hondt AM et al (1993) Selection of the optimal nonexercise stress for the evaluation of ischemic regional myocardial dysfunction and malperfusion. Comparison of dobutamine and adenosine using echocardiography and 99mTc-MIBI single photon emission computed tomography. Circulation 87(2):345–354
51. Amanullah AM, Kiat H, Friedman JD, Berman DS (1996) Adenosine technetium-99m sestamibi myocardial perfusion SPECT in women: diagnostic efficacy in detection of coronary artery disease. J Am Coll Cardiol 27(4):803–809
52. Miller DD, Younis LT, Chaitman BR, Stratmann H (1997) Diagnostic accuracy of dipyridamole technetium 99m-labeled sestamibi myocardial tomography for detection of coronary artery disease. J Nucl Cardiol 4(1 Pt 1):18–24
53. Schillaci O, Moroni C, Scopinaro F et al (1997) Technetium-99m sestamibi myocardial tomography based on dipyridamole echocardiography testing in hypertensive patients with chest pain. Eur J Nucl Med 24(7):774–778
54. Soman P, Khattar R, Senior R, Lahiri A (1997) Inotropic stress with arbutamine is superior to vasodilator stress with dipyridamole for the detection of reversible ischemia with Tc-99m sestamibi single-photon emission computed tomography. J Nucl Cardiol 4(5):364–371
55. Amanullah AM, Berman DS, Kiat H, Friedman JD (1997) Usefulness of hemodynamic changes during adenosine infusion in predicting the diagnostic accuracy of adenosine technetium-99m sestamibi single-photon emission computed tomography (SPECT). Am J Cardiol 79(10):1319–1322
56. Ogilby JD, Kegel JG, Heo J, Iskandrian AE (1998) Correlation between hemodynamic changes and tomographic sestamibi imaging during dipyridamole-induced coronary hyperemia. J Am Coll Cardiol 31(1):75–82
57. Jamil G, Ahlberg AW, Elliott MD et al (1999) Impact of limited treadmill exercise on adenosine Tc-99m sestamibi single-photon emission computed tomographic myocardial perfusion imaging in coronary artery disease. Am J Cardiol 84(4):400–403
58. Smart SC, Bhatia A, Hellman R et al (2000) Dobutamine-atropine stress echocardiography and dipyridamole sestamibi scintigraphy for the detection of coronary artery disease: limitations and concordance. J Am Coll Cardiol 36(4):1265–1273
59. Onbasili OA, Erdogan S, Tekten T, Ceyhan C, Yurekli Y (2004) Dipyridamole stress echocardiography and ultrasonic myocardial tissue characterization in predicting myocardial ischemia, in comparison with dipyridamole stress Tc-99m MIBI SPECT myocardial imaging. Jpn Heart J 45(6):937–948
60. Fan ZJ, Chen LB, Li F, Chen HY, Shen ZJ, Zhang SY (2006) The application of adenosine stress myocardial perfusion tomographic imaging in detecting coronary artery disease. Zhonghua Nei Ke Za Zhi 45(2):112–115
61. Gunalp B, Dokumaci B, Uyan C et al (1993) Value of dobutamine technetium-99m-sestamibi SPECT and echocardiography in the detection of coronary artery disease compared with coronary angiography. J Nucl Med 34(6):889–894
62. Forster T, McNeill AJ, Salustri A et al (1993) Simultaneous dobutamine stress echocardiography and technetium-99m isonitrile single-photon emission computed tomography in patients with suspected coronary artery disease. J Am Coll Cardiol 21(7):1591–1596
63. Marwick T, D'Hondt AM, Baudhuin T et al (1993) Optimal use of dobutamine stress for the detection and evaluation of coronary artery disease: combination with echocardiography or scintigraphy, or both? J Am Coll Cardiol 22(1):159–167
64. Mairesse GH, Marwick TH, Vanoverschelde JL et al (1994) How accurate is dobutamine stress electrocardiography for detection of coronary artery disease? Comparison with two-dimensional echocardiography and technetium-99m methoxyl isobutyl isonitrile (mibi) perfusion scintigraphy. J Am Coll Cardiol 24(4):920–927

5 Myocardial Perfusion Scintigraphy with 99mTc-MIBI

65. Marwick TH, D'Hondt AM, Mairesse GH et al (1994) Comparative ability of dobutamine and exercise stress in inducing myocardial ischaemia in active patients. Br Heart J 72(1):31–38
66. Senior R, Sridhara BS, Anagnostou E, Handler C, Raftery EB, Lahiri A (1994) Synergistic value of simultaneous stress dobutamine sestamibi single-photon-emission computerized tomography and echocardiography in the detection of coronary artery disease. Am Heart J 128(4):713–718
67. Di Bello V, Bellina CR, Gori E et al (1996) Incremental diagnostic value of dobutamine stress echocardiography and dobutamine scintigraphy (technetium 99m-labeled sestamibi single-photon emission computed tomography) for assessment of presence and extent of coronary artery disease. J Nucl Cardiol 3(3):212–220
68. Iftikhar I, Koutelou M, Mahmarian JJ, Verani MS (1996) Simultaneous perfusion tomography and radionuclide angiography during dobutamine stress. J Nucl Med 37(8):1306–1310
69. Kisacik HL, Ozdemir K, Altinyay E et al (1996) Comparison of exercise stress testing with simultaneous dobutamine stress echocardiography and technetium-99m isonitrile single-photon emission computerized tomography for diagnosis of coronary artery disease. Eur Heart J 17(1):113–119
70. Slavich GA, Guerra UP, Morocutti G et al (1996) Feasibility of simultaneous Tc99m sestamibi and 2D-echo cardiac imaging during dobutamine pharmacologic stress. Preliminary results in a female population. Int J Card Imaging 12(2):113–118
71. Elhendy A, Geleijnse ML, van Domburg RT et al (1998) Comparison of dobutamine stress echocardiography and technetium-99m sestamibi single-photon emission tomography for the diagnosis of coronary artery disease in hypertensive patients with and without left ventricular hypertrophy. Eur J Nucl Med 25(1):69–78
72. Schwaiger M, Schricke U (2000) Hibernating and stunned myocardium. Pathophysiological consideration. In: Iskandrian AE, Van der Wall EE (eds) Myocardial viability, 2nd edn., pp 1–20
73. Udelson JE, Coleman PS, Metherall J et al (1994) Predicting recovery of severe regional ventricular dysfunction. Comparison of resting scintigraphy with 201Tl and 99mTc-sestamibi. Circulation 89(6):2552–2561
74. Kauffman GJ, Boyne TS, Watson DD, Smith WH, Beller GA (1996) Comparison of rest thallium-201 imaging and rest technetium-99m sestamibi imaging for assessment of myocardial viability in patients with coronary artery disease and severe left ventricular dysfunction. J Am Coll Cardiol 27(7):1592–1597
75. Medrano R, Lowry RW, Young JB et al (1996) Assessment of myocardial viability with 99mTc sestamibi in patients undergoing cardiac transplantation. A scintigraphic/pathological study. Circulation 94(5):1010–1017
76. Maes AF, Borgers M, Flameng W et al (1997) Assessment of myocardial viability in chronic coronary artery disease using technetium-99m sestamibi SPECT. Correlation with histologic and positron emission tomographic studies and functional follow-up. J Am Coll Cardiol 29(1):62–68
77. Dilsizian V, Arrighi JA, Diodati JG et al (1994) Myocardial viability in patients with chronic coronary artery disease. Comparison of 99mTc-sestamibi with thallium reinjection and [18F] fluorodeoxyglucose. Circulation 89(2):578–587
78. Altehoefer C, Kaiser HJ, Dorr R et al (1992) Fluorine-18 deoxyglucose PET for assessment of viable myocardium in perfusion defects in 99mTc-MIBI SPET: a comparative study in patients with coronary artery disease. Eur J Nucl Med 19(5):334–342
79. Siebelink HM, Blanksma PK, Crijns HJ et al (2001) No difference in cardiac event-free survival between positron emission tomography-guided and single-photon emission computed tomography-guided patient management: a prospective, randomized comparison of patients with suspicion of jeopardized myocardium. J Am Coll Cardiol 37(1):81–88
80. Barrington SF, Chambers J, Hallett WA, O'Doherty MJ, Roxburgh JC, Nunan TO (2004) Comparison of sestamibi, thallium, echocardiography and PET for the detection of hibernating myocardium. Eur J Nucl Med Mol Imaging 31(3):355–361
81. Bisi G, Sciagra R, Santoro GM, Fazzini PF (1994) Rest technetium-99m sestamibi tomography in combination with short-term administration of nitrates: feasibility and reliability for prediction of postrevascularization outcome of asynergic territories. J Am Coll Cardiol 24(5):1282–1289

82. Sciagra R, Bisi G, Santoro GM et al (1997) Comparison of baseline-nitrate technetium-99m sestamibi with rest-redistribution thallium-201 tomography in detecting viable hibernating myocardium and predicting postrevascularization recovery. J Am Coll Cardiol 30(2):384–391

83. Germano G, Erel J, Lewin H, Kavanagh PB, Berman DS (1997) Automatic quantitation of regional myocardial wall motion and thickening from gated technetium-99m sestamibi myocardial perfusion single-photon emission computed tomography. J Am Coll Cardiol 30(5):1360–1367

84. Smanio PE, Watson DD, Segalla DL, Vinson EL, Smith WH, Beller GA (1997) Value of gating of technetium-99m sestamibi single-photon emission computed tomographic imaging. J Am Coll Cardiol 30(7):1687–1692

85. Klocke FJ, Baird MG, Lorell BH et al (2003) ACC/AHA/ASNC guidelines for the clinical use of cardiac radionuclide imaging–executive summary: a report of the American College of Cardiology/American Heart Association Task Force on Practice Guidelines (ACC/AHA/ASNC Committee to Revise the 1995 Guidelines for the Clinical Use of Cardiac Radionuclide Imaging). J Am Coll Cardiol 42(7):1318–1333

86. Gibbons RJ, Abrams J, Chatterjee K et al (2003) ACC/AHA 2002 guideline update for the management of patients with chronic stable angina–summary article: a report of the American College of Cardiology/American Heart Association Task Force on Practice Guidelines (Committee on the Management of Patients With Chronic Stable Angina). Circulation 107(1):149–158

87. Yusuf S, Zucker D, Peduzzi P et al (1994) Effect of coronary artery bypass graft surgery on survival: overview of 10-year results from randomised trials by the coronary artery bypass graft surgery trialists collaboration. Lancet 344(8922):563–570

88. The Bypass Angioplasty Revascularization Investigation (BARI) Investigators (1996) Comparison of coronary bypass surgery with angioplasty in patients with multivessel disease. N Engl J Med 335(4):217–225

89. Leslie WD, Tully SA, Yogendran MS, Ward LM, Nour KA, Metge CJ (2005) Prognostic value of lung sestamibi uptake in myocardial perfusion imaging of patients with known or suspected coronary artery disease. J Am Coll Cardiol 45(10):1676–1682

90. Sharir T, Germano G, Kang X et al (2001) Prediction of myocardial infarction versus cardiac death by gated myocardial perfusion SPECT: risk stratification by the amount of stress-induced ischemia and the poststress ejection fraction. J Nucl Med 42(6):831–837

91. Gibbons RJ, Hodge DO, Berman DS et al (1999) Long-term outcome of patients with intermediate-risk exercise electrocardiograms who do not have myocardial perfusion defects on radionuclide imaging. Circulation 100(21):2140–2145

92. Hachamovitch R, Berman DS, Shaw LJ et al (1998) Incremental prognostic value of myocardial perfusion single photon emission computed tomography for the prediction of cardiac death: differential stratification for risk of cardiac death and myocardial infarction. Circulation 97(6):535–543

93. Germano G, Kavanagh PB, Waechter P et al (2000) A new algorithm for the quantitation of myocardial perfusion SPECT. I: technical principles and reproducibility. J Nucl Med 41(4):712–719

94. Sharir T, Germano G, Waechter PB et al (2000) A new algorithm for the quantitation of myocardial perfusion SPECT. II: validation and diagnostic yield. J Nucl Med 41(4):720–727

95. Kirac S, Wackers FJ, Liu YH (2000) Validation of the Yale circumferential quantification method using 201Tl and 99mTc: a phantom study. J Nucl Med 41(8):1436–1441

96. Liu YH, Sinusas AJ, DeMan P, Zaret BL, Wackers FJ (1999) Quantification of SPECT myocardial perfusion images: methodology and validation of the Yale-CQ method. J Nucl Cardiol 6(2):190–204

97. Faber TL, Cooke CD, Folks RD et al (1999) Left ventricular function and perfusion from gated SPECT perfusion images: an integrated method. J Nucl Med 40(4):650–659

98. Germano G, Kiat H, Kavanagh PB et al (1995) Automatic quantification of ejection fraction from gated myocardial perfusion SPECT. J Nucl Med 36(11):2138–2147

99. Berman DS, Kang X, Van Train KF et al (1998) Comparative prognostic value of automatic quantitative analysis versus semiquantitative visual analysis of exercise myocardial perfusion single-photon emission computed tomography. J Am Coll Cardiol 32(7):1987–1995

100. Germano G (2006) Quantitative analysis in myocardial SPECT imaging. In: Zaidi H (ed) Quantitative analysis in nuclear medicine imaging. Springer, New York, pp 471–493
101. Kakhki VR, Sadeghi R, Zakavi SR (2007) Assessment of transient left ventricular dilation ratio via 2-day dipyridamole Tc-99m sestamibi nongated myocardial perfusion imaging. J Nucl Cardiol 14(4):529–536
102. Bacher-Stier C, Sharir T, Kavanagh PB et al (2000) Postexercise lung uptake of 99mTc-sestamibi determined by a new automatic technique: validation and application in detection of severe and extensive coronary artery disease and reduced left ventricular function. J Nucl Med 41(7):1190–1197
103. Hachamovitch R, Hayes S, Friedman JD et al (2003) Determinants of risk and its temporal variation in patients with normal stress myocardial perfusion scans: what is the warranty period of a normal scan? J Am Coll Cardiol 41(8):1329–1340
104. Elhendy A, Schinkel A, Bax JJ, van Domburg RT, Poldermans D (2003) Long-term prognosis after a normal exercise stress Tc-99m sestamibi SPECT study. J Nucl Cardiol 10(3):261–266
105. Gibson PB, Demus D, Noto R, Hudson W, Johnson LL (2002) Low event rate for stress-only perfusion imaging in patients evaluated for chest pain. J Am Coll Cardiol 39(6):999–1004
106. Soman P, Parsons A, Lahiri N, Lahiri A (1999) The prognostic value of a normal Tc-99m sestamibi SPECT study in suspected coronary artery disease. J Nucl Cardiol 6(3):252–256
107. Alkeylani A, Miller DD, Shaw LJ et al (1998) Influence of race on the prediction of cardiac events with stress technetium-99m sestamibi tomographic imaging in patients with stable angina pectoris. Am J Cardiol 81(3):293–297
108. Boyne TS, Koplan BA, Parsons WJ, Smith WH, Watson DD, Beller GA (1997) Predicting adverse outcome with exercise SPECT technetium-99m sestamibi imaging in patients with suspected or known coronary artery disease. Am J Cardiol 79(3):270–274
109. Geleijnse ML, Elhendy A, van Domburg RT et al (1996) Prognostic value of dobutamine-atropine stress technetium-99m sestamibi perfusion scintigraphy in patients with chest pain. J Am Coll Cardiol 28(2):447–454
110. Berman DS, Hachamovitch R, Kiat H et al (1995) Incremental value of prognostic testing in patients with known or suspected ischemic heart disease: a basis for optimal utilization of exercise technetium-99m sestamibi myocardial perfusion single-photon emission computed tomography. J Am Coll Cardiol 26(3):639–647
111. Brown KA, Altland E, Rowen M (1994) Prognostic value of normal technetium-99m-sestamibi cardiac imaging. J Nucl Med 35(4):554–557
112. Iskander S, Iskandrian AE (1998) Risk assessment using single-photon emission computed tomographic technetium-99m sestamibi imaging. J Am Coll Cardiol 32(1):57–62
113. Delcour KS, Khaja A, Chockalingam A, Kuppuswamy S, Dresser T (2009) Outcomes in patients with abnormal myocardial perfusion imaging and normal coronary angiogram. Angiology 60(3):318–321
114. Alqaisi F, Albadarin F, Jaffery Z et al (2008) Prognostic predictors and outcomes in patients with abnormal myocardial perfusion imaging and angiographically insignificant coronary artery disease. J Nucl Cardiol 15(6):754–761
115. Bilodeau L, Theroux P, Gregoire J, Gagnon D, Arsenault A (1991) Technetium-99m sestamibi tomography in patients with spontaneous chest pain: correlations with clinical, electrocardiographic and angiographic findings. J Am Coll Cardiol 18(7):1684–1691
116. Varetto T, Cantalupi D, Altieri A, Orlandi C (1993) Emergency room technetium-99m sestamibi imaging to rule out acute myocardial ischemic events in patients with nondiagnostic electrocardiograms. J Am Coll Cardiol 22(7):1804–1808
117. Hilton TC, Fulmer H, Abuan T, Thompson RC, Stowers SA (1996) Ninety-day follow-up of patients in the emergency department with chest pain who undergo initial single-photon emission computed tomographic perfusion scintigraphy with technetium 99m-labeled sestamibi. J Nucl Cardiol 3(4):308–311
118. Kontos MC, Schmidt KL, Nicholson CS, Ornato JP, Jesse RL, Tatum JL (1999) Myocardial perfusion imaging with technetium-99m sestamibi in patients with cocaine-associated chest pain. Ann Emerg Med 33(6):639–645

119. Wackers FJ, Brown KA, Heller GV et al (2002) American Society of Nuclear Cardiology position statement on radionuclide imaging in patients with suspected acute ischemic syndromes in the emergency department or chest pain center. J Nucl Cardiol 9(2):246–250

120. Abbott BG, Jain D (2003) Impact of myocardial perfusion imaging on clinical management and the utilization of hospital resources in suspected acute coronary syndromes. Nucl Med Commun 24(10):1061–1069

121. Abbott BG, Wackers FJ (1998) Emergency department chest pain units and the role of radionuclide imaging. J Nucl Cardiol 5(1):73–79

122. Abbott BG, Jain D (2000) Nuclear cardiology in the evaluation of acute chest pain in the emergency department. Echocardiography 17(6 Pt 1):597–604

123. Gibbons RJ, Verani MS, Behrenbeck T et al (1989) Feasibility of tomographic 99mTc-hexakis-2-methoxy-2-methylpropyl-isonitrile imaging for the assessment of myocardial area at risk and the effect of treatment in acute myocardial infarction. Circulation 80(5): 1277–1286

124. Christian TF, Behrenbeck T, Pellikka PA, Huber KC, Chesebro JH, Gibbons RJ (1990) Mismatch of left ventricular function and infarct size demonstrated by technetium-99m isonitrile imaging after reperfusion therapy for acute myocardial infarction: identification of myocardial stunning and hyperkinesia. J Am Coll Cardiol 16(7):1632–1638

125. Kristensen J, Mortensen UM, Nielsen SS et al (2004) Myocardial perfusion imaging with 99mTc sestamibi early after reperfusion reliably reflects infarct size reduction by ischaemic preconditioning in an experimental porcine model. Nucl Med Commun 25(5):495–500

126. Rizzello V, Poldermans D, Bax JJ (2005) Assessment of myocardial viability in chronic ischemic heart disease: current status. Q J Nucl Med Mol Imaging 49(1):81–96

127. Williams KA, Borer JS, Supino P (2003) Radionuclide angiography. In: Iskandrian AE, Verani MS, eds. Nuclear cardiac imaging principles & applications. 3 ed, p 323

128. Boucher CA, Wackers FJ, Zaret BL, Mena IG (1992) Technetium-99m sestamibi myocardial imaging at rest for assessment of myocardial infarction and first-pass ejection fraction. Multicenter Cardiolite Study Group. Am J Cardiol 69(1):22–27

129. Iskandrian AE, Germano G, VanDecker W et al (1998) Validation of left ventricular volume measurements by gated SPECT 99mTc-labeled sestamibi imaging. J Nucl Cardiol 5(6): 574–578

130. Sharir T, Kang X, Germano G et al (2006) Prognostic value of poststress left ventricular volume and ejection fraction by gated myocardial perfusion SPECT in women and men: gender-related differences in normal limits and outcomes. J Nucl Cardiol 13(4):495–506

131. Jones RH, Borges-Neto S, Potts JM (1990) Simultaneous measurement of myocardial perfusion and ventricular function during exercise from a single injection of technetium-99m sestamibi in coronary artery disease. Am J Cardiol 66(13):68E–71E

132. Williams KA, Taillon LA, Draho JM, Foisy MF (1993) First-pass radionuclide angiographic studies of left ventricular function with technetium-99m-teboroxime, technetium-99m-sestamibi and technetium-99m-DTPA. J Nucl Med 34(3):394–399

133. Borges-Neto S, Coleman RE, Potts JM, Jones RH (1991) Combined exercise radionuclide angiocardiography and single photon emission computed tomography perfusion studies for assessment of coronary artery disease. Semin Nucl Med 21(3):223–229

134. Lee KL, Pryor DB, Pieper KS et al (1990) Prognostic value of radionuclide angiography in medically treated patients with coronary artery disease. A comparison with clinical and catheterization variables. Circulation 82(5):1705–1717

135. Sharir T, Germano G, Kavanagh PB et al (1999) Incremental prognostic value of post-stress left ventricular ejection fraction and volume by gated myocardial perfusion single photon emission computed tomography. Circulation 100(10):1035–1042

136. Acampa W, Caprio MG, Nicolai E et al (2010) Assessment of poststress left ventricular ejection fraction by gated SPECT: comparison with equilibrium radionuclide angiocardiography. Eur J Nucl Med Mol Imaging 37(2):349–356

137. DePuey EG, Rozanski A (1995) Using gated technetium-99m-sestamibi SPECT to characterize fixed myocardial defects as infarct or artifact. J Nucl Med 36(6):952–955

5 Myocardial Perfusion Scintigraphy with 99mTc-MIBI

138. Johnson LL, Verdesca SA, Aude WY et al (1997) Postischemic stunning can affect left ventricular ejection fraction and regional wall motion on post-stress gated sestamibi tomograms. J Am Coll Cardiol 30(7):1641–1648
139. Ben-Haim S, Gips S, Merdler A, Front A, Tamir A (2004) Myocardial stunning demonstrated with rest and post-stress measurements of left ventricular function using dual-isotope gated myocardial perfusion SPECT. Nucl Med Commun 25(7):657–663
140. Tanaka H, Chikamori T, Hida S et al (2005) Comparison of post-exercise and post-vasodilator stress myocardial stunning as assessed by electrocardiogram-gated single-photon emission computed tomography. Circ J 69(11):1338–1345
141. Sobic-Saranovic DP, Pavlovic SV, Jovanovic IV et al (2010) Evaluation of myocardial perfusion and function by gated single-photon emission computed tomography technetium-99m methoxyisobutylisonitrile in children and adolescents with severe congenital heart disease. Nucl Med Commun 31(1):12–21
142. Kiratli PO, Tuncel M, Ozkutlu S, Caglar M (2008) Gated myocardial perfusion scintigraphy in children with myocarditis: Can it be considered as an indicator of clinical outcome? Nucl Med Commun 29(10):907–914

^{99m}Tc-Sestamibi Scintimammography

Jan Bucerius

6

6.1   Introduction

From an anatomical point of view, the mammary gland is part of the female secondary sexual characteristics. The primary biological function of the mammary glands is the feeding of infants with breast milk. The mammary glands belong to the major glands of the cutis (*glandulae cutis*) and develop from epithelial cones, which grow in the surrounding connective tissue. Initially, the mammary glands are established in the same way in both genders.

The female mammary glands are located on the major and minor pectoral muscles (*M. pectoralis major, M. pectoralis minor*) between the third and the seventh rib and between the sternal- and axillary line. The arterial blood supply of the mammary glands is provided by vascular branches (*R. mammarii mediales and laterales*) of the internal and lateral thoracic arteries (*A. thoracica interna, A. thoracica lateralis*) as well as by branches (*R. preforantes and R. mammarii laterales*) of the anterior and posterior intercostal arteries (*Aa. intercostales anterior and posterior*). The venous drain follows from superficial veins into the lateral and internal thoracic veins (*Vv. thoracica lateralis and interna*). The mammary glands are characterized by numerous lymphatic vessels, which build a superficial and deep lymphatic mesh with several directions of lymphatic drainage. From a clinical point of view, the main and most important lymphatic drainage reaches the axillary lymph nodes. Additional lymphatic drains flow off to the cervical lymph nodes superior to the clavicles and via the interpectoral lymphatic nodes (*N. lymphatici interpectorales*) between the pectoral muscles to the axillary lymph nodes, via the parasternal lymph nodes (*N. lymphatici parasternales*) along the internal thorac vein, and via the

---

J. Bucerius
Department of Nuclear Medicine and Cardiovascular Research Institute Maastricht (CARIM),
Maastricht University Medical Center, P. Debyelaan 25, 6229 HX Maastricht, The Netherlands
e-mail: jan.bucerius@mumc.nl

J. Bucerius et al. (eds.), *^{99m}Tc-Sestamibi*,
DOI 10.1007/978-3-642-04233-1_6, © Springer-Verlag Berlin Heidelberg 2012

intercostal lymph nodes (*N. lymphatici intercostales*) even across the median line to the contralateral side of the chest.

With a relative number of 28% of all newly diagnosed malignant diseases, breast cancer is still the most common malignancy in females. Based on data from Germany one in eight to ten women suffers from breast cancer throughout her life time accounting for a total of about 57,000 initial diagnoses of malignancies of the breast per year or 135 cases per 100,000 a year. According to data from the WHO, about 1,050,000 initial diagnoses are estimated per year of which 580,000 are observed in the industrial nations. Breast cancer is the most common type of malignancy in females and accounts for the common cause of death in that population [1, 2]. The worldwide annual death rate per year is specified with 370,000. Based on a total of 17,197 (2.0% of all deaths) breast cancer-related deaths in 2009, malignancies of the mammary glands ranked number ten in the overall mortality statistic in Germany [3]. In females only, based on 17,066 cases (3.8% of all deaths in females), breast cancer-related death ranked number four in the German annual statistic of mortality in Germany [3]. Age distribution revealed females between the age of 45 and 50 years at high risk for primary diagnosis of breast cancer with a further increasing risk at the age of 60 years and more (incidence about 500/100,000 females in females aged >70 years). Diagnosis of breast cancer in younger females (<35 years) is rare. Hereditary disease accounts for about 5% of cases. Male subjects account for approximately 1% of cases (400 cases per year in Germany, ratio males versus females 1:100).

Histology differentiates between ductal- (origin from the lactiferous ducts, 65% of cases), lobular carcinomas (origin from the lobuli or acini of the mammary glands, 15% of cases), and combined forms of both types as well as invasive and noninvasive growth. The left mammary gland is statistically more often (5–7%) affected compared to the right breast. Fifty-five percent of carcinomas are located in the upper outer quadrant of the breast (lower outer: 10%, upper inner: 15%, lower inner: 5%, central 15%) and in 5–25% of cases a multicenter localization can be observed. Unfortunately, a common and early metastatic spread has to be taken into account during primary staging of patients with breast cancer. It is estimated that at primary diagnosis, about 50% of patients already suffer from metastatic disease. Lymphogenic spread occurs mainly into the ipsilateral axillary lymph nodes, the parasternal lymph nodes, and, more rarely, into the supraclavicullary and retrosternal lymph nodes as well as into the contralateral mammary gland. Hematogenous metastatic spread is most commonly observed in the skeletal system, the pleura, the lungs, the skin/soft tissue, the liver, the brain, the ovaries, the uterus, and the adrenal glands. Classification of breast cancer disease according to the TNM classification and the UICC staging is depicted by Tables 6.1 and 6.2 [4].

Diagnosis of breast cancer includes breast self-examination as well as clinical breast examination by an experienced physician on a routine basis. The importance of this clinical-based evaluation of the breasts is emphasized by the fact, that it is well known, that some cancers not identified by mammography can be detected by

Table 6.1 TNM classification for breast cancer disease 2009 [4]

Primary tumor (T)

Tx	Primary tumor cannot be assessed
T0	No evidence of primary tumor
Tis	Carcinoma in situ
Tis (DCIS)	Ductal carcinoma in situ
Tis (LICIS)	Labular carcinoma in situ
Tis (Paget)	Paget's disease of the nipple with no detectable tumor
T1	≤2.0 cm in greatest dimension
T1mic	Microinvasion ≤0.1 cm in greatest dimension
• T1a	>0.1≤0.5 cm in greatest dimension
• T1b	>0.5≤1.0 cm in greatest dimension
• T1c	>1.0≤2.0 cm in greatest dimension
T2	>2.0≤5.0 cm in greatest dimension
T3	>5.0 cm in greatest dimension
T4	Tumor of any size with direct extension to (T4a) chest wall or (T4b) skin (edema including peau d'orange, or ulceration of the skin of the breast or satellite skin nodules confined to the same breast), (T4c = T4a + T4b), T4d: inflammatory carcinoma

Regional lymph nodes (N)

NX	Regional lymph nodes cannot be assessed
N0	No regional lymph node metastases
N1	Metastasis to moveable ipsilateral axillary lymph node(s) of Level I and II
N2	N2a or N2b
• N2a	Metastasis to ipsilateral axillary lymph node(s) fixed to each other or to other structures
• N2b	Metastasis in clinically detectable ipsilateral lymph node(s) along of the internal mammary artery in absence of clinically detectable axillary lymph node metastases
N3	N3a or N3b or N3c
• N3a	Metastasis in ipsilateral internal mammary lymph node(s)
• N3b	Metastasis in clinically detectable ipsilateral lymph node(s) along the internal mammary artery in presence axillary lymph node metastases
• N3c	Metastasis in ipsilateral supraclavicullary lymph node(s)

Pathological lymph node classification (pN)

pNx	Regional lymph nodes cannot be assessed (not removed for pathologic study or previously removed)
pNx (sn)	Sentinel lymph node cannot be histologically assessed
pN0	No regional lymph node metastasis
pN0 (sn)	Sentinel lymph node with no histologically proven metastasis
pN0(i−)	Histologically no metastasis in lymph node(s) and no morphological proof of isolated tumor cells
pN0(i+)	Histologically no metastasis in lymph node(s) but morphological proof of isolated tumor cells

(continued)

Table 6.1 (continued)

pN0(mol−)	Histologically no metastasis in lymph node(s) and no nonmorphological proof of isolated tumor cells
pN0(mol+)	Histologically no metastasis in lymph node(s) but nonmorphological proof of isolated tumor cells
pN1mic	Micrometastasis(ses) [>0.2 mm (and/or >200 tumor cells) and ≤0.2 cm]
pN1	pN1a or pN1b or pN1c
• pN1a	Metastasis(ses) in 1–3 ipsilateral axillary lymph nodes, at least one >0.2 cm
• pN1b	Lymph nodes along the internal mammary artery with microscopically proven metastasis(ses), detected by examination of the sentinel lymph node but not clinically detectable
• pN1c	pN1a and pN1b
pN2	pN2a or pN2b
• pN2a	Metastasis(ses) in 4–9 axillary lymph nodes, at least one >2.0 cm
• pN2b	Clinically detectable metastasis(ses) in lymph nodes along the internal mammary artery without axillary lymph node metastases
pN3	pN3a or pN3b or pN3c
• pN3a	Metastasis(ses) in ten or more ipsilateral axillary lymph nodes, at least one >2.0 cm or in ipsilateral infraclavicullary lymph nodes
• pN3b	Metastasis(ses) in clinically detectable lymph nodes along the internal mammary artery with at least one axillary lymph node metastasis or lymph node metastases in more than 3 axillary lymph nodes and in lymph nodes along the internal mammary artery, detected by examination of the sentinel lymph node(s) but not clinically detectable
• pN3c	Metastasis(ses) in ipsilateral supraclavicullary lymph nodes
Distant metastasis (M)	
Mx	Presence of distant metastasis cannot be assessed
M0	No distant metastasis
M1	Distant metastasis present

Clinically detectable are metastases, which have been diagnosed by clinical examination or by imaging (exclusive of sentinel lymph node scintigraphy)

Table 6.2 UICC staging for breast cancer disease 2009 [4]

Stage 0		Tis	N0	M0
Stage I	A	T1, T1mic	N0	M0
	B	T0[a], T1	N1mi	M0
Stage II	A	T0[a], T1, T1mic	N1	M0
		T2	N0	M0
	B	T2	N1	M0
		T3	N0	M0
Stage III	A	T0[a], T1, T1mic, T2	N2	M0
		T3	N1, N2	M0
	B	T4	N0, N1, N2	M0
	C	All T	N3	M0
Stage IV		All T	All N	M1

[a] Occult breast cancer

physical examination. Mammography in two views depicts a radiological diagnostic tool able to identify masses of the breasts about 5 mm in size. Furthermore, mammography currently remains the only imaging modality that is recommended for routine screening for breast cancer in the general population [5]. Breast ultrasonography is presently considered primarily a diagnostic tool. It is most commonly used to characterize lesions initially detected through mammographic screening or to evaluate patients who present with clinical findings, such a palpable mass [5]. Routine screening with breast ultrasonography is not currently recommended [5–7]. Breast magnetic resonance imaging (MRI) has become a commonly used imaging modality and, in skilled hands, MRI is often helpful in patients with a newly diagnosed mass of the breast. MRI may be especially useful in cases where the mammographic, ultrasonographic, and clinical findings are inconclusive and no focal finding is apparent (e. g., spontaneous bloody single-duct nipple discharge, silicone injections, subtle architectural distortions, etc.) [5]. Furthermore, breast MRI can be useful as a screening modality for a certain group of patients, mainly those at high risk of developing breast cancer. However, based on the current knowledge, breast MRI should not replace careful diagnostic mammographic views or ultrasonography in the setting of an abnormal clinical examination or screening mammography [5]. Nowadays, percutaneous needle biopsy has demonstrated accuracy equivalent to open surgical biopsy and is the optimal initial tissue-acquisition procedure for image-detected breast abnormalities. Image-guided percutaneous breast biopsy helps in establishing a definitive benign diagnosis for the majority of image-detected abnormalities, eliminating the need for the patient to undergo an open surgical diagnostic procedure [5]. For those with malignant diagnoses, needle biopsy permits preoperative staging as well as acquisition of histologic and biomarker data [5].

Molecular imaging tools for breast cancer detection include technetium-99m sestamibi scintigraphy (^{99m}Tc-sestamibi) and positron emission tomography with ^{18}F-fluordeoxyglucose (^{18}F-FDG PET). Data available on the diagnostic performance of these tools indicate that they might have equivalent sensitivity and even improved specificity when compared to breast MRI [5]. It is recommended to use these adjunctive tools only after standard imaging procedures. Furthermore, their results should not prevent performing a biopsy recommended after conventional imaging. Either ^{99m}Tc-sestamibi or ^{18}F-FDG PET may be used as an alternative to breast MRI when high-quality MRI is not available or contraindicated in particular patients. Both diagnostic tools may be valuable in preoperative surgical staging. Finally, ^{99m}Tc-sestamibi scintimammography may be useful as an additional problem-solving tool in some situation were conventional imaging of suspected masses of the breast remains inconclusive [5]. This chapter focuses on indications and data on the diagnostic performance of ^{99m}Tc-sestamibi scintimammography in different clinical settings of breast cancer disease.

Treatment regimes of breast cancer disease are constantly under evaluation and focus of numerous experimental and clinical trials. Therefore, establishing treatment protocols and schemes is a permanently ongoing process. Depending on the stage of disease, different therapeutic approaches need to be considered. These consist of surgical treatment of the primary malignancy with or without lymph node dissection frequently followed by external radiation therapy. Surgical treatment with adjuvant therapeutic measures like postoperative polychemotherapy, hormone therapy, or external radiation therapy, either alone or combined, are treatment options in more advanced or high-risk stages of disease. External radiation therapy only can be applied as a palliative therapy in patients with advanced, inoperable disease stages.

About 50% of females suffering from breast cancer die due to this disease. Statistically, every woman with breast cancer loses 6 years of her life time expectancy. The overall 5 years survival rate based on an optimal treatment regime is 79% (T1: 85%; T2: 75%; T3N1: 55%, T4N1-3: 40%, M1: 15%; mean survival in residual disease with bone metastases: 2 years, with organ metastases 6–12 months), the 10 years survival rate decreases to 50%.

6.2 ^{99m}Tc-Sestamibi Scintimammography

6.2.1 Background

In the early 1990s ^{99m}Tc-sestamibi became commercially available and was proposed as an alternative agent to ^{201}thallium for myocardial perfusion studies. One of the first reports on ^{99m}Tc-sestamibi for breast cancer detection was published by Aktolun et al. in 1992 during its evaluation as a cardiac imaging agent [8, 9]. Four of thirty-four patients with histologically proven cancers had breast carcinomas all of which showed ^{99m}Tc-sestamibi uptake [8]. Two years later, Khalkhali et al. were among the first to report its use in patients with suspected breast cancer [10]. Afterwards, in June 1997, ^{99m}Tc-sestamibi has been the first radiopharmaceutical, which was approved by the Food and Drug Administration in the USA for radionuclide breast imaging [11]. Nowadays, ^{99m}Tc-sestamibi is licensed for identification of breast cancer in most European countries as well [12, 13]. It was the group by Khalkhali, which consecutively devised and popularized the technique of ^{99m}Tc-sestamibi scintimammography [10, 14]. Since that time multiple techniques that used both planar and single photon emission computed tomography (SPECT) for the detection of breast cancer have been evaluated.

Over the past decades, investigations were continuously performed on the mechanisms of cellular uptake of ^{99m}Tc-sestamibi by cancer cells. In 1990, Chiu et al. demonstrated ^{99m}Tc-sestamibi, a small lipophilic cation, to be sequestered within the cytoplasm and mitochondria of cultured mouse fibroblasts. Furthermore, they could also show that its net cellular uptake and retention occurred in response to the electrical potentials generated across the membrane bilayers of both the cell and the mitochondria [15]. ^{99m}Tc-sestamibi uptake is driven by a negative transmembrane potential and as much as 90% of the radiotracer activity is found in the mitochondria. This uptake is energy dependent because energy-consuming biochemical reactions control these transmembrane potentials [11, 15]. Delmon-Moingeon et al. were the first who could demonstrate an increased uptake of ^{99m}Tc-sestamibi by carcinoma cells [16]. Three years later, Piwnica-Worms et al. reported on ^{99m}Tc-sestamibi being a substrate if the transmembrane P-glycoprotein (Pgp-170), which is present in the cells, which overexpress the multidrug resistance gene (MDR1) and which acts as a protective pump by extruding a wide range of molecules out of the tumor cells, including ^{99m}Tc-sestamibi [17]. This observation is of clinical importance, as it may allow the *in vivo* visualization of the level of the MDR1 expression, which can be of interest in patients on chemotherapy [18, 19]. Studies performed in humans showed that in tumors with high levels of Pgp, ^{99m}Tc-sestamibi efflux was significantly faster than in the control group or in the group with no Pgp [11]. It is known that several factors may impact the degree of ^{99m}Tc-sestamibi uptake by carcinomas of the mammary glands. Papantoniou et al. evaluated the relationship between the histological type and grade of the tumor and the uptake and washout of ^{99m}Tc-sestamibi. They found that the ^{99m}Tc-sestamibi uptake ratios were significantly higher in ductal than in lobular carcinomas [20]. Furthermore, grade II carcinomas also showed a significantly faster washout (i. e., lower retention index values) than that observed in grade III tumors [20].

6.2.2 Clinical Indications

Currently, most of the guidelines on screening and diagnostic imaging of breast cancer do not recommend ^{99m}Tc-sestamibi scintimammography as part of routine diagnostic cascade [6, 7, 21, 22]. However, in a 2009 consensus conference on image-detected breast cancer, the use of molecular breast imaging, including ^{99m}Tc-sestamibi and ^{18}F-FDG PET, was recommended as an adjunctive tool after standard imaging and as an alternative to breast MRI when MRI is not available or contraindicated [5] (Fig.6.1). It was also pointed out that their results should not prevent performing a biopsy recommended after conventional imaging and that breast-specific gamma imaging may also be useful in cases of inconclusive results of the standard imaging procedures. Furthermore, the consensus panel stated molecular imaging to be of value in preoperative surgical staging in patients with breast cancer [5].

The procedure guidelines on breast scintigraphy published 2003 by the European Association of Nuclear Medicine (EANM) defined four indications in which breast scintigraphy has a role:

1. Detection of breast cancer when mammography is doubtful, inadequate, or indeterminate. In particular, it may serve as a complementary procedure in patients with doubtful microcalcifications or parenchymal distortions, in the presence of scar tissue in the breast following surgery or biopsy, in mammographically dense breast tissue, and in breasts with implants.

Fig. 6.1 (a) Lateral view of the left breast. (b) Lateral view of the right breast. Female patient with a malignant mass in the right breast depicted by an intense focal ^{99m}Tc-sestamibi uptake. No indication of any pathological MIBI uptake in the left breast

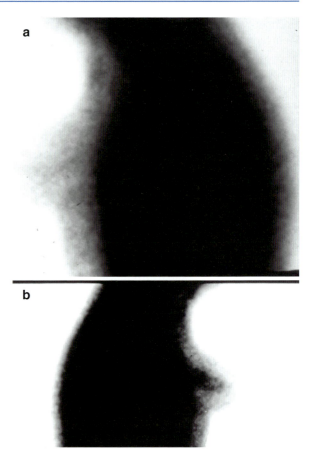

2. Assistance in identifying multicentric, multifocal, or bilateral breast cancer in patients with a diagnosis of breast cancer
3. Study of multidrug resistance
4. Evaluation and prediction of tumor response to chemotherapy for breast carcinoma [12]

The more recently published Society of Nuclear Medicine (SNM) practice guidelines for breast scintigraphy with breast-specific γ-camera indicated an even broader spectrum of common clinical indications for the use of breast scintigraphy (Table 6.3) [23]. However, one has to be aware that this recently published (December 2010) guideline assumes using a state of the art high-resolution small-field-of-view, breast-optimized γ-camera [23]. This assumption needs to be taken into account when performing breast scintigraphies based on the recommendations stated in the SNM practice guideline.

Table 6.3 Clinical indication for breast scintigraphy provided by the SNM practice guidelines for breast scintigraphy [23]

A. Breast scintigraphy was addressed by the American College of Radiology Appropriateness Criteria Panel on Breast Imaging, the American College of Surgeons Consensus Conference III, and the Institute for Clinical Systems Improvement in its guideline on diagnosis of breast disease [5, 24]

B. In patients with recently detected breast malignancy, breast scintigraphy is used to:
  1. Evaluate the extent of disease (initial staging)
  2. Detect multicentric, multifocal, or bilateral disease
  3. Assess response to neoadjuvant chemotherapy [11, 25, 26]

C. In patients at high risk for breast malignancy, breast scintigraphy is used when:
  1. Recurrence is suspected
  2. Only a limited mammogram was obtained or previous malignancy was occult on mammography [13, 27, 28]

D. In patients with indeterminate breast abnormalities and remaining diagnostic concerns, breast scintigraphy is used to:
  1. Evaluate nipple discharge in patients with abnormal mammography or sonographic findings, with or without contrast ductography
  2. Evaluate bloody nipple discharge in patients with normal mammography or ductography findings
  3. Evaluate significant nipple discharge in patients who underwent ductography unsuccessfully
  4. Evaluate lesions when patient reassurance is warranted (Breast Imaging Reporting and Data System [BIRADS])
  5. Evaluate lesions – whether palpable or nonpalpable – identified by other breast imaging techniques
  6. Evaluate palpable abnormalities not demonstrated on mammography or ultrasound
  7. Evaluate multiple masses demonstrated on breast imaging
  8. Aid in biopsy targeting
  9. Evaluate diffuse or multiple clusters of microcalcifications
  10. Evaluate breasts for occult disease in cases of axillary lymph node metastases with an unknown primary
  11. Evaluate unexplained architectural distortion
  12. Evaluate a suggestive mammographic finding seen on one view only
  13. Increase specificity by evaluating enhancing areas seen on MRI [11, 25, 29, 30]

E. In patients with technically difficult breast imaging, breast scintigraphy is used in cases of:
  1. Radiodense breast tissue
  2. Implants, free silicone, or paraffin injections compromising the mammogram [9, 11, 27–29, 31]

F. In patients for whom breast MRI would be indicated, breast scintigraphy is used if:
  1. MRI is diagnostically indicated but not possible:
    a. Implanted pacemakers or pumps
    b. Ferromagnetic surgical implants
    c. Risk of a nephrogenic systemic fibrotic response to gadolinium
    d. Body habitus exceeding the inside diameter of the MRI bore
    e. Patients with breasts too large to be evaluated within the breast coil
    f. Patients with acute claustrophobia
    g. Other factors limiting compliance with a prescribed MRI study

(continued)

Table 6.3 (continued)

    2. An alternative is needed for patients who meet MRI screening criteria: breast cancer susceptibility gene 1 or 2; parent, sibling, or child with breast cancer; lifetime risk of 20–25%; chest radiation performed between ages of 10 and 30 year [5, 32–34]

G. In patients undergoing preoperative chemotherapy who require monitoring of neoadjuvant tumor response, breast scintigraphy is used to:

    1. Determine the impact of therapy

    2. Plan surgery for residual disease [35–37]

All of the guidelines considering breast scintigraphy as part of the diagnostic cascade of breast cancer evaluation share the recommendation that the use of molecular imaging with ^{99m}Tc-sestamibi scintimammography may be valuable to provide additional and complementary information but should not replace standard diagnostic procedures like mammography or, consequently, biopsy neither for screening nor for further evaluation of suspicious masses of the breasts.

6.2.3 Methods/Image Acquisition

Patients should remove all clothing and jewelry above the waist and should wear a hospital gown open in front. It is important to have results of previous diagnostic measures like mammograms, ultrasound studies, physical examinations, etc. available at the time of the breast scintigraphy procedure and analysis. Because of the possibility of unspecific ^{99m}Tc-sestamibi uptake, it is recommended that scintimammography is performed before or at least 7–10 days after fine needle aspiration, 4–6 weeks after a breast biopsy, and at least 2–3 months after breast surgery or radiotherapy [11]. These recommendations are based on experience in clinical practice, which showed these time intervals to be appropriate most of the time without influencing the specificity of the procedure. However, no clinical studies are available at this time to confirm these time intervals [11]. By now it is not clear at which phase of the menstrual cycle scintimammograms should be preferably performed. Until serial studies evaluating scintimammographies obtained in the same patients show a clinically relevant difference between phases of the menstrual cycle, no general recommendations about the best time to image can be made [11]. However, the SNM guidelines recommend breast specific γ-imaging to be performed between days 2 and 12 of the menstrual cycle if possible [23].

The following information summarizes the recommendations of the practice guidelines for breast scintigraphy published by the SNM in 2010 and by the EANM in 2003 [12, 23]. Both guidelines are attached to this chapter and can also be downloaded from the websites of both societies. Differences with regard to the recommendations of both societies are pointed out and described. Furthermore, it has to be emphasized that all of the statements made in this chapter are related to the recommendations of the two societies and should be considered only as general indications. Additionally, all recommendations, and this is mainly due with regard to the administered activity of the radiotracer, need to respect the rules stated by the law of the individual country. The radiotracer will be used for the purpose of evaluation of the mammary glands.

6.2.4 Precautions

Based on the EANM guideline, in case of female patients with suspected or confirmed pregnancy a clinical decision is necessary to consider the benefits against the possible harm of carrying out any procedure [12]. The SNM guidelines state pregnancy as a contraindication against performing ^{99m}Tc-sestamibi breast scintigraphy. The SNM recommendations include determining the date of last menses or the pregnancy and lactation status of the patient. They furthermore state a known hypersensitivity to ^{99m}Tc-sestamibi as a contraindication as well [23]. In patients who are breastfeeding, the breastfeeding should be interrupted for 24 h following the administration of the radiopharmaceutical when possible) [12].

6.2.5 Tracer Injection, Dosage and Administration

[99m]Tc-sestamibi should be administered by intravenous injection in an arm vein contralateral to the breast with the suspected abnormality [12, 23]. If the disease is bilateral, the injection is ideally administered in a dorsal vein of the foot [12]. The ^{99m}Tc-sestamibi activity required for good quality imaging should range between 740 and 1110 MBq [20–30 mCi; SNM: 925 MBq (25 mCi)] [12, 23]. Injection of activities greater than local Diagnostic Reference Levels (DRL) for radiopharmaceuticals should be justified [12].

Table 6.4 depicts doses of ^{99m}Tc-sestamibi used in several international studies on breast scintimammography. With regard to the applied dose it has to be pointed out that a certain range of radioactivity has to be applied in order to take account of clinical and patient-related circumstances. An appropriate dose of the applied radioactivity with regard to diagnostic reference values (DRV) is calculated under consideration of the ALARA-principle (As Low As Reasonably Achievable) and, in addition, of the fact, that a certain amount of activity has to be applied to the patient in order to achieve a valuable image quality [81]. DRVs refer on patients with a standard body weight of 70 kg. Besides the application of a weight-adapted dose calculation the concept of DRV permits also exceeding of the reference activities in cases of, for example, severely ill or restless patients or in cases of reduced organ function.

The applied dose of ^{99m}Tc-sestamibi for diagnosis of breast cancer within the above named published literature is within the range of the recommended ^{99m}Tc-sestamibi doses and as such in accordance to the above-mentioned dosages recommended by the guidelines of the SNM and EANM for ^{99m}Tc-sestamibi breast scintigraphy. In only four of the cited studies applied doses were below the recommended minimal dose of 740 MBq, in none of the studies, higher doses as recommended were applied (1,110 MBq).

Table 6.4 Dosage of [99mTc]-sestamibi used in clinical studies

Author	Continent	Country	Dosage (MBq)
Alonso [38]	America	Uruguay	740-1,110
Alonso [36]	America	Uruguay	740-1,110
Clifford [39]	America	USA	740
Cutrone [40]	America	USA	740
Dunnwald [35]	America	USA	740-1,110
Khalkhali [10]	America	USA	740
Khalkhali [41]	America	USA	740
Khalkhali [42]	America	USA/Canada	740-1,110
Sampalis [43]	America	Canada	740-1,110
Taillefer [44]	America	Canada	900-1,100
Tolmos [45]	America	USA	740
Villanueva-Meyer [46]	America	USA	740
Arslan [47]	Europe	Turkey	740
Becherer [48]	Europe	Austria	630–740
Buscombe [49]	Europe	UK	740
Buscombe [50]	Europe	UK	740
Cwikla [51]	Europe	UK	740
Cwikla [52]	Europe	UK	740
Cwikla [53]	Europe	UK	740
Fondrinier [54]	Europe	France	740
Helbich [55]	Europe	Austria	629–740
Imbriaco [56]	Europe	Italy	555
Maffioli [57]	Europe	Italy	740
Marshall [58]	Europe	UK	750
Mathieu [59]	Europe	Belgium	740
Maublant [60]	Europe	France	740
Moretti [19]	Europe	France	500
Myslivecek [61]	Europe	Czech Republic	740
Palmedo [62]	Europe	Germany	740
Palmedo [63]	Europe	Germany	740
Papantoniou [64]	Europe	Greece	925-1,110
Prats [65]	Europe	Spain	740
Prats [66]	Europe	Spain	740
Sanidas [67]	Europe	Greece	740
Tiling [68]	Europe	Germany	740
Tiling [69]	Europe	Germany	740
Uriarte [70]	Europe	Spain	740
Chen [71]	Asia	China	740
Kao [72]	Asia	Taiwan	740
Kim [73]	Asia	South Korea	750
Kim [74]	Asia	South Korea	925
Kim [75]	Asia	South Korea	750

Table 6.4 (continued)

Author	Continent	Country	Dosage (MBq)
Mekhmandarov [76]	Asia	Israel	740
Melloul [77]	Asia	Israel	740–925
Massardo [78]	America/Asia/Europe (Multicenter)		740-1,110
Massardo [79]	America/Europe (Multicenter)		740–925
Howarth [80]	Australia	Australia	740

6.2.6   Physiological ^{99m}Tc-Sestamibi Distribution

Several organs show *in vivo* ^{99m}Tc-sestamibi tracer uptake on a physiological basis. In particular, normal tracer uptake can be observed in the salivary glands, the thyroid, the myocardium, the liver, the gallbladder, the small and large intestine, the kidneys, the bladder, the choroids plexuses, and in skeletal muscles. About 8% of the injected ^{99m}Tc-sestamibi dose remains in circulation at 5 min post-injection. The effective half-life of clearance is approximately 3 h for the heart and approximately 30 min for the liver. A faint homogeneous uptake of the radiopharmaceutical in the breast or axilla is normal. Physiological tracer uptake may be observed in the nipples [12].

6.2.7   Image Acquisition

A single- or multiple-head gamma camera is needed to acquire planar and/or tomographic (SPECT) images. A low-energy, high-resolution collimator should be used. The energy window for image collection should be 10% (±5%) centered over the 140 keV photopeak of ^{99m}Tc [12]. For planar imaging a 256 × 256 or larger matrix should be used [12].

Acquisition for planar images should start 5–10 min after injection of ^{99m}Tc-sestamibi and should last for 10 min (SNM: 10 min or 175,000 counts) [12, 23]. However few anecdotal reports indicate an improved target-to-background ratio by starting the data acquisition 60–90 min after injection of the tracer [82]. Despite these data, it is currently recognized that high diagnostic accuracy can be achieved by starting imaging 5–15 min after injection of ^{99m}Tc-sestamibi, which is in accordance to the time line recommended by both the EANM as well as the SNM. Furthermore, delayed imaging may result in false-negative studies if there is an increased washout of ^{99m}Tc-sestamibi from a primary breast cancer expressing the MDR1 gene [11]. However, delayed imaging can be applied for assessment of chemoresistance of tumors since for this purpose it is recommended to acquire images at various time points.

Khalkhali et al. were the first to propose the use of the prone position instead of supine imaging [10]. Prone-dependent breast imaging can be performed with either a special table with lateral cutouts or foam cushion (with a lateral semicircular aperture) placed over the imaging table [11]. Prone imaging is known to provide several advantages over the supine or upright position. Separation from the myocardium and the liver is advantageous in avoiding a spillover from the very high ^{99m}Tc-sestamibi uptake in both organs. This overlay might mask the breast activity. Furthermore, the evaluation of deep breast tissue adjacent to the thoracic wall is also facilitated by imaging the patient in the prone position. Finally, the distance between the detector and the breast is minimized in the prone position. However, supine can still be useful mainly for better localization of the primary tumor, especially those in the inner quadrants, and also to visualize axillae and possible internal mammary lymph node involvement [11]. Therefore, a combination of prone and supine images should be carried out whenever possible. These suggestions gained entrance to the guidelines as in accordance to the EANM; lateral views in prone position and anterior view in supine position must be acquired in all circumstances. The detector should touch the patient's side to improve the resolution. Prone lateral breast images should be acquired with the patient lying prone with her heads resting on her arms on a breast scintigraphy mattress. The axilla must be included in the lateral and anterior views in all circumstances: the arms should be raised to provide clear imaging of the axilla [12]. The SNM guideline recommends that the patient should be seated for the entire scan and that the views of the scintimammography should duplicate standard mammographic views according to the most recent mammogram [23].

Based on the recommendations published in the EANM practice guidelines, images must be acquired in sequence starting with a prone lateral scintigraphy of the breast with the suspected lesion followed by a the same image acquisition of the contralateral breast. Afterward, a supine (or upright) anterior scintigraphy should be performed [12]. In this regard, the SNM guidelines provide more detailed recommendations by starting with right craniocaudal, left craniocaudal, right mediolateral oblique, left mediolateral oblique planar images for the breast with the suspected abnormality followed by the same image acquisition of the contralateral breast [23]. Optional SPECT images (360°, 120 steps, 20 s per step) should be acquired after the planar imaging [12]. Furthermore, a prone posterior oblique scintigraphy might be useful to acquire as well as images with markers over the nipple or breast lesion(s) [12]. In order to evaluate multidrug resistance, delayed images (1 h after injection) should be collected in the same conditions like the initial data acquisition [12].

Over the past years, the use of routine SPECT imaging for breast cancer detection was a matter of debate. Even though it might be useful to provide a better contrast resolution, accurate localization and characterization of the lesion can sometime be more difficult to obtain [11]. In 1996, Palmedo et al. demonstrated planar imaging slightly more sensitive and specific than SPECT imaging for detection of breast cancer [62]. In a more recent study including 303 patients, Myslivecek et al. found an overall sensitivity in the detection of breast cancer of 92% for SPECT and 82% for planar imaging (p=n.s.), respectively. The overall specificity was 91% for SPECT and 91% for planar scans (p=n.s.), respectively. Metastatic axillary lymph node involvement was seen in 35 patients; per-axilla overall sensitivity was 66% for SPECT and 54% for planar images (p=n.s.), respectively; overall specificity was 76% and 86%, respectively (p=n.s.) [61]. In general, routine use of SPECT imaging alone cannot be recommended but may be able to provide additional information to planar imaging and might therefore be of value when planar images are inconclusive, to better characterize multicentric or multifocal lesions, or in the detection of axillary metastases [11, 48, 83].

6.2.8 Sources of Error

One has to be aware of potential sources of errors, which might impair the image quality and/or the interpretation of the images. Among these a small lesion size (lesions <1 cm may be missed) has to be taken into account and, if data on the lesion size are available in advance of the scheduled breast scintimammography, it should be considered whether one has to expect reliable data from breast scintigraphy in case of a known small lesion [12].

Additional sources of error [12]:
- Extravasation following tracer injection in the contralateral arm potentially leading to an abnormal uptake in the axillary region
- Couch scatter
- Patient motion; wrong patient positioning
- If both breasts are dependent, cross-talk of activity may result in a false positive result in the contralateral breast
- Local pathological or physiological uptakes asking or confounding cancer lesions
- Interfering cytostatic treatments that decrease tumor uptake
- Postsurgery uptakes
- Postradiotherapy uptakes

6.2.9 Radiation Dosimetry

The estimated adsorbed radiation dose to various organs in healthy subjects following administration of ^{99m}Tc-sestamibi is given in Table 6.5. The data are quoted from ICRP no. 80 [12].

The dosimetry to the gall bladder is 0.039 mGy/MBq (0.14 rads/mCi) and the effective dose is 0.0085 mSv/MBq (0.031 rem/mCi). More detailed information about the dosimetry of ^{99m}Tc-sestamibi breast scintigraphy can be obtained from the EANM- and SNM guidelines [12, 23].

No recommendations are made for usage of the radiopharmaceutical for diagnosis of breast masses in children.

6.3 Clinical Studies

6.3.1 ^{99m}Tc-Sestamibi Scintimammography in Detecting Breast Cancer

A clear evidence exists that ^{99m}Tc-sestamibi scintimammography has a primary use in identifying the presence of breast cancer when mammogram or ultrasound is unhelpful [84]. Though this may represent a small number of patients it does include those who are premenopausal, the very group in which mammography is most unhelpful because of high breast density leading to poor positive predictive value [85]. It is also in this group that there is the largest increase in the incidence of breast

Table 6.5 Radiation dosimetry as quoted ICRP no. 80

Organ	Absorbed dose per unit activity administered (mGy/MBq)	
	Adult	15 years
Adrenals	0.0075	0.0099
Bladder	0.011	0.014
Bone surfaces	0.0082	0.010
Brain	0.0052	0.0071
Breast	0.0038	0.0053
Gallbladder	0.039	0.045
Stomach	0.0065	0.0090
Small intestine	0.015	0.018
Colon	0.024	0.031
Heart	0.0063	0.0082
Kidneys	0.036	0.043
Liver	0.011	0.014
Lungs	0.0046	0.0064
Muscles	0.0029	0.0037
Esophagus	0.0041	0.0057
Ovaries	0.0091	0.012
Pancreas	0.0077	0.010
Salivary glands	0.014	0.017
Skin	0.0031	0.0041
Red marrow	0.0055	0.0071
Spleen	0.0065	0.0086
Testes	0.0038	0.0050
Thymus	0.0041	0.0057
Thyroid	0.0053	0.0079
Uterus	0.0078	0.010
Remaining organs	0.0031	0.0039
Effective dose (mSv/MBq)	0.0085	0.011

cancer so that accurate identification of not just the presence of a breast cancer but also its extent is most useful. Another group has patients in whom biopsy material is sought but in whom only benign tissue has been removed but clinical suspicion of malignancy remains. A ^{99m}Tc-sestamibi scintimammogram can direct further biopsy. False-positive uptake can be seen in fibrocystic disease and fibroadenomas with epithelial hyperplasia as well as tumor phylloides [86]. It is interesting to note that in some patients these can be considered as premalignant conditions [84].

Fifty-one studies (1994–2005) investigating the diagnostic value of ^{99m}Tc-sestamibi scintimammography for evaluation of breast lesions in different study designs have been reviewed. The reported studies included patients with palpable and nonpalpable breast lesions, patients with abnormal mammograms as the only inclusion criteria, and studies including data concerning planar and/or SPECT imaging. The majority (80%) of the named studies' results yielded a sensitivity over 80%. Even 90% of all studies still revealed a sensitivity of over 75% (90%). Fourteen studies (27.5%) had sensitivity estimates of more than 90%. A rather small number of stud-

6   99mTc-Sestamibi Scintimammography   103

ies revealed sensitivities lower than 80% ($n = 10$; 20%). Of these, three were reported with sensitivities of 60% or less. The lowest sensitivity of 99mTc-scintimammography was found in a study on 24 patients and was reported to be as low as 50%. With regard to specificity, the majority (71.4%) of the studies reported estimates of 80% or more, whereas 16 studies (32.7%) reported specificity estimates of 90% or more. The lowest specificity of 33.3% was reported in a study of 18 investigated breast lesions of which 15 had been confirmed as cancer (Table 6.6).

The use of scintimammography as an adjuvant test to mammography is both sensitive and specific. In case 99mTc-sestamibi breast scintigraphy is used as an adjuvant to physical examinations and mammograms, the rates of negative biopsies and breast surgery could be significantly reduced. In this multimodality diagnostic approach scintimammography would be recommended only for those lesions where additional information is required in order to reach a definitive diagnosis. Patients with equivocal or unremarkable mammograms that have other risk factors including a positive physical examination, family history, and previous cancer may benefit from the additional information provided by breast scintigraphy (Fig. 6.2). In addition, younger women with dense breasts and women with implants may also benefit from scintimammography since the latter technique is not affected by breast density and is permeable to implants.

Currently, the most beneficial use of 99mTc-sestamibi scintimammography is reported for patients with equivocal physical examination and mammography in order to identify women who are at high or low risk for breast cancer. This benefit is mainly due when decisions need to be made which patients would require immediate definitive invasive diagnostic evaluation [27]. By now, the value of 99mTc-sestamibi scintigraphy as a screening method has to be doubted since its sensitivity for lesions less than 10 mm is rather poor with virtually no lesion detected below 6 mm. There is a broad consensus that morphological imaging with mammography, ultrasound, and/or MRI has a clear advantage in the screening setting for breast cancer disease as compared to scintimammography. Therefore, these diagnostic tools, mainly mammography, but not 99mTc-sestamibi mammography are currently recommended in the diagnostic algorithm for screening of breast cancer disease (Tables 6.8–6.10).

6.3.2 Diagnostic Value of 99mTc-Sestamibi Scintimammography in Comparison to Other Noninvasive Diagnostic Modalities

6.3.2.1 Functional Imaging with FDG PET

18F-fluorodeoxyglucose positron emission tomography (FDG PET) has been introduced as a method with a very high sensitivity and specificity for imaging the breast [105, 106]. The reported sensitivity for FDG PET was found to be in the high range of 85-95% with a specificity ranging from 80% to 100% and a positive predictive value greater than 90% [106, 107]. Secondary goals for PET are related to staging of axillary and internal lymph nodes, the detection of metastatic disease, the detection of local or distant recurrence, and the assessment of the response of the tumor to treatment. Various studies showed a diagnostic accuracy of FDG PET between 70% and 97% and a sensitivity and specificity of 64–96% and 73–100%, respectively

Table 6.6 Diagnostic value of ^{99m}Tc-sestamibi scintimammography for the evaluation of breast lesions

Author	Year	Age	N (lesions)	Malignant	Benign	TP	TN	FP	FN	Sens (%)	Spec (%)	PPV (%)	NPV (%)	ACC (%)
Alonso [38]	2001	50	245	189	56	157	43	13	32	83	77			
Ambrus [87]	1997		51	40	11	38	8	3	2	95	73	93	80	90
Arslan [47]	1998	50	105	52	53	42	46	7	10	80.8	86.8	85.7	82.1	83.8
Becherer [48]	1997	50	174	52	122	40	106	16	12	76.9	86.9	71.4	89.8	83.9
Burak [88]	1994	51	41	27	14	25	12	2	2	92.6	85.7	92.6	85.7	90.2
Buscombe [49]	1999		48	26	22	25	18	4	1	96.2	81.8	86.2	94.7	89.6
Buscombe [50]	2001	53	374	204	170	181	122	49	23	89	71	79	84	
Carril [89]	1997	35–81	41	22	19	19	11	8	3	86.4	57.9	70.4	78.6	73.2
Chen [71]	1997	48.8	63	32	31	25	28	3	7	78.1	90.3	89.3	80.0	84.1
Clifford [39]	1996	23–78	148	43	105	36	100	5	7	83.7	95.2	87.8	93.5	91.9
Cutrone [40]	1999		68	23	45	22	41	4	1	95.7	91.1	84.6	97.6	92.6
Cwikla [53]	2001	53		40								96.0		
Cwikla [90]	2000	52	298	228	70	202	45	25	26	89	64	89	63	
Danielson [91]	1999	54.4	121	86	35	72	26	9	14	83.7	74.3	88.9	65.0	81.0
De Vincentis [92]	1997		14	8	6	6	6	0	2	75.0	100.0	100.0	75.0	85.7
De Vincentis [93]	1998	71	36	32	4	26	4	0	6	81.3	100.0	100.0	40.0	83.3
Flanagan [94]	1998	52.5	80	21	59	17	48	11	4	81.0	81.4	60.7	92.3	81.3
Fondrinier [54]	2004		45	24	21					58.3	81	78	63	
Helbich [55]	1997	47	150	52	98	36	82	16	16	69.2	83.7	69.2	83.7	78.7
Howarth [80]	1999	23–87	123	103	20	87	16	4	16	84	80			84
Imbriaco [56]	2001	49	49	25	24	20	21	3	5	80	88			84
Kao [72]	1994	31–79	38	32	6	27	6	0	5	84.4	100.0	100.0	54.5	86.8

Author	Year	Age												
Khalkhali [95]	1997	47.9	164	52	112	48	98	14	4	92.3	87.5	77.4	96.1	89.0
Lam [96]	1996	20–88	52	38	14	37	11	3	1	97.4	78.6	92.5	91.7	92.3
Lu [82]	1995		44							91	83	67	96	85
Maffioli [57]	1996	49.8	24	14	10	7	9	1	7	50.0	90.0	87.5	56.3	66.7
Mathieu [59]	2005	57	118	69	49					88.4	67	79	80.5	80
Maublant [60]	1996	57	18	16	2	14	0	2	2	87.5		87.5		77.8
Mekhmandarov [76]	1998	61.4	140	85	55	71	47	8	14	83.5	85.5	89.9	77.0	84.3
Melloul [77]	1999	53	121	18	103	16	91	12	2	88.9	88.3	57.1	97.8	88.4
Mirzaei [97]	2000	51	94	30	64	26	52	12	4	87	93	68	93	83
Moretti [19]	1996	37–76	15	13	2	10	2	0	3	76.9	100.0	100.0	40.0	80.0
Myslivecek [61]	2004		308	85	223	78	204	19	7	92	91			
Palmedo [62]	1996	55	108	48	60	41	51	9	7	85.4	85.0	82.0	87.9	85.2
Palmedo [63]	1996		56	27	29	23	19	10	4	85	66	70	83	
Palmedo [98]	1998	54.5	253	165	88	100	71	17	65	60.6	80.7	85.5	52.2	67.6
Prats [65]	1999	55	97	41	56	35	44	12	6	85.4	78.6	74.5	88.0	81.4
Prats [66]	2001	21–86	268	155	113	141	80	33	14	91	71	81	85	
Sampalis [43]	2003	56	1243	201	1042	186	906	136	15	93	87	58	98	88
Schillaci [99]	1997	57	198	126	72	105	65	7	21	83.3	90.3	93.8	75.6	85.9
Scopinaro [100]	1997	52	449	355	94	301	85	9	54	84.8	90.4	97.1	61.2	86.0
Sillar [101]	1997	37–84	18	15	3	14	1	2	1	93.3	33.3	87.5	50.0	83.3
Sommer [102]	1997		81	33	48	29	44	4	4	87.9	91.7	87.9	91.7	90.1
Taillefer [44]	1995	56	65	47	18	43	17	1	4	91.5	94.4	97.7	81.0	92.3

(continued)

Table 6.6 (continued)

Author	Year	Age	N (lesions)	Malignant	Benign	TP	TN	FP	FN	Sens (%)	Spec (%)	PPV (%)	NPV (%)	ACC (%)
Tiling [68]	1998	52	44	24	20	19	16	4	5	79.2	80.0	82.6	76.2	79.5
Tiling [69]	2005		252	143	109	120	93	16	23	84	85			
Tolmos [45]	1998	51	70	9	61	5	53	8	4	55.6	86.9	38.5	93.0	82.9
Uriarte [70]	1998	35–81	78	41	37	38	18	19	3	92.7	48.6	66.7	85.7	71.8
Villanueva-Meyer [46]	1996	52	66	35	31	29	29	2	6	82.9	93.5	93.5	82.9	87.9
Waxman [103]	1994		149							89	72			
Yuen-Green [104]	1996	53.9	21	6	15	5	14	1	1	83.3	93.3	83.3	93.3	90.5

TP True positive, *TN* true negative, *FP* false positive, *FN* false negative, *Sens* sensitivity, *Spec* specificity, *PPV* positive predictive value, *NPV* negative predictive value, *Acc* accuracy

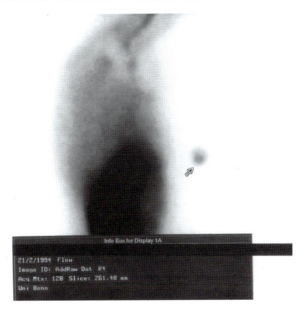

Fig. 6.2 Right lateral view of the right breast. Female patient with the diagnosis of a carcinoma in the right mamma depicted by ^{99m}Tc-sestamibi breast scintigraphy

(Table 6.7). However, most of these studies included only a small number of patients with a high prevalance of malignancy. In a meta-analysis published 2002, Samson et al. found a sensitivity of 88%, a specificity of 82%, an accuracy of 87%, a positive predictive value of 94%, and a negative predictive value of 69% for FDG PET in the differential diagnosis of benign from malignant lesions among patients with abnormal mammograms or a palpable breast mass [120]. In a further meta-analysis, Gambhir et al. summarized the diagnostic value of PET for various indications in diagnosis of breast cancer disease [121]. On a patient basis, they reported a sensitivity of 91%, a specificity of 93%, and a diagnostic accuracy of 95% for FDG-PET in diagnosing breast cancer disease. On a lesions basis, reported values for diagnostic performance of FDG PET are slightly lower (sensitivity: 90%; specificity: 92%, diagnostic accuracy: 88%) [121]. With regard to staging of breast cancer disease, FDG PET showed a sensitivity of 91%, a specificity of 88%, and a diagnostic accuracy of 90% on a patient basis (lesion basis: sensitivity: 95%, specificity: 88%, diagnostic accuracy: 88%) [121].

The low sensitivity of PET in lesions <1 cm limits its use for screening. Furthermore, study costs are high, PET scanners have still limited availability and patient throughput is low. Furthermore, it has been reported that FDG PET may yield false-negative results following chemotherapy, which is mainly due to chemotherapy-induced changes in tumor metabolism. False negative results yielded by FDG PET were also reported for ductal carcinoma in situ, dependent of the tumor size, whereas false-positive results were seen in cases of inflammation and fibrous dysplasia [122].

It is anticipated that fusion of morphological and functional data will boost sensitivity and specificity compared with the individual imaging technique. The CT portion of PET/CT provides anatomical mapping images for PET as well as attenuation correction data. Thus, PET/CT offers PET, CT, and high-quality fused images of both

Table 6.7 Diagnostic value of functional imaging with FDG PET in suspicious breast lesions

Authors	Year	No. of patients	No. of lesions	Sens (%)	Spec (%)	Acc (%)	PPV (%)	NPV (%)
Heinisch [108]	2003	36	40	68	73	70	81	58
Schirrmeister [109]	2001	117	117	93	75	89	92	78
Avril [110]	2000	144	185	64–80	76–94	73–79	89–87	52–61
Palmedo [111]	1997	20	22	92	86	82	92	67
Avril [112]	1996	51	72	83	84	83	87	79
Scheidhauer [106]	1996	30	30	91	86	90	95	75
Dehdashti [113]	1995	32	32	88	100	91	100	73
Adler [114]	1993	28	35	96	100	97	100	89
Nitzsche [115]	1993	37	n. a.	94	100	95	100	80
Wahl [116]	1991		10	100		100		
Tse [117]	1992		35	80	100	86		
Nieweg [118]	1993		19	91	100	97		
Kole [119]	1997		13	100	67	92		

No. number, *Sens* sensitivity, *Spec* specificity, *Acc* accuracy, *PPV* positive predictive value, *NPV* negative predictive value

functional and anatomy at the same location of the body. This yields a clear improvement in diagnostic accuracy. In a study published by Tatsumi et al. evaluating the diagnostic value of PET/CT in the evaluation of breast cancer, an overall of 69 malignant and 13 benign regions with confirmation was found and sensitivity, specificity, and accuracy of 87%, 62%, and 83% for PET/CT and 68%, 69%, and 68% for CT were reported [123]. Staging evaluation was performed in 69 patients. In eight patients in whom initial staging was performed, PET/CT and CT accurately evaluated seven and six patients, respectively. Of the other 61 patients (with suspected recurrence or undergoing follow-up), PET/CT accurately staged 52, while CT accurately evaluated 47. The reported sensitivity, specificity, and accuracy for the total study population were 84%, 88%, and 86% for PET/CT and 73%, 83%, and 77% for CT [123].

Radan et al. reported about the role of FDG PET/CT in suspected recurrence of breast cancer [124]. In this study, 47 consecutive FDG PET/CT studies of 46 women with a history of breast cancer presented with elevated serum tumor markers 1–21 years after their initial diagnosis. Sensitivity, specificity, and accuracy were 90%, 71%, and 83%, respectively. PPV and NPV were 84% and 80%, respectively. PET/CT had a higher sensitivity (85% vs 70%), specificity (76% vs 47%), and accuracy (81% vs 59%) as contrast-enhanced CT.

6.3.2.2 Morphological Imaging with Mammography, MRI, and Ultrasound

Mammography is still the number one diagnostic tool for the assessment of the breasts. For evaluation of breast lesions mammography is reported to be associated with a sensitivity of 65–100% and with a specificity of 14–96%. The major drawback of mammographic breast assessment is surely related to its rather low specificity since only two studies revealed specificity estimates over 75% (75% and 96%) whereas in contrast 7 out of 9 studies revealed values lower than 70% (Table 6.8).

Table 6.8 Morphological imaging measures in breast cancer disease

Authors	Year	Purpose	No. of patients	No. of lesions	Sens (%)	Spec (%)	Acc (%)	PPV (%)	NPV (%)
Mammography									
Arslan [47]	1999	Diagnosis	77	105	94	56			
Alonso [38]	2001	Diagnosis	238	245	85	66			
Buscombe [50]	2001	Diagnosis	353	374	70	69		73	66
Cwikla [90]	2000	Diagnosis	273	298	68	69		88	40
Cutrone [40]	1999	Diagnosis	67	68	73.9	53.3	63.2	44.7	80.0
Howarth [80]	1999	Diagnosis	117	123	65	63	64		
Palmedo [64]	1996	Diagnosis	56	56	89	14		49	57
Kaiser [125]	2002	Diagnosis	123		100	96			100
Lorenzen [126]	2005	Diagnosis		632	92	75			
Rissanen [127]	1993	Recurrence	67		45				
Cwikla [128]	2000	Recurrence	63	33	42				
Berg [129]	2004	CA	111	258	67.8	75	70.2	85.7	
Hata [130]	2004	CA	183		22.2	85.7	50		
Satake [131]	2000	CA		46	55	100	72		
Kuhl [132]	2000	Screening	192		33				
Kuhl [133]	2005	Screening	529		32.6	96.8		23.7	
Kriege [134]	2004	Screening	1909		40	95			
Kolb [135]	2002	Screening	27,825		77.6	98.8	98.6	35.8	99.8
Warner [136]	2004	Screening	236		36				
Warner [137]	2001	Screening	196		33	99.5		66	97
Zonderland [138]	1999	Screening	4,811		83	97		72	99
Lam [139]	1996	ALNM	64		20	95			
Magnetic resonance imaging									
Heinisch [108]	2003	Diagnosis	36	40	92	73	85	85	85

(continued)

Table 6.8 (continued)

Authors	Year	Purpose	No. of patients	No. of lesions	Sens (%)	Spec (%)	Acc (%)	PPV (%)	NPV (%)
Walter [122]	2003	Diagnosis	40	42	89	91	90	89	91
Heywang-Koebrunner [140]	2001	Diagnosis	n. a.	519	96–90	71–64	n. a.	89–83	88–75
Leinsinger [141]	2001	Diagnosis	40	40	86	96	93	92	93
Tiling [69]	2005	Diagnosis	68		84	51			
Kvistad [142]	2000	Diagnosis	130	130	89	67	79	77	83
Helbich [55]	1997	Diagnosis	66	75	96	82	87	74	98
Buemke [143]	2004	Diagnosis	821		88.1	67.7		72.4	85.4
Imbriaco [56]	2001	Diagnosis	49	49	96	75	86	80	95
Palmedo [63]	1996	Diagnosis	56	56	93	21		52	75
Tiling [68]	1998	Diagnosis	68		84	49		49	84
Kuhl [144]	1999	Screening	230	266	91	83	86	77	94
Kuhl [133]	2005	Screening	529		90.7	97.2		50.0	
MARBIS [145]	2005	Screening	649		77	81			
Kriege [134]	2004	Screening	1909		71.1	89.8			
Warner [137]	2001	Screening	196		100	91		26	100
Berg [129]	2004	CA	111	258	94.4	26	72.9	73.6	
Hata [130]	2004	CA	183		66.7	64.2	65.6		
Satake [131]	2000	CA		25	93	90	92		
Murray [146]	2002	ALNM	47		100	56	89	38	100
Michel [147]	2002	ALNM	20		82	100		100	78
Kvistad [148]	2000	ALNM	65		83	90	88		
Ultrasound									
Howarth [80]	1999	Diagnosis		76	68	65	67		
Kaiser [119]	2002	Diagnosis	77		100	96			100
Cha [149]	2005	Diagnosis	67	75	62	80		55	84

	Year	Purpose			Sens	Spec	Acc	PPV	NPV
Lorenzen [126]	2005	Diagnosis		632	86	76			
Raza [150]	1997	Diagnosis		86	68	95		85	88
Moon [151]	2002	Diagnosis		77	100	51		64	100
Rissanen [127]	1993	Recurrence	67		91				
Berg [129]	2004	CA	111	258	83	34	67.8	73.5	
Hata [130]	2004	CA	183		20.6	85.2	50		
Satake [131]	2000	CA		46	89	76	85		
Kuhl [133]	2005	Screening	529		39.5	90.5		11.3	
Kuhl [132]	2000	Screening	192		33				
Kolb [135]	2002	Screening	27,825		75.3	96.8	96.6	20.5	99.7
Warner [136]	2004	Screening	236		33				
Podo [152]	2002	Screening	105		13				
Warner [137]	2001	Screening	186		60	93		19	99
Buchberger [153]	2000	Screening	8,970		100	31			
Strauss [154]	1998	ALNM	78	90	91.7				
Verbanck [155]	1997	ALNM	144		92	95		96	91
Lam [139]	1996	ALNM	36	72.7	95				

ALNM Axillary lymph node metastases, *CA* cancer assessment, *Sens* sensitivity, *Spec* specificity, *Acc* accuracy, *PPV* positive predictive value, *NPV* negative predictive value

This is also for breast assessment with MRI since its high diagnostic value based on a sensitivity, within the range of 84% and 96% for the diagnosis of breast lesions, is diminished by its specificity estimates within the range of 21% and 96%. This is even emphasized by the fact that 8 out of 11 studies revealed specificity estimates of only 75% and lower (Table 6.8).

Sonographically evaluation of breast lesions yielded a sensitivity of 62–100% and a specificity of 51–95%. However, 50% of cited studies revealed sensitivity estimates lower than 70%, and 66.7% of cited studies specificity values of 80% and lower (Table 6.8). This clearly needs to be taken into account when applying ultrasound for evaluation of breast lesions that led to the fact that it is not valued as a stand-alone diagnostic measure neither for screening nor for the assessment of breast cancer disease.

Based on the results on the diagnostic value of ^{99m}Tc-sestamibi breast scintigraphy and those of the morphological imaging modalities mentioned above, scintimammography was shown to be a valuable adjunct to one or more of these diagnostic measures. Several studies evaluated the use of ^{99m}Tc-sestamibi scintigraphy as an adjunct to mammography for the diagnosis of breast cancer and showed it to be useful, in particular for assessing dense breasts. In contrast to mammography, the sensitivity of breast scintigraphy was found not to be reduced when dense breasts were imaged. In dense breasts, ultrasound was reported to be more sensitive than scintimammography but at the cost of decreases specificity [59]. Breast MRI has high sensitivity but only moderate specificity independent of breast density, tumor type, and menopausal status [143].

6.3.3 ^{99m}Tc-Sestamibi for Particular Diagnostic Situations

6.3.3.1 Diagnostic Value of ^{99m}Tc-Sestamibi in the Detection of Axillary Lymph Node Involvement in Primary Breast Cancer Patients

Locoregional lymph node involvement in the axilla has a major bearing on the prognosis of the disease. Surgical biopsy and clearance are the standard methods used for establishing the presence of axillary disease but there is often a significant morbidity. It was hoped that ^{99m}Tc-sestamibi scintimammography could accurately predict the presence of axillary lymph node involvement (Fig 6.3). In a series of patients from Canada, planar ^{99m}Tc-sestamibi scintimammography was associated with a sensitivity of 84% and a specificity of 91% for axillary lymph node disease [44]. However, some other groups have failed to obtain such good results with the lowest reported sensitivity being only 57%. The lowest sensitivity was reported by Massardo et al. in a multicenter study including 149 patients. They found a sensitivity of planar data acquisition of only 27.8% [79]. The lowest reported sensitivity for SPECT imaging with ^{99m}Tc-sestamibi was 62% and the lowest specificity could be shown to be 64% (SPECT). However, the majority (83.3%) of studies reported specificities of 85% and over (Table 6.9). Comparative studies have demonstrated that SPECT acquisition significantly improves the sensitivity and

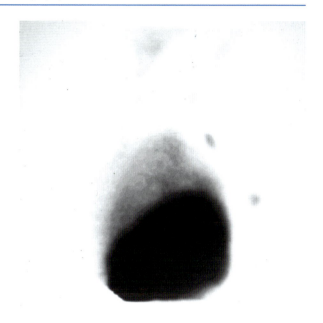

Fig. 6.3 Right lateral view of the right breast. Focal ^{99m}Tc-sestamibi uptake according to a carcinoma in the right mamma. This uptake corresponds to the primary malignant lesion in the breast. Additional focal MIBI uptake in the right axilla of the patient indicating a lymph node metastasis of the malignant mass in the right breast

accuracy achieved with planar scintimammography [166]. Thus, SPECT should be preferred to planar imaging, particularly in those patients without clinical suspicion of axillary metastatic involvement given its high negative predictive value [166]. However, false negative results have been reported due to the small size of lymph nodes and/or to partial or micrometastatic involvement. As such, since axillae are imaged in the standard protocol, abnormal lymph node uptake should be reported and acted on but a negative ^{99m}Tc-sestamibi study in the axilla however does not exclude lymph node involvement and all such axillae should still be explored (Table 6.9).

Magnetic resonance imaging is becoming an increasingly valuable tool in selected groups of patients with breast cancer. The sensitivity for diagnosis of axillary lymph node metastases has been shown to be between 82% and 100% with a specificity of 56–100% (accuracy: 88–89%; PPV: 38–100%; NPV: 78–100%; Table 6.8). Although ultrasound has long been the first method in radiological examination of the axilla, it has not been considered as especially important. But, in breast imaging, ultrasound has gained acceptance, and today it is an important adjunct to mammography. Sensitivity of ultrasound for diagnosis of axillary lymph node metastases was 92–95% and specificity was reported to be 95% (Table 6.8). In mammography, lymph nodes are visible on standard projections, and it is possible to differentiate between normal and pathological nodes. Pathological nodes are of greater density than normal nodes, and the hilus disappears. The form also becomes more expansive – oval to round – but the size is not necessarily increased. However, in the standard projections, only part of the axilla can be seen, and during exposure

Table 6.9 Diagnostic value of ^{99m}Tc scintimammography in the diagnosis of axillary lymph node metastases

Authors	Year	No. of patients	Method	Sens (%)	Spec (%)	Accuracy (%)	PPV (%)	NPV (%)
Burak [88]	1994	27	Planar	57				
Kao [72]	1994	12	Planar	67				
Taillefer [44]	1995	41	Planar	84	91		89	87
Lu [82]	1995	11	Planar	100	100		100	100
Lam [139]	1996	36	Planar	64	90		78	82
Palmedo [156]	1996	11	Planar	82				
			SPECT	82				
Schillaci [99]	1997	49	Planar	81	93		89	87
			SPECT	62	96		93	77
Perre [157]	1997	36	Planar	91	64		80	82
Chiti [158]	1997	27	SPECT	82	100		100	89
Clifford [39]	1996	147	Planar	44	83		80	50
Taillefer [159]	1998	100	Planar	79	85		83	81
Kubo [160]	1997		SPECT	100	83.3	90		
Tiling [161]	1998	113	SPECT	64.7	90.5			
			Planar	41.2	95.2			
Myslivecek [61]	2004	35	SPECT	66	76			
			Planar	54	86			
Mulero [162]	2000	84	Planar	36	100		100	48
Nishiyama [163]	2001	50	Planar	73				
Lumachi [164]	2001	239	Planar	82.3	94.1			
Chen [165]	2003	60	Planar	83.3	86.1			
Massardo [79]	2005	149	Planar	27.8	91.7			

No. Number, *Sens* sensitivity, *Spec* specificity, *PPV* positive predictive value, *NPV* negative predictive value

of the mammogram, pathological nodes can be pushed outside the mammographic image. Mammography is therefore not a reliable method in axillary lymph node imaging [167]. In a study by Lam et al., sensitivity of mammography for diagnosis of malignant axillary lymph nodes was as low as 20% with a specificity of 95% [139] (Table 6.8).

Whereas mammography was shown not to be a reliable method for assessment of axillary lymph node metastases, MRI and ultrasound were reported to be associated with a high sensitivity in diagnosing malignant axillary lymph nodes as already mentioned above. In contrast, data regarding specificity for this purpose, mainly for MRI, remain inconclusive. With regard to scintimammography with ^{99m}Tc-sestamibi, several studies reported a low sensitivity for assessment of axillary lymph node disease especially with planar data acquisition. Therefore, if applied to the diagnostic cascade of the assessment of the axillae in patients with breast cancer,

SPECT data acquisition should be assured. However, nowadays, FDG PET might be the more reliable functional imaging tool in the assessment of the lymph node status in breast cancer patients since a recently published meta-analysis revealed sensitivities ranging from as low as 20% but up to 100% and specificities ranging from 65% to 100%. Moreover, the additional benefit of an assessment of distal metastatic spread provided by FDG PET in one single session needs also to be taken into account [168]. FDG-PET may therefore play a role for axillary lymph node evaluation under particular circumstances but one has to be aware that even FDG PET cannot replace axillary dissection in axillary lymph gland staging due to the high number of false-positives results.

6.3.3.2 Diagnostic Value of ^{99m}Tc-Sestamibi in Recurrence of Breast Cancer Disease

The number of recurrence of breast cancer with local recurrence remains small – less than 5%, but may increase with the trend toward breast conservation surgery. Early identification and assessment of recurrence should be of clinical benefit [169]. The interpretation of mammograms may be problematic due to alterations of previous surgery or radiotherapy leading to a change of breast density. In a study by Cwikla et al., a similar sensitivity has been reported for ^{99m}Tc-sestamibi in finding recurrent cancer within the breast and in primary breast cancer [51]. One has to mention that the uptake can be quite low grade and diffuse, and this is probably due to the fact that there is no mass of tumor cells but an area with diffuse cancer involvement throughout the breast tissue. A further advantage of ^{99m}Tc-sestamibi is that, in contrast to mammography, it can identify recurrence in other adjacent tissues. In a more recently published study (2005), Mathieu et al. reported a sensitivity of 81% and a specificity of 65.6% in diagnosis of suspicion of breast cancer recurrence [59]. Cwikla et al. showed a sensitivity of mammography of only about 50% in recurrent breast cancer increasing to 70% for ^{99m}Tc-sestamibi. Additionally, six sites of cancer outside the breast could be identified which were not seen on mammography (Table 6.10) [51].

FDG-PET is associated with a sensitivity of 80–85% in diagnosis of recurrence of breast cancer disease. Its specificity is reported to be 79–85% and the accuracy is 82% [121].

Table 6.10 Diagnostic value of ^{99m}Tc-sestamibi scintimammography in the diagnosis of recurrent breast cancer disease

Authors	Year	No. of patients	No. of lesions	Sens (%)	Spec (%)	Acc (%)	PPV (%)	NPV (%)
Cwikla [51]	1998			88.9	70.0	78.9	72.7	87.5
Cwikla [128]	2000	63	33	78				
Mathieu [59]	2005	48	48	81	65.6	71	54	87.5

No. Number, *Sens* sensitivity, *Spec* specificity, *Acc* accuracy, *PPV* positive predictive value, *NPV* negative predictive value

Due to altered density of the breast after surgical treatment, chemotherapy and/or radiation therapy sensitivity of mammography for diagnosis of recurrence of breast cancer was shown to be only 42–45%, whereas sonographically examination was associated with a sensitivity of 91% for diagnosis of breast cancer recurrence (Table 6.8).

Therefore, ^{99m}Tc-sestamibi scintimammography demonstrated its usefulness for detection of recurrence of breast cancer mainly in cases where triple diagnosis with conventional mammography, ultrasound, and fine needle aspiration is doubtful or discordant [59]. However, FDG-PET may be a more reliable method due to the reported higher specificity.

6.3.4 ^{99m}Tc-Sestamibi for the Evaluation of Response to Chemotherapy

[99m]Tc-sestamibi scintimammography might be a reliable diagnostic tool in assessing the response to chemotherapy. Marshall et al. found a positive MIBI scan highly predictive of the presence of significant residual disease on completion of chemotherapy [58]. In contrast, a negative MIBI scan did not rule out the presence of considerable residual tumor. Whereas ultrasound and clinical assessment may underestimate the response to chemotherapy, MIBI imaging tends to overestimate the response. Maini et al. reported a specificity for prediction of tumor presence at the completion of chemotherapy (measured after three cycles) of 100% for scintimammography, 67% for clinical evaluation, and 33% for mammography [170]. Dunnwald et al. observed that patients with high residual MIBI uptake in breast tumors after 2 months of chemotherapy and posttreatment had a significantly increased risk of breast cancer recurrence and an increased risk of death due to breast carcinoma [35]. These data suggest that serial MIBI imaging may provide a useful quantitative surrogate end point for chemotherapy trials. Given the association between MIBI uptake and tumor blood flow, this prognostic capability may be related to retained tumor vascularity after treatment [35].

In 1997, Alonso et al. performed a study in order to investigate the clinical value of a standard ^{99m}Tc-sestamibi scintimammography technique in the prediction of response to chemotherapy in advanced breast cancer patients. They found sensitivities, specificities, positive, and negative predictive values of 88%, 92%, 97%, and 71% and 91%, 100%, 100%, and 77% for early and delayed tumor/background ratios, respectively, and conclude that ^{99m}Tc-sestamibi scintigraphy may be a clinically valuable tool for guiding chemotherapy in advanced breast cancer patients [36].

For monitoring of response to chemotherapy, FDG PET has been reported to be associated with a sensitivity of 81–90%, a specificity of 74–96%, and an accuracy of 92% [121].

Scintimammography seems therefore to be a clinically valuable tool for guiding chemotherapy. It may be even advantageous compared to conventional mammography due to a higher sensitivity especially if FDG-PET imaging is not available.

6.3.5 Recent Studies Evaluating ⁹⁹ᵐTc-Sestamibi Breast Scintigraphy in Various Settings

Most of the studies evaluating the diagnostic impact of ⁹⁹ᵐTc-sestamibi in breast cancer disease have been published between 1995 and 2005. After that time, with numerous published studies, the efforts in evaluating ⁹⁹ᵐTc-scintimammography declined to some degree. However, over the past 5 years, several published studies indicate that there is still an interest in investigating and improving as well as in identifying new or broader indications for this noninvasive diagnostic tool. This is not only for primary diagnosis of breast cancer with ⁹⁹ᵐTc-sestamibi but also for the evaluation of the axillary lymph node status of patients with breast cancer disease as well as for identification of patients with recurrence of disease. Most of the recently published studies compared the diagnostic value of ⁹⁹ᵐTc-sestamibi scintigraphy with those of other diagnostic measures in the named settings.

In a retrospective study published in 2008 by Brem et al, of 146 women who underwent ⁹⁹ᵐTc-sestamibi breast scintigraphy and breast biography, scintimammography helped to detect cancer in 80 of 83 malignant lesions yielding a sensitivity of 96.4%. Fifty out of eighty-four nonmalignant lesions were correctly identified as negative for cancer with a specificity of 59.5% [9]. The positive predictive value was 68.8%, the negative predictive value 94.3%. Notably, the smallest invasive cancer and ductal carcinoma in situ were both 1 mm. Scintimammography helped to detect occult cancer not visualized by mammography or ultrasonography in six patients [9]. Gupta et al. compared the diagnostic accuracy of ⁹⁹ᵐTc-sestamibi with those of the combined use of mammography and ultrasound in the detection of breast lesions. Histopathology was the gold standard. Sensitivity, specificity, positive predictive value, negative predictive value, and diagnostic accuracy of scintimammography were found to be 92%, 72%, 58%, 96%, and 78% respectively and 89%, 94%, 86%, 95%, and 92% for the combined use of mammography and ultrasound. Based on these results, breast scintigraphy with ⁹⁹ᵐTc-sestamibi showed a slightly better sensitivity whereas specificity was clearly higher in combined mammography and ultrasound [171]. Similar results with regard to the sensitivity (93.3%) and the specificity (71.4%) of scintimammography were reported by Habib et al. in 2009 in 22 patients presenting with breast lesions [172]. Ozülker et al. compared the diagnostic efficacy of ⁹⁹ᵐTc-sestamibi with mammography, ultrasonography, and MRI. They found a sensitivity of 93%, 68%, 81%, and 81%, respectively for the above named imaging modalities. The specificities were 86%, 87%, 63%, and 73%, respectively [173]. Interestingly, Usmani et al. found slightly contrary results in a study published 2008. In a total of 36 patients with breast lesions with histopathological evaluation they found a sensitivity of 86% and a slightly higher specificity of 88% [174]. Their results might be influenced by six patients with nonpalpable breast lesions as Gommans et al. also observed a higher specificity (92.8%, sensitivity 82.2%) of ⁹⁹ᵐTc-sestamibi as compared to histopathology, clinical, and radiological follow-up in 101 patients with nonpalpable breast lesions [175]. They concluded that ⁹⁹ᵐTc-sestamibi scintimammography could be of incremental value in the workup of patients with nonpalpable breast lesions [175]. In some patients with nonpalpable breast cancer, microcalcifications might be the only indication of tumor presence. Although mammography has high sensitivity in detecting these microcalcifications, its specificity is too low for diagnostic purposes. Grosso et al. investigated the impact of ^{99m}Tc-sestamibi breast scintigraphy on the differential diagnosis between benign and malignant clusters of microcalcifications as compared to mammography [176]. Including a total of 283 patients with microcalcifications identified by mammography, they found a better diagnostic value of combined mammography and ^{99m}Tc-sestamibi scintimammography as revealed by receiver operating characteristics (ROC; 0.86) compared to mammography alone (ROC 0.72). Furthermore, the combination of mammography and scintimammography provided a significant improvement of the negative predictive value (98%) for microcalcifications with low suspicion of malignancy revealed by mammography [176].

Accurately diagnosing the axillary lymph node status in breast cancer patients still remains a challenge. In a prospective study published in 2006, Lumachi et al. compared the diagnostic values of ultrasonographi and scintigraphicy assessment of the axillary lymph node status in a series of 77 consecutive women [177]. The results of the imaging studies were compared against pathology. The sensitivity, specificity, and accuracy were 67.6%, 80.0%, and 74.0% for ultrasound, 78.4%, 85.0%, and 81.8% for ^{99m}Tc-scintigraphy, and 91.9%, 92.5%, and 92.2% for combined ultrasound and scintigraphy, respectively. They found a significant difference ($p < 0.05$) in the number of metastasized axillary lymph nodes between patients with metastases correctly detected and undetected by both ultrasound and scintigraphy [177]. It seems to be therefore obvious that, even though the result of each diagnostic test is strictly dependent on the number of the metastasized axillary lymph nodes, combined ultrasound and scintigraphy depict a sensitive low-costs procedure in the assessment of the axillary lymph node status of breast cancer patients [177]. One year later, a study including 159 women with confirmed breast cancer undergoing curative surgery and preoperative ^{99m}Tc-sestamibi scintimammography for the assessment of the axillary lymph node status was published by the same group [178]. Again, results of the imaging procedure were compared against the final histopathology of the axillary nodes. The reported sensitivity, specificity, positive predictive value, negative predictive value, and accuracy of scintimammography in detecting axillary lymph node metastases were 81.4%, 91.0%, 84.2%, 91.0%, and 87.4%, respectively. Confirming their results from the previous study, they found a higher sensitivity in patients with three or more positive lymph nodes (96.4%) while in patients with two or one positive nodes, the sensitivity decreased to 80% and 28.6%, respectively [178]. Whereas they judged scintimammography to be potentially useful in patients undergoing surgery for breast cancer disease in case a preoperative assessment of the axillary lymph node status is required, they also see the need to use another imaging technique in conjunction with the scintigraphically assessment because of its low sensitivity in detecting lymph node metastases when the number of involved nodes is two or less [178].

In 2007, Rajkovaca et al. published their results on the diagnostic accuracy of ^{99m}Tc-scintimammography in detection of suspected recurrent breast cancer in the breast or locoregional tissues [179]. They included 19 patients with recurrent tumors (15 with locoregional recurrence and 4 in the contralateral breast). Mammography identified 13 of these cancers whereas scintimammography was able to detect 17 of recurrent breast cancers. Scintimammography showed higher sensitivity, specificity, and accuracy per patient as compared to mammography (90.9% vs 63.6%, 71.4% vs 57.1%, and 83.3% vs 61.1%, respectively) and seems therefore more reliable in identifying recurrent breast cancer disease [179]. Between 2007 and 2010, the group of Usmani et al. published four studies on the diagnostic impact of ^{99m}Tc-sestamibi breast scintigraphy in the evaluation of recurrence of breast cancer [180–183]. First, they evaluated the role of scintimammography and mammography in the diagnosis of locoregional recurrence of breast cancer and observed a sensitivity, specificity, positive predictive value, negative predictive value, and diagnostic accuracy of 87.5%, 91.7%, 94.7%, 78.6%, and 87.8%, respectively [180]. In general, diagnostic performance of mammography was lower compared to ^{99m}Tc-sestamibi scintigraphy (sensitivity 52.9%, specificity 66.7%, positive predictive value 75.0%, negative predictive value 42.9%, and accuracy 57.7%) [180]. In the same year, they also published their results on chest wall recurrence of breast cancer as demonstrated on ^{99m}Tc-sestamibi scintimammography [181]. They included 26 patients with suspected chest wall recurrence of breast cancer as revealed by clinical evaluation. All patients underwent planar and SPECT scintimammography as well as excision biopsy or fine needle aspiration cytology for tissue diagnosis. The sensitivity, specificity, positive predictive value, negative predictive value, and accuracy were 78%, 87.5%, 93%, 64%, and 81% for planar imaging. SPECT showed a significantly higher overall sensitivity than planar imaging (89% vs 78%, $p < 0.001$) but showed the same specificity (87.5%). SPECT however showed a significantly higher negative predictive value and diagnostic accuracy (78% vs 64% and 88% vs 81%, respectively; $p < 0.05$) [181]. They concluded that scintimammography is a reliable diagnostic tool in detecting chest wall recurrence and that SPECT aids in the diagnosis of the chest wall recurrence with greater confidence. One year later, they evaluated the diagnostic impact of ^{99m}Tc-sestamibi breast scintigraphy for identifying residual or multifocal disease in patients with breast cancer after excision biopsy. This is of interest, since evaluation of a postinterventional breast may be complex and difficult because masses, calcifications, and structural changes due to the intervention might mimic residual or additional masses. In 21 included patients, the sensitivity, specificity, positive predictive values, negative predictive value, and accuracy were 92.6%, 85.7%, 92.6%, 85.7%, and 90.5%, respectively [182]. Despite the rather small study population, scintimammography seems therefore to be of value in assessing residual or multifocal breast cancer disease in patients after excision biopsy. The most recent publication by the group of Usmani et al. was published in 2010 [183]. Including 41 consecutive postmastectomy patients with clinical suspicion of breast cancer recurrence, they evaluated the diagnostic performance of scintimammography and ultrasound for further assessment of suspected local recurrence. Compared against histology, ultrasound alone revealed a sensitivity of 86%, a specificity of 77%, a positive predictive value of 89%, a negative predictive value of 71%, and a diagnostic accuracy of 83%. All of these diagnostic parameters were found to be higher for ^{99m}Tc-scintimammography (89%, 92%, 96%, 80%, and 80%, respectively). By using a combination of both imaging modalities, the sensitivity and the negative predictive value improved to 100%, whereas the specificity declined to 77% compared to the single imaging approach using scintimammography [183]. It is mainly due to the high negative predictive value that the combined application of ultrasound and breast scintigraphy might be useful to exclude recurrence of disease in patients with a low initial index of suspicion and/or inconclusive histological evaluation.

Investigating the incremental diagnostic value of quantified indices of double phase ^{99m}Tc-sestamibi breast scintigraphy additive to magnetic resonance imaging, Kim et al. imaged 239 patients with highly suspected breast 10 min and 3 h after injection of the radiotracer [184]. Double phase scintimammography was analyzed by visual and quantitative methods. Sensitivity and specificity of visual analysis of scintimammography were 86.4% and 100%, respectively, and 96.1% and 58.8%, respectively, for contrast-enhanced MRI. The optimal lesion to nonlesion ratios (L/N) were 1.84 for early and 1.04 for delayed image acquisition [183]. Using early L/N of 1.84 as cutoff, they found a sensitivity and specificity of ^{99m}Tc-scintimammography of 67.8% and 97.1%, respectively, and 88.3% and 55.9%, respectively, when using the delayed L/N of 1.04. Among various variables of double phase scintimammography and MRI, early L/N was the potent predictor for breast cancer. Based on their results, early phase breast scintigraphy and MRI showed similar diagnostic accuracy for breast cancer and early L/N was shown to be a potent predictor for breast cancer [184]. In 2009, applying the double phase approach of ^{99m}Tc-sestamibi scintimammography, Zaman et al. determined its role in predicting chemotherapeutic response in breast cancer [185]. Despite the fact that this is not a new approach and was already applied by others more than 10 years before, this study not only confirms the value of double phase scintimammography in assessing the response to chemotherapy but also adds new insights to this interesting topic as Zaman et al. included patients on anthracycline-based neoadjuvant chemotherapy [36, 185]. MIBI washout was scored >30% as a positive prognostic test (predicting a poor response to chemotherapy) and <30% as negative prognostic test (accordingly, predicting a good response). The criterion for good and bad responses was a reduction of tumor burden >50% or <50%, respectively. By applying this approach to 32 included patients, they found a sensitivity of 72%, a specificity of 90%, a positive predictive value of 80%, and a negative predictive value of 86.5%. Receiver operating curve (ROC) analysis demonstrated 30% as a cutoff for the washout in quantitative dual phase ^{99m}Tc-sestamibi scintigraphy for the prediction of the chemotherapeutic response [185]. Based on their data, they concluded scintimammography to be a reliable and effective diagnostic approach for predicting the response to neoadjuvant chemotherapy.

Two studies on the impact of hybrid imaging in the evaluation of breast cancer disease have been published in 2007 [186, 187]. This is of importance since, as already mentioned above, scintimammography has drawbacks in identifying lesions less than 1 cm mainly because of its limited spatial resolution. By fusing functional information provided by ^{99m}Tc-sestamibi imaging to anatomical information by CT or MRI, this limitation might be overcome. Interestingly, despite the fact that fused imaging with hybrid SPECT/CT devices becomes more and more popular over the past years, up to now, Schillaci et al. published the only data on using SPECT/CT in breast cancer disease [186]. In 53 patients with mammographically suspicious lesions, they found planar ^{99m}Tc-sestamibi scintimammography to be associated with an overall sensitivity of 73% when compared to histopathological diagnosis. Overall sensitivity increased to 89.2% by using SPECT/CT acquisition [186]. This discrepancy was even higher when narrowing the analysis to only lesions ≤ 10 mm (sensitivity planar: 42.9% vs SPECT/CT: 71.4%). However, in lesions >10 mm, the gap between planar- and SPECT/CT imaging became at least more wide as the observed sensitivity was 91.3% (planar) and 100% (SPECT/CT), respectively. Therefore, hybrid imaging with SPECT/CT was able to more sensitively detect breast cancer compared to planar imaging, mainly in small cancers. Also combining functional and morphological imaging data, Duarte et al. used a software-based approach to fuse ^{99m}TC-sestamibi scintimammography and MRI [187]. In their pilot study they included 20 consecutive breast cancer patients prior to mastectomy. All of them underwent scintimammography and contrast-enhanced MRI 2–10 days before surgery. To evaluate the accuracy of software-fused scintimammography/MRI in estimating the size of breast cancer, it was compared to MRI alone, mammography, and clinical examination, employing pathologic sizing as gold standard. Tumor size was evaluated in three diameters and correlated with pathological measurements. The scintimammography/MRI cancer measurements correlated better with pathology than MRI, mammography, and clinical exam in all diameters analyzed and appeared therefore to be more accurate than other examinations to measure breast cancer size [187].

References

1. WHO/IARC: World Cancer Report (2003) Lyon
2. Ärzte-Zeitung 1. Sept 2008 Brustkrebs bei Frauen häufigste Todesursache
3. Todesursachen (2009) Statistisches Bundesamt Wiesbaden. http://www.destatis.de/jetspeed/portal/cms/Sites/destatis/Internet/DE/Content/Statistiken/Gesundheit/Todesursachen/Tabellen/Content75/SterbefaelleInsgesamt,templateId=renderPrint.psml
4. Sobin LH, Gospodarowicz MK, Wittekind C (2009) TNM classification of malignant tumours, 7th edition (UICC International Union Against Cancer). Wiley, Oxford/NJ
5. Silverstein MJ, Recht A, Lagios MD, Bleiweiss IJ, Blumencranz PW, Gizienski T, Harms SE, Harness J, Jackman RJ, Klimberg VS, Kuske R, Levine GM, Linver MN, Rafferty EA, Rugo H, Schilling K, Tripathy D, Vicini FA, Whitworth PW, Willey SC (2009) Special report: consensus conference III. Image-detected breast cancer: state-of-the-art diagnosis and treatment. J Am Coll Surg 209:504–520
6. Albert US, Altland H, Duda V, Engel J, Geraedts M, Heywang-Köbrunner S, Hölzel D, Kalbheim E, Koller M, König K, Kreienberg R, Kühn T, Lebeau A, Nass-Griegoleit I, Schlake W, Schmutzler R, Schreer I, Schulte H, Schulz-Wentland R, Wagner U, Kopp I (2009) 2008 update of the guideline: early detection of breast cancer in Germany. J Cancer Res Clin Oncol 135:339–354

7. Perry N, Broeders M, de Wolf C, Törnberg S, Holland R, von Karsa L (2008) European guidelines for quality assurance in breast cancer screening and diagnosis. Fourth edition–summary document. Ann Oncol 19:614–622
8. Aktolun C, Bayhan H, Kir M (1992) Clinical experience with Tc-99m MIBI imaging in patients with malignant tumors: preliminary results and comparison with Tl-201. Clin Nucl Med 17:171–176
9. Brem RF, Floerke AC, Rapelyea JA, Teal C, Kelly T, Mathur V (2008) Breast-specific gamma imaging as an adjunct imaging modality for the diagnosis of breast cancer. Radiology 247:651–657, Erratum in: Radiology 2009; 251: 308
10. Khalkhali I, Mena I, Jouanne E, Diggles L, Venegas R, Block J, Alle K, Klein S (1994) Prone scintimammography in patients with suspicion of carcinoma of the breast. J Am Coll Surg 178:491–497
11. Taillefer R (2005) Clinical applications of 99mTc-sestamibi scintimammography. Semin Nucl Med 35:100–115
12. EANM Breast scintigraphy procedure guideline for tumour imaging (2003) https://www.eanm.org/scientific_info/guidelines/guidelines_intro.php?navId=54
13. Hussain R, Buscombe JR (2006) A meta-analysis of scintimammography: an evidence-based approach to its clinical utility. Nucl Med Commun 27:589–594
14. Khalkhali I, Diggles LE, Taillefer R, Vandestreek PR, Peller PJ, Abdel-Nabi HH (1999) Procedure guideline for breast scintigraphy. Society of Nuclear Medicine. J Nucl Med 40:1233–1235
15. Chiu ML, Kronange JF, Piwnica-Worms D (1990) Effect of mitochondrial and plasma membrane potentials on accumulation of hexakis (2 methoxyisobutyl isonitrile) technetium in cultured mouse fibroblasts. J Nucl Med 31:1646–1653
16. Delmon-Moingeon LI, Piwnica-Worms D, Van den Abbeele AD, Holman BL, Davison A, Jones AG (1990) Uptake of the cation hexakis (2-methoxy isobutylisonitrile)-technetium-99m by human carcinoma cell lines in vitro. Cancer Res 50:2198–2202
17. Piwnica-Worms D, Chiu ML, Budding M, Kronauge JF, Kramer RA, Croop JM (1993) Functional imaging of multidrug resistant P-glycoprotein with an organotechnetium complex. Cancer Res 53:977–984
18. Cordobes MD, Starzec A, Delmon-Moingeon L, Blanchot C, Kouyoumdjian JC, Prévost G, Caglar M, Moretti JL (1996) Technetium-99m-sestamibi uptake by human benign and malignant breast tumor cells: correlation with mdr gene expression. J Nucl Med 37:286–289
19. Moretti JL, Azaloux H, Boisseron D, Kouyoumdjian JC, Vilcoq J (1996) Primary breast cancer imaging with technetium-99m sestamibi and its relation with P-glycoprotein overexpression. Eur J Nucl Med 23:980–986
20. Papantoniou V, Christodoulidou J, Papadaki E, Valotassiou V, Souvatzoglou M, Louvrou A, Feida H, Sotiropoulou M, Pampouras G, Michalas S, Zerva C (2002) Uptake and washout of 99mTcV-dimercaptosuccinic acid and 99mTc-sestamibi in the assessment of histological type and grade in breast cancer. Nucl Med Commun 23:461–467
21. Smith RA, Cokkinides V, Brooks D, Saslow D, Brawley OW (2010) Cancer screening in the United States, 2010: a review of current American Cancer Society guidelines and issues in cancer screening. CA Cancer J Clin 60:99–119
22. Lee CH, Dershaw DD, Kopans D, Evans P, Monsees B, Monticciolo D, Brenner RJ, Bassett L, Berg W, Feig S, Hendrick E, Mendelson E, D'Orsi C, Sickles E, Burhenne LW (2010) Breast cancer screening with imaging: recommendations from the Society of Breast Imaging and the ACR on the use of mammography, breast MRI, breast ultrasound, and other technologies for the detection of clinically occult breast cancer. J Am Coll Radiol 7:18–27
23. Goldsmith SJ, Parsons W, Guiberteau MJ, Stern LH, Lanzkowsky L, Weigert J, Heston TF, Jones E, Buscombe J, Stabin MG, Society of Nuclear Medicine (2010) SNM practice guideline for breast scintigraphy with breast-specific gamma-cameras 1.0. J Nucl Med Technol 38:219–224
24. Institute for Clinical Systems Improvement (ICSI) (2010) Diagnosis of breast disease. Institute for Clinical Systems Improvement, Bloomington, MN, pp 1–47
25. Zhou M, Johnson N, Gruner S, Ecklund GW, Meunier P, Bryn S, Glissmeyer M, Steinbock K (2009) The clinical utility of breast specific gamma imaging for evaluating disease extent in the newly diagnosed breast cancer patient. Am J Surg 197:159–163

26. Killelea BK, Gillego A, Kirstein LJ, Asad J, Shpilko M, Shah A, Feldman S, Boolbol SK (2009) George Peters Award: How does breast-specific gamma imaging affect the management of patients with newly diagnosed breast cancer? Am J Surg 198:470–474
27. Liberman M, Sampalis F, Mulder D, Sampalis J (2003) Breast cancer diagnosis by scintimammography: a meta-analysis and review of the literature. Breast Cancer Res Treat 80: 115–126
28. Brem RF, Rapelyea JA, Zisman G, Mohtashemi K, Raub J, Teal CB, Majewski S, Welch BL (2005) Occult breast cancer: scintimammography with high-resolution breast-specific gamma camera in women at high risk for breast cancer. Radiology 237:274–280
29. Schillaci O, Buscombe JR (2004) Breast scintigraphy today: indications and limitations. Eur J Nucl Med Mol Imaging 31(Suppl):S35–S45
30. (2007) Scintimammography as an adjunctive breast imaging technology: an evidence based analysis. Ontario Health Technol Assess Ser 7:1–46
31. Rhodes DJ, O'Connor MK, Phillips SW, Smith RL, Collins DA (2005) Molecular breast imaging: a new technique using technetium Tc99m scintimammography to detect small tumors of the breast. Mayo Clin Proc 80:24–30
32. Brem RF, Fishman M, Rapelyea J (2007) Detection of ductal carcinoma in situ with mammography, breast specific gamma imaging, and magnetic resonance imaging: a comparative study. Acad Radiol 14:945–950
33. Brem RF, Petrovitch I, Rapelyea JA, Young H, Teal C, Kelly T (2007) Breast-specific gamma imaging with 99m Tc-sestamibi and magnetic resonance imaging in the diagnosis of breast cancer: a comparative study. Breast J 13:465–469
34. Tiling R, Khalkhali I, Sommer H, Moser R, Meyer G, Willemsen F, Pfluger T, Tatsch K, Hahn K (1997) Role of technetium-99m sestamibi scintimammography and contrast-enhanced magnetic resonance imaging for the evaluation of indeterminate mammograms. Eur J Nucl Med 24:1221–1229
35. Dunnwald LK, Gralow JR, Ellis GK, Livingston RB, Linden HM, Lawton TJ, Barlow WE, Schubert EK, Mankoff DA (2005) Residual tumor uptake of [99mTc]-sestamibi after neoadjuvant chemotherapy for locally advanced breast carcinoma predicts survival. Cancer 103:680–688
36. Alonso O, Delgado L, Núñez M, Vargas C, Lopera J, Andruskevicius P, Sabini G, Gaudiano J, Musé IM, Roca R (2002) Predictive value of 99mTc sestamibi scintigraphy in the evaluation of doxorubicin based chemotherapy response in patients with advanced breast cancer. Nucl Med Commun 23:765–771
37. Mezi S, Primi F, Capoccetti F, Scopinaro F, Modesti M, Schillaci O (2003) In vivo detection of resistance to anthracycline based neoadjuvant chemotherapy in locally advanced and inflammatory breast cancer with technetium-99m sestamibi scintimammography. Int J Oncol 22:1233–1240
38. Alonso O, Massardo T, Delgado LB, Horvath J, Kabasakal L, Llamas-Olier A, Maunda KK, Morales R, Padhy AK, Shankar UR (2001) Is 99mTc-sestamibi scintimammography complementary to conventional mammography for detecting breast cancer in patients with palpable masses? J Nucl Med 42:1614–1621
39. Clifford EJ, Lugo-Zamudio C (1996) Scintimammography in the diagnosis of breast cancer. Am J Surg 172:483–486
40. Cutrone JA, Khalkhali I, Yospur LS, Diggles L, Weinberg I, Pong EM, Tolmos J, Vargas MP, Vargas HI (1999) Tc99m sestamibi scintimammography for the evaluation of breast masses in patients with radiographically dense breasts. Breast J 5:383–388
41. Khalkhali I, Cutrone J, Mena I, Diggles L, Venegas R, Vargas H, Jackson B, Klein S (1995) Technetium-99m-sestamibi scintimammography of breast lesions: clinical and pathological follow-up. J Nucl Med 36:1784–1789
42. Khalkhali I, Baum JK, Villanueva-Meyer J, Edell SL, Hanelin LG, Lugo CE, Taillefer R, Freeman LM, Neal CE, Scheff AM, Connolly JL, Schnitt SJ, Houlihan MJ, Sampalis JS, Haber SB (2002) (99m)Tc sestamibi breast imaging for the examination of patients with dense and fatty breasts: multicenter study. Radiology 222:149–155

43. Sampalis FS, Denis R, Picard D, Fleiszer D, Martin G, Nassif E, Sampalis JS (2003) International prospective evaluation of scintimammography with [99m]Technetium sestamibi. Am J Surg 185:544–549
44. Taillefer R, Robidoux A, Lambert R, Turpin S, Laperrière J (1995) Technetium-99m-sestamibi prone scintimammography to detect primary breast cancer and axillary lymph node involvement. J Nucl Med 36:1758–1765
45. Tolmos J, Cutrone JA, Wang B, Vargas HI, Stuntz M, Mishkin FS, Diggles LE, Venegas RJ, Klein SR, Khalkhali I (1998) Scintimammography analysis of nonpalpable breast lesions previously identified by conventional mammography. J Natl Cancer Inst 90:846–849
46. Villanueva-Meyer J, Leonard MH Jr, Briscoe E, Cesani F, Ali SA, Rhoden S, Hove M, Cowan D (1996) Mammoscintigraphy with technetium-99m-sestamibi in suspected breast cancer. J Nucl Med 37:926–930
47. Arslan N, Oztürk E, Ilgan S, Urhan M, Karaçalioglu O, Pekcan M, Tufan T, Bayhan H (1999) 99Tcm-MIBI scintimammography in the evaluation of breast lesions and axillary involvement: a comparison with mammography and histopathological diagnosis. Nucl Med Commun 20:317–325
48. Becherer A, Helbich T, Staudenherz A, Jakesz R, Kubista E, Lehner R, Rudas M, Teleky B, Kletter K, Leitha T (1997) The diagnostic value of planar and SPET scintimammography in different age groups. Nucl Med Commun 18:710–718
49. Buscombe JR, Cwikla JB, Thakrar DS, Parbhoo SP, Hilson AJ (1999) Prone SPET scintimammography. Nucl Med Commun 20:237–245
50. Buscombe JR, Cwikla JB, Holloway B, Hilson AJ (2001) Prediction of the usefulness of combined mammography and scintimammography in suspected primary breast cancer using ROC curves. J Nucl Med 42:3–8
51. Cwikla JB, Buscombe JR, Parbhoo SP, Kelleher SM, Thakrar DS, Hinton J, Crow J, Deery A, Hilson AJ (1998) Use of [99]Tc[m]-MIBI in the assessment of patients with suspected recurrent breast cancer. Nucl Med Commun 19:649–655
52. Cwikla JB, Buscombe JR, Kolasinska AD, Parbhoo SP, Thakrar DS, Hilson AJ (1999) Correlation between uptake of Tc-99m sestaMIBI and prognostic factors of breast cancer. Anticancer Res 19:2299–2304
53. Cwikla JB, Buscombe JR, Holloway B, Parbhoo SP, Davidson T, McDermott N, Hilson AJ (2001) Can scintimammography with 99mTc-MIBI identify multifocal and multicentric primary breast cancer? Nucl Med Commun 22:1287–1293
54. Fondrinier E, Muratet JP, Anglade E, Fauvet R, Berger V, Lorimier G, Jallet P (2004) Clinical experience of ^{99m}Tc-MIBI scintimammography in patients with breast microcalcifications. Breast 13:316–320
55. Helbich TH, Becherer A, Trattnig S, Leitha T, Kelkar P, Seifert M, Gnant M, Staudenherz A, Rudas M, Wolf G, Mostbeck GH (1997) Differentiation of benign and malignant breast lesions: MR imaging versus Tc-99m sestamibi scintimammography. Radiology 202:421–429
56. Imbriaco M, Del Vecchio S, Riccardi A, Pace L, Di Salle F, Di Gennaro F, Salvatore M, Sodano A (2001) Scintimammography with ^{99m}Tc-MIBI versus dynamic MRI for non-invasive characterization of breast masses. Eur J Nucl Med 28:56–63
57. Maffioli L, Agresti R, Chiti A, Crippa F, Gasparini M, Greco M, Bombardieri E (1996) Prone scintimammography in patients with non-palpable breast lesions. Anticancer Res 16:1269–1273
58. Marshall C, Eremin J, El-Sheemy M, Eremin O, Griffiths PA (2005) Monitoring the response of large (> 3 cm) and locally advanced (T3-4, N0-2) breast cancer to neoadjuvant chemotherapy using 99mTc-Sestamibi uptake. Nucl Med Commun 26:9–15
59. Mathieu I, Mazy S, Willemart B, Destine M, Mazy G, Lonneux M (2005) Inconclusive triple diagnosis in breast cancer imaging: Is there a place for scintimammography? J Nucl Med 46:1574–1581
60. Maublant J, de Latour M, Mestas D, Clemenson A, Charrier S, Feillel V, Le Bouedec G, Kaufmann P, Dauplat J, Veyre A (1996) Technetium-99m-sestamibi uptake in breast tumor and associated lymph nodes. J Nucl Med 37:922–925

61. Myslivecek M, Koranda P, Kamínek M, Husák V, Hartlová M, Dusková M, Cwiertka K (2004) Technetium-99m-MIBI scintimammography by planar and SPECT imaging in the diagnosis of breast carcinoma and axillary lymph node involvement. Nucl Med Rev Cent East Eur 7:151–155
62. Palmedo H, Schomburg A, Grünwald F, Mallmann P, Krebs D, Biersack HJ (1996) Technetium-99m-MIBI scintimammography for suspicious breast lesions. J Nucl Med 37:626–630
63. Palmedo H, Grünwald F, Bender H, Schomburg A, Mallmann P, Krebs D, Biersack HJ (1996) Scintimammography with technetium-99m methoxyisobutylisonitrile: comparison with mammography and magnetic resonance imaging. Eur J Nucl Med 23:940–946
64. Papantoniou V, Tsiouris S, Koutsikos J, Sotiropoulou M, Mainta E, Lazaris D, Valsamaki P, Melissinou M, Zerva C, Antsaklis A (2006) Scintimammographic detection of usual ductal breast hyperplasia with increased proliferation rate at risk for malignancy. Nucl Med Commun 27:911–917
65. Prats E, Aisa F, Abós MD, Villavieja L, García-López F, Asenjo MJ, Razola P, Banzo J (1999) Mammography and ^{99m}Tc-MIBI scintimammography in suspected breast cancer. J Nucl Med 40:296–301
66. Prats E, Banzo J, Meroño E, Herranz R, Carril JM, SMCSTMS (2001) ^{99m}Tc-MIBI scintimammography as a complement of the mammography in patients with suspected breast cancer. A multicentre experience. Breast 10:109–116
67. Sanidas EE, Koukouraki S, Velidaki A, Manios A, Stathopoulos E, De Bree E, Kafousi M, Kodogiannis E, Karkavitsas N, Tsiftsis DD (2003) Contribution of 99mTc-anti-carcinoembryonic antigen antibody and 99mTc-sestamibi scintimammography in the evaluation of high risk palpable breast lesions. Nucl Med Commun 24:291–296
68. Tiling R, Khalkhali I, Sommer H, Linke R, Moser R, Willemsen F, Pfluger T, Tatsch K, Hahn K (1998) Limited value of scintimammography and contrast-enhanced MRI in the evaluation of microcalcification detected by mammography. Nucl Med Commun 19:55–62
69. Tiling R, Kessler M, Untch M, Sommer H, Linke R, Hahn K (2005) Initial evaluation of breast cancer using Tc-99m sestamibi scintimammography. Eur J Radiol 53:206–212
70. Uriarte I, Carril JM, Quirce R, Gutiérrez-Mendiguchía C, Blanco I, Banzo I, Vega A, Hernández A (1998) Optimization of X-ray mammography and technetium-99m methoxyisobutylisonitrile scintimammography in the diagnosis of non-palpable breast lesions. Eur J Nucl Med 25: 491–496
71. Chen SL, Yin YQ, Chen JX, Sun XG, Xiu Y, Liu WG, Liu M, Zhu WM, Zhang YB (1997) The usefulness of technetium-99m-MIBI scintimammography in diagnosis of breast cancer: using surgical histopathological diagnosis as the gold standard. Anticancer Res 17:1695–1698
72. Kao CH, Wang SJ, Liu TJ (1994) The use of technetium-99m methoxyisobutylisonitrile breast scintigraphy to evaluate palpable breast masses. Eur J Nucl Med 21:432–436
73. Kim SJ, Kim IJ, Bae YT, Kim YK, Kim DS (2004) Incremental diagnostic value of quantitative analysis of double phase Tc-99m MIBI scintimammography for the detection of primary breast cancer additive to visual analysis. Breast Cancer Res Treat 83:129–138
74. Kim SJ, Kim IJ, Bae YT, Kim YK, Kim DS (2005) Comparison of early and delayed quantified indices of double-phase ^{99m}Tc MIBI scintimammography in the detection of primary breast cancer. Acta Radiol 46:148–154
75. Kim SJ, Kim IJ, Bae YT, Kim YK, Kim DS (2005) Comparison of quantitative and visual analysis of Tc-99m MIBI scintimammography for detection of primary breast cancer. Eur J Radiol 53:192–198
76. Mekhmandarov S, Sandbank J, Cohen M, Lelcuk S, Lubin E (1998) Techentium-99m-MIBI scintimammography in palpable and non-palpable breast lesions. J Nucl Med 39:86–91
77. Melloul M, Paz A, Ohana G, Laver O, Michalevich D, Koren R, Wolloch Y, Gal R (1999) Double-phase ^{99m}Tc-sestamibi scintimammography and trans-scan in diagnosing breast cancer. J Nucl Med 40:376–380
78. Massardo T, Alonso O, Kabasakal L, Llamas-Olier A, Shankar UR, Zhu H, Delgado L, González P, Mut F, Padhy AK (2002) Diagnostic value of 99mTc-methylene diphosphonate

and 99mTc-pentavalent DMSA compared with 99mTc-sestamibi for palpable breast lesions. J Nucl Med 43:882–888

79. Massardo T, Alonso O, Llamas-Ollier A, Kabasakal L, Ravishankar U, Morales R, Delgado L, Padhy AK (2005) Planar Tc99m-sestamibi scintimammography should be considered cautiously in the axillary evaluation of breast cancer protocols: results of an international multicenter trial. BMC Nucl Med 5:4

80. Howarth D, Sillar R, Clark D, Lan L (1999) Technetium-99m sestamibi scintimammography: the influence of histopathological characteristics, lesion size and the presence of carcinoma in situ in the detection of breast carcinoma. Eur J Nucl Med 26:1475–1481

81. Noßke D, Minkov V, Brix G (2004) Establishment and application of diagnostic reference levels for nuclear medicine procedures in Germany. Nuklearmedizin 43:79–84

82. Lu G, Shih WJ, Huang HY, Long MQ, Sun Q, Liu YH, Chou C (1995) 99mTc-MIBI mammoscintigraphy of breast masses: early and delayed imaging. Nucl Med Commun 16: 150–156

83. Waxman AD (1997) The role of 99mTc methoxyisobutylisonitrile in imaging breast cancer. Semin Nucl Med 27:40–54

84. Buscombe JR, Cwikla JB, Thakrar DS, Hilson AJ (1999) Scintimammography: a review. Nucl Med Rev Cent East Eur 2:36–41

85. Kopans DB (1992) The positive predictive value of mammography. AJR Am J Roentgenol 26:521–526

86. Cwikla JB, Buscombe JR, Kelleher SM, Parbhoo SP, Thakrar DS, Hinton J, Deery AR, Crow J, Hilson AJ (1998) Comparison of accuracy of scintimammography and X-ray mammography in the diagnosis of primary breast cancer in patients selected for surgical biopsy. Clin Radiol 53:274–280

87. Ambrus E, Rajtár M, Ormándi K, Séra T, Tószegi A, Láng J, Pávics L, Csernay L (1997) Value of 99m-Tc MIBI and 99m-Tc(V) DMAS scintigraphy in evaluation of breast mass lesions. Anticancer Res 17:1599–1605

88. Burak Z, Argon M, Memiş A, Erdem S, Balkan Z, Duman Y, Ustün EE, Erhan Y, Ozkiliç H (1994) Evaluation of palpable breast masses with 99Tcm-MIBI: a comparative study with mammography and ultrasonography. Nucl Med Commun 15:604–612

89. Carril JM, Gómez-Barquín R, Quirce R, Tabuenca O, Uriarte I, Montero A (1997) Contribution of 99mTc-MIBI scintimammography to the diagnosis of non-palpable breast lesions in relation to mammographic probability of malignancy. Anticancer Res 17:1677–1681

90. Cwikła JB, Buscombe JR, Chaberek S, Holloway B, Parbhoo S, Hilson AJ (2000) Diagnostic accuracy of mammography and scintimammography in detection of primary breast cancer related size of the tumour. Nucl Med Rev Cent East Eur 3:127–132

91. Danielsson R, Boné B, Gad A, Sylvan M, Aspelin P (1999) Sensitivity and specificity of planar scintimammography with 99mTc-sestamibi. Acta Radiol 40:394–399

92. De Vincentis G, Scopinaro F, Pani R, Pellegrini R, Soluri A, Ierardi M, Ballesio L, Weinberg IN, Pergola A (1997) 99mTc MIBI scintimammography with a high resolution single tube gamma camera: preliminary study. Anticancer Res 17:1627–1630

93. De Vincentis G, Gianni W, Pani R, Cacciafesta M, Pellegrini R, Soluri A, Troisi G, Marigliano V, Scopinaro F (1998) Role of 99mTc-sestamibi scintimammography by SPEM camera in the management of breast cancer in the elderly. Breast Cancer Res Treat 48:159–163

94. Flanagan DA, Gladding SB, Lovell FR (1998) Can scintimammography reduce "unnecessary" biopsies? Am Surg 64:670–673

95. Khalkhali I, Iraniha S, Cutrone JA, Diggles LE, Klein SR (1997) Scintimammography with Tc-99m sestamibi. Acta Med Austriaca 24:46–49

96. Lam WW, Yang WT, Chan YL, Stewart IE, King W, Metreweli C (1996) Role of MIBI breast scintigraphy in evaluation of palpable breast lesions. Br J Radiol 69:1152–1158

97. Mirzaei S, Zajicek SM, Knoll P, Lipp C, Lipp RW, Salzer H, Umek H, Kohn H (2000) Scintimammography enhances negative predictive value of non-invasive pre-operative assessment of breast lesions. Eur J Surg Oncol 26:738–741

6 ^{99m}Tc-Sestamibi Scintimammography

98. Palmedo H, Biersack HJ, Lastoria S, Maublant J, Prats E, Stegner HE, Bourgeois P, Hustinx R, Hilson AJ, Bischof-Delaloye A (1998) Scintimammography with technetium-99m methoxy-isobutylisonitrile: results of a prospective European multicentre trial. Eur J Nucl Med 25:375–385
99. Schillaci O, Scopinaro F, Danieli R, Tavolaro R, Picardi V, Cannas P, Colella AC (1997) 99Tcm-sestamibi scintimammography in patients with suspicious breast lesions: comparison of SPET and planar images in the detection of primary tumours and axillary lymph node involvement. Nucl Med Commun 18:839–845
100. Scoparino F, Schillaci O, Ussof W et al (1997) A three center study on the diagnostic accuracy of 99mTc-MIBI scintimammography. Anticancer Res 17:1631–1634
101. Sillar R, Howarth D, Clark D (1997) The initial Australian experience of technetium-99m sestamibi scintimammography: a complementary test in the management of breast cancer. Aust NZ J Surg 67:433–437
102. Sommer H, Tiling R, Pechmann M, Kindermann G, Kress K, Moser R, Tatsch K, Hahn K, Pfluger T, Assemi C (1997) Evaluation of mammographic lesions with Tc-99m sestamibi scintimammography and contrast enhanced MRI. Zentralbl Gynakol 119:6–11
103. Waxman A, Nagaraj N, Ashok G et al (1994) Sensitivity and specificity of Tc-99m methoxy isobutyle isonitrile (MIBI) in the evaluation of primary carcinoma of the breast: comparison of palpable and nonpalpable lesions with mammography. J Nucl Med 35:22P
104. Yuen-Green M, Wasnich R, Caindec-Ranchez S, Davis J (1996) New method for breast cancer detection using Tc-99m sestamibi scintimammography. Hawaii Med J 55:26–28
105. Avril N, Bense S, Ziegler SI, Dose J, Weber W, Laubenbacher C, Römer W, Jänicke F, Schwaiger M (1997) Breast imaging with fluorine-18-FDG PET: quantitative image analysis. J Nucl Med 38:1186–1191
106. Scheidhauer K, Scharl A, Pietrzyk U, Wagner R, Göhring UJ, Schomäcker K, Schicha H (1996) Qualitative ^{18}F-FDG PET in primary breast cancer: clinical relevance and practicability. Eur J Nucl Med 23:618–623
107. Flanagan FL, Dehdashti F, Siegel BA (1998) PET in breast cancer. Semin Nucl Med 28:290–302
108. Heinisch M, Gallowitsch HJ, Mikosch P, Kresnik E, Kumnig G, Gomez I, Lind P, Umschaden HW, Gasser J, Forsthuber EP (2003) Comparison of FDG-PET and dynamic contrast-enhanced MRI in the evaluation of suggestive breast lesions. Breast 12:17–22
109. Schirrmeister H, Kühn T, Guhlmann A, Santjohanser C, Hörster T, Nüssle K, Koretz K, Glatting G, Rieber A, Kreienberg R, Buck AC, Reske SN (2001) Fluorine-18 2-deoxy-2-fluoro-D-glucose PET in the preoperative staging of breast cancer: comparison with the standard staging procedures. Eur J Nucl Med 28:351–358
110. Avril N, Rosé CA, Schelling M, Dose J, Kuhn W, Bense S, Weber W, Ziegler S, Graeff H, Schwaiger M (2000) Breast imaging with positron emission tomography and fluorine-18 fluorodeoxyglucose: use and limitations. J Clin Oncol 18:3495–3502
111. Palmedo H, Bender H, Grünwald F, Mallmann P, Zamora P, Krebs D, Biersack HJ (1997) Comparison of fluorine-18 fluorodeoxyglucose positron emission tomography and technetium-99m methoxyisobutylisonitrile scintimammography in the detection of breast tumors. Eur J Nucl Med 24:1138–1145
112. Avril N, Dose J, Jänicke F, Bense S, Ziegler S, Laubenbacher C, Römer W, Pache H, Herz M, Allgayer B, Nathrath W, Graeff H, Schwaiger M (1996) Metabolic characterization of breast tumors with positron emission tomography using ^{18}F fluorodeoxyglucose. J Clin Oncol 14:1848–1857
113. Dehdashti F, Mortimer JE, Siegel BA, Griffeth LK, Bonasera TJ, Fusselman MJ, Detert DD, Cutler PD, Katzenellenbogen JA, Welch MJ (1995) Positron emission tomographic assessment of estrogen receptors in breast cancer: comparison with FDG-PET and *in vitro* receptor assays. J Nucl Med 36:1766–1774
114. Adler LP, Crowe JP, al-Kaisi NK, Sunshine JL (1993) Evaluation of breast masses and axillary lymph nodes with (^{18}F)2-deoxy-2-fluoro-D-glucose PET. Radiology 187:743–750

115. Nitzsche EU, Hoh CK, Dalbohm NM, Glaspy JA, Phelps ME, Moser EA, Hawkins RA (1993) Whole body positron emission tomography in breast cancer. Rofo 158:293–298
116. Wahl RL, Cody RL, Hutchins GD, Mudgett EE (1991) Primary and metastatic breast carcinoma: initial clinical evaluation with PET with the radiolabelled glucose analog 2-(F-18)-fluoro-deoxy-2-D-glucose (FDG). Radiology 179:765–770
117. Tse NY, Hoh CK, Hawkins RA, Zinner MJ, Dahlbom M, Choi Y, Maddahi J, Brunicardi FC, Phelps ME, Glaspy JA (1992) The application of positron emission tomographic imaging with fluorodeoxyglucose to the evaluation of breast disease. Ann Surg 216:27–34
118. Nieweg OE, Kim EE, Wong WH, Broussard WF, Singletary SE, Hortobagyi GN, Tilbury RS (1993) Positron emission tomography with fluorine-18-deoxyglucose in the detection and staging of breast cancer. Cancer 71:3920–3925
119. Kole AC, Nieweg OE, Pruim J, Paans AM, Plukker JT, Hoekstra HJ, Schraffordt Koops H, Vaalburg W (1997) Standardized uptake value and quantification of metabolism for breast cancer imaging with FDG and L-[1-11 C]tyrosine PET. J Nucl Med 38:692–696
120. Samson DJ, Flamm CR, Pisano ED, Aronson N (2002) Should FDG PET be used to decide whether a patient with an abnormal mammogram or breast finding at physical examination should undergo biopsy? Acad Radiol 9:773–783
121. Gambhir SS, Czernin J, Schwimmer J, Silverman DH, Coleman RE, Phelps ME (2001) A tabulated summary of the FDG PET literature. J Nucl Med 42:1S–93S
122. Walter C, Scheidhauer K, Scharl A, Goering UJ, Theissen P, Kugel H, Krahe T, Pietrzyk U (2003) Clinical and diagnostic value of preoperative MR mammography and FDG-PET in suspicious breast lesions. Eur Radiol 13:1651–1656
123. Tatsumi M, Cohade C, Mourtzikos KA, Fishman EK, Wahl RL (2006) Initial experience with FDG-PET/CT in the evaluation of breast cancer. Eur J Nucl Med Mol Imaging 33:254–262
124. Radan L, Ben-Haim S, Bar-Shalom R, Guralnik L, Israel O (2006) The role of FDG-PET/CT in suspected recurrence of breast cancer. Cancer 107:2545–2551
125. Kaiser JS, Helvie MA, Blacklaw RL, Roubidoux MA (2002) Palpable breast thickening: role of mammography and US in cancer detection. Radiology 223:839–844
126. Lorenzen J, Wedel AK, Lisboa BW, Löning T, Adam G (2005) Diagnostische Mammographie und Sonographie: Korrelation von diagnostischer BI-RADS-Einstufung mit dem histologischen und klinischen Endbefund. Fortschr Röntgenstr 177:1545–1551
127. Rissanen TJ, Mäkäräinen HP, Mattila SI, Lindholm EL, Heikkinen MI, Kiviniemi HO (1993) Breast cancer recurrence after mastectomy: diagnosis with mammography and US. Radiology 188:463–467
128. Cwikla JB, Kolasinska A, Buscombe JR, Hilson AJ (2000) Tc-99m MIBI in suspected recurrent breast cancer. Cancer Biother Radiopharm 15:367–372
129. Berg WA, Gutierrez L, NessAiver MS, Carter WB, Bhargavan M, Lewis RS, Ioffe OB (2004) Diagnostic accuracy of mammography, clinical examination, US, and MR imaging in preoperative assessment of breast cancer. Radiology 233:830–849
130. Hata T, Takahashi H, Watanabe K, Takahashi M, Taguchi K, Itoh T, Todo S (2004) Magnetic resonance imaging for preoperative evaluation of breast cancer: a comparative study with mammography and ultrasonography. J Am Coll Surg 198:190–197
131. Satake H, Shimamoto K, Sawaki A, Niimi R, Ando Y, Ishiguchi T, Ishigaki T, Yamakawa K, Nagasaka T, Funahashi H (2000) Role of ultrasonography in the detection of intraductal spread of breast cancer: correlation with pathologic findings, mammography, and MR imaging. Eur Radiol 10:1726–1732
132. Kuhl CK, Schmutzler RK, Leutner CC, Kempe A, Wardelmann E, Hocke A, Maringa M, Pfeifer U, Krebs D, Schild HH (2000) Breast MR imaging screening in 192 women proved or suspected to be carriers of a breast cancer susceptibility gene: preliminary results. Radiology 215:267–279
133. Kuhl CK, Schrading S, Leutner CC, Morakkabati-Spitz N, Wardelmann E, Fimmers R, Kuhn W, Schild HH (2005) Mammography, breast ultrasound, and magnetic resonance imaging for surveillance of women at high familial risk for breast cancer. J Clin Oncol 23:8469–8476

134. Kriege M, Brekelmans CT, Boetes C, Besnard PE, Zonderland HM, Obdeijn IM, Manoliu RA, Kok T, Peterse H, Tilanus-Linthorst MM, Muller SH, Meijer S, Oosterwijk JC, Beex LV, Tollenaar RA, de Koning HJ, Rutgers EJ, Klijn JG, Magnetic Resonance Imaging Screening Study Group (2004) Efficacy of MRI and mammography for breast-cancer screening in women with a familial or genetic predisposition. N Engl J Med 351:427–437

135. Kolb TM, Lichy J, Newhouse JH (2002) Comparison of the performance of screening mammography, physical examination, and breast US and evaluation of factors that influence them: an analysis of 27,825 patient evaluations. Radiology 225:165–175

136. Warner E, Plewes DB, Hill KA, Causer PA, Zubovits JT, Jong RA, Cutrara MR, DeBoer G, Yaffe MJ, Messner SJ, Meschino WS, Piron CA, Narod SA (2004) Surveillance of *BRCA1* and *BRCA2* mutation carriers with magnetic resonance imaging, ultrasound, mammography, and clinical breast examination. JAMA 292:1317–1325

137. Warner E, Plewes DB, Shumak RS, Catzavelos GC, Di Prospero LS, Yaffe MJ, Goel V, Ramsay E, Chart PL, Cole DE, Taylor GA, Cutrara M, Samuels TH, Murphy JP, Murphy JM, Narod SA (2001) Comparison of breast magnetic resonance imaging, mammography, and ultrasound for surveillance of women at high risk for hereditary breast cancer. J Clin Oncol 19:3524–3531

138. Zonderland HM, Coerkamp EG, Hermans J, van de Vijver MJ, van Voorthuisen AE (1999) Diagnosis of breast cancer: contribution of US as an adjunct to mammography. Radiology 213:413–422

139. Lam WW, Yang WT, Chan YL, Stewart IE, Metreweli C, King W (1996) Detection of axillary lymph node metastases in breast carcinoma by technetium-99m sestamibi breast scintigraphy, ultrasound and conventional mammography. Eur J Nucl Med 23:498–503

140. Heywang-Köbrunner SH, Bick U, Bradley WG Jr, Boné B, Casselman J, Coulthard A, Fischer U, Müller-Schimpfle M, Oellinger H, Patt R, Teubner J, Friedrich M, Newstead G, Holland R, Schauer A, Sickles EA, Tabar L, Waisman J, Wernecke KD (2001) International investigation of breast MRI: results of a multicentre study (11 sites) concerning diagnostic parameters for contrast-enhanced MRI based on 519 histopathologically correlated lesions. Eur Radiol 11:531–546

141. Leinsinger GL, Friedl L, Tiling R, Scherr MK, Heiss DT, Kandziora C, Camerer B, Sommer H, Pfluger T, Hahn K (2001) Comparison of dynamic MR imaging of the breast and sestamibi for evaluation indeterminate mammographic lesions. Eur Radiol 11:2050–2057

142. Kvistad KA, Rydland J, Vainio J, Smethurst HB, Lundgren S, Fjøsne HE, Haraldseth O (2000) Breast lesions: evaluation with dynamic contrast-enhanced T1-weighted MR imaging and with T2*-weighted first-pass perfusion MR imaging. Radiology 216:545–553

143. Bluemke DA, Gatsonis CA, Chen MH, DeAngelis GA, DeBruhl N, Harms S, Heywang-Köbrunner SH, Hylton N, Kuhl CK, Lehman C, Pisano ED, Causer P, Schnitt SJ, Smazal SF, Stelling CB, Weatherall PT, Schnall MD (2004) Magnetic resonance imaging of the breast prior to biopsy. JAMA 292:2735–2742

144. Kuhl CK, Mielcareck P, Klaschik S, Leutner C, Wardelmann E, Gieseke J, Schild HH (1999) Dynamic breast MR imaging: Are signal time course data useful for differential diagnosis of enhancing lesions? Radiology 211:101–110

145. MARBIS study group (2005) Screening with magnetic resonance imaging and mammography at high familial risk of breast cancer: a prospective multi-centre trial. Lancet 365:1769–1778

146. Murray AD, Staff RT, Redpath TW, Gilbert FJ, Ah-See AK, Brookes JA, Miller ID, Payne S (2002) Dynamic contrast enhanced MRI of the axilla in women with breast cancer: comparison with pathology of excised nodes. Br J Radiol 75:220–228

147. Michel SC, Keller TM, Fröhlich JM, Fink D, Caduff R, Seifert B, Marincek B, Kubik-Huch RA (2002) Preoperative breast cancer staging: MR imaging of the axilla with ultrasmall superparamagnetic iron oxide enhancement. Radiology 225:527–536

148. Kvistad KA, Rydland J, Smethurst HB, Lundgren S, Fjøsne HE, Haraldseth O (2000) Axillary lymph node metastases in breast cancer: preoperative detection with dynamic contrast-enhanced MRI. Eur Radiol 10:1464–1471

149. Cha JH, Moon WK, Cho N, Chung SY, Park SH, Park JM, Han BK, Choe YH, Cho G, Im JG (2005) Differentiation of benign from malignant solid breast masses: conventional US versus spatial compound imaging. Radiology 237:841–846
150. Raza S, Baum JK (1997) Solid breast lesions: evaluation with power Doppler US. Radiology 203:164–168
151. Moon WK, Noh DY, Im JG (2002) Multifocal, multicentric, and contralateral breast cancers: bilateral whole-breast US in the preoperative evaluation of patients. Radiology 224: 569–576
152. Podo F, Sardanelli F, Canese R, D'Agnolo G, Natali PG, Crecco M, Grandinetti ML, Musumeci R, Trecate G, Bergonzi S, De Simone T, Costa C, Pasini B, Manuokian S, Spatti GB, Vergnaghi D, Morassut S, Boiocchi M, Dolcetti R, Viel A, De Giacomi C, Veronesi A, Coran F, Silingardi V, Turchett D, Cortesi L, De Santis M, Federico M, Romagnoli R, Ferrari S, Bevilacqua G, Bartolozzi C, Caligo MA, Cilotti A, Marini C, Cirillo S, Marra V, Martincich L, Contegiacomo A, Pensabene M, Capuano I, Burgazzi GB, Petrillo A, Bonomo L, Carriero A, Mariani-Constantini R, Battista P, Cama A, Palca G, Di Maggio C, D'Andrea E, Bazzocchi M, Francescutti GE, Zuiani C, Londero V, Zunnui I, Gustavino C, Centurioni MG, Iozzelli A, Panizza P, Del Maschio A (2002) The Italian multi-centre project on evaluation of MRI and other imaging modalities in early detection of breast cancer in subjects at high genetic risk. J Exp Clin Cancer Res 21:115–124
153. Buchberger W, Niehoff A, Obrist P, DeKoekkoek-Doll P, Dünser M (2000) Clinically and mammographically occult breast lesions: detection and classification with high-resolution sonography. Semin Ultrasound CT MR 21:325–336
154. Strauss HG, Lampe D, Methfessel G, Buchmann J (1998) Preoperative axilla sonography in breast tumor suspected of malignancy- a diagnostic advantage? Ultraschall Med 19:70–77
155. Verbanck J, Vandewiele I, De Winter H, Tytgat J, Van Aelst F, Tanghe W (1997) Value of axillary ultrasonography and sonographically guided puncture of axillary lymph nodes: a prospective study in 144 consecutive patients. J Clin Ultrasound 25:53–56
156. Palmedo H, Schomburg A, Grünwald F, Mallmann P, Boldt I, Biersack HJ (1996) Scintimammography with Tc-99m MIBI in patients with suspicion of primary breast cancer. Nucl Med Biol 23:681–684
157. Perre CI, Rütter JE, Vos PA, de Hooge P (1997) Technetium-99m-sestamibi uptake in axillary lymph node metastases in breast cancer patients. Eur J Surg Oncol 23:142–144
158. Chiti A, Maffioli LS, Agresti R, Spinelli A, Savelli G, Casteliani MR, Giovanazzi R, Greco M, Bombardieri E (1997) Axillary node metastasis detection in breast cancer with 99mTc-Sestamibi and 111In-Pentetroide. Tumori 83:537–538
159. Taillefer R, Robidoux A, Turpin S, Lambert R, Cantin J, Léveillé J (1998) Metastatic axillary lymph node technetium-99m-MIBI imaging in primary breast cancer. J Nucl Med 39: 459–464
160. Kubo H, Fukumitsu N, Nagata T, Tomita H, Tabei II, Uchida K, Yamazaki Y (1997) ^{99m}Tc SPECT compared with ^{201}Tl-SPECT for the detection of breast cancer and lymph node metastases. Breast Cancer 4:297–302
161. Tiling R, Tatsch K, Sommer H, Meyer G, Pechmann M, Gebauer K, Münzing W, Linke R, Khalkhali I, Hahn K (1998) Technetium-99m-sestamibi scintimammography for the detection of breast carcinoma: comparison between planar and SPECT imaging. J Nucl Med 39:849–856
162. Mulero F, Nicolás F, Castellón MI, Claver MA, Abad L, de la Rosa JA Nuño (2000) Scintigraphy with 99mTc-MIBI in the diagnosis of axillary lymph node invasion of breast cancer. Rev Esp Med Nucl 19:416–422
163. Nishiyama Y, Yamamoto Y, Ono Y, Irie A, Yamauchi A, Satoh K, Ohkawa M (2001) Comparative evaluation of 99mTc-MIBI and 99mTc-HMDP scintimammography for the diagnosis of breast cancer and its axillary metastases. Eur J Nucl Med 28:522–528
164. Lumachi F, Ferretti G, Povolato M, Marzola MC, Zucchetta P, Geatti O, Bui F, Brandes AA (2001) Usefulness of 99m-Tc-sestamibi in suspected breast cancer and in axillary lymph node metastases detection. Eur J Surg Oncol 27:256–259

165. Chen J, Wu H, Zhou J, Hu J (2003) Using Tc-99m MIBI scintimammography to differentiate nodular lesions in breast and detect axillary lymph node metastases from breast cancer. Chin Med J 116:620–624
166. Madeddu G, Spanu A (2004) Use of tomographic nuclear medicine procedures, SPECT and pinhole SPECT, with cationic lipophilic radiotracers for the evaluation of axillary lymph node status in breast cancer patients. Eur J Nucl Med Mol Imaging 31(Suppl 1):S23–S34
167. Lernevall A (2000) Imaging of axillary lymph nodes. Acta Oncol 39:421–422
168. Peare R, Staff RT, Heys SD (2010) The use of FDG-PET in assessing axillary lymph node status in breast cancer: a systematic review and meta-analysis of the literature. Breast Cancer Res Treat 123:281–290
169. Saphner T, Tormey DC, Gray R (1996) Annual hazard rates of recurrence for breast cancer after primary therapy. J Clin Oncol 14:2738–2746
170. Maini CL, Tofani A, Sciuto R, Semprebene A, Cavaliere R, Mottolese M, Benevolo M, Ferranti F, Grandinetti ML, Vici P, Lopez M, Botti C (1997) Technetium-99m-MIBI scintigraphy in the assessment of neoadjuvant chemotherapy in breast cancer. J Nucl Med 38:1546–1551
171. Gupta R, Collier D, Abdeen S, Roberts L, Hussein AY, Al-Bader I, Syed GM (2006) Usefulness of scintimammography as an adjunct to mammography and ultrasound in the diagnosis of breast diseases. Australas Radiol 50:539–542
172. Habib S, Maseeh-uz-Zaman, Hameed A, Niaz K, Hashmi H, Kamal S (2009) Diagnostic accuracy of Tc-99m-MIBI for breast carcinoma in correlation with mammography and sonography. J Coll Physicians Surg Pak 19:622–626
173. Ozülker T, Ozülker F, Ozpaçaci T, Bender O, Değirmenci H (2010) The efficacy of (99m) Tc-MIBI scintimammography in the evaluation of breast lesions and axillary involvement: a comparison with X-rays mammography, ultrasonography and magnetic resonance imaging. Hell J Nucl Med 13:144–149
174. Usmani S, Khan HA, Javed A, Al Mohannadi S, Al Huda FA, Al Shammary I (2008) Functional breast imaging with Tc 99m Mibi for detection of primary breast lesion and axillary lymph node metastases. Gulf J Oncolog 4:52–57
175. Gommans GM, van der Zant FM, van Dongen A, Boer RO, Teule GJ, de Waard JW (2007) (99M)Technetium-sestamibi scintimammography in non-palpable breast lesions found on screening X-ray mammography. Eur J Surg Oncol 33:23–27
176. Grosso M, Chiacchio S, Bianchi F, Traino C, Marini C, Cilotti A, Manca G, Volterrani D, Roncella M, Rampin L, Marzola MC, Rubello D, Mariani G (2009) Comparison between 99mTc-sestamibi scintimammography and X-ray mammography in the characterization of clusters of microcalcifications: a prospective long-term study. Anticancer Res 29:4251–4257
177. Lumachi F, Tregnaghi A, Ferretti G, Povolato M, Marzola MC, Zucchetta P, Cecchin D, Bui F (2006) Accuracy of ultrasonography and 99mTc-sestamibi scintimammography for assessing axillary lymph node status in breast cancer patients. A prospective study. Eur J Surg Oncol 32:933–936
178. Lumachi F, Ferretti G, Povolato M, Bui F, Cecchin D, Marzola MC, Zucchetta P, Basso U (2007) Axillary lymph node metastases detection with 99mTc-sestamibi scintimammography in patients with breast cancer undergoing curative surgery. Anticancer Res 27:2949–2952
179. Rajkovaca Z, Vuleta G, Matavulj A, Kovacević P, Ponorac N (2007) 99m Tc-sestamibi scintimammography in detection of recurrent breast cancer. Bosn J Basic Med Sci 7:256–260
180. Usmani S, Niaz K, Maseeh-Uz-Zaman, Kamal S, Niyaz K, Mehboob J, Hashmi A, Habib S, Hashmi H (2007) Role of 99mTc-MIBI scintimammography and X-ray mammography in the diagnosis of locoregional recurrence of breast cancer. J Pak Med Assoc 57:172–175
181. Usmani S, Niaz K, Maseeh-Uz-Zaman, Niyaz K, Khan HA, Habib S, Kamal S (2007) Chest wall recurrence of breast cancer demonstrated on 99mTc-MIBI scintimammography. Nucl Med Commun 28:842–846
182. Usmani S, Khan HA, Niaz K, Uz-Zaman M, Niyaz K, Javed A, al Mohannadi S, al Abu Huda F, Kamal S (2008) Tc-99m-methoxy isobutyl isonitrile scintimammography: imaging postexcision biopsy for residual and multifocal breast tumor. Nucl Med Commun 29:826–829

183. Usmani S, Khan H, Ahmed N, Marafi F, Garvie N (2010) Scintimammography in conjunction with ultrasonography for local breast cancer recurrence in post-mastectomy breast. Br J Radiol 83:934–939
184. Kim IJ, Kim YK, Kim SJ (2009) Detection and prediction of breast cancer using double phase Tc-99m MIBI scintimammography in comparison with MRI. Onkologie 32:556–560
185. Zaman MU, Nasir Z, Raza T, Hashmi H, Hashmi A, Fatima N (2009) Dual phase qualitative and quantitative 99mTc-MIBI scintimammography for predicting response to neoadjuvant chemotherapy in breast cancer. J Coll Physicians Surg Pak 19:173–178
186. Schillaci O, Danieli R, Filippi L, Romano P, Cossu E, Manni C, Simonetti G (2007) Scintimammography with a hybrid SPECT/CT imaging system. Anticancer Res 27: 557–562
187. Duarte GM, Cabello C, Torresan RZ, Alvarenga M, Telles GH, Bianchessi ST, Caserta N, Segala SR, de Lima Mda C, Etchebehere EC, Camargo EE, Tinois E (2007) Fusion of magnetic resonance and scintimammography images for breast cancer evaluation: a pilot study. Ann Surg Oncol 14:2903–2910

Tc-99m-MIBI for Thyroid Imaging

7

Matthias Schmidt

7.1 Thyroid: Basic Anatomy and Physiology

The thyroid is an endocrine gland mostly located in the neck anterior to the trachea and just below the larynx consisting of two lateral lobes which are connected by an isthmus. The thyroid gland is closely attached to the cartilage of the larynx and to the proximal trachea and moves on swallowing. The embryologic origin of the thyroid gland is the base of the tongue from which it descends to the middle of the neck. Sometimes, remnants of thyroid tissue can be found at the base of the tongue as a lingual thyroid or along the line of descent. There exist a number of morphological variations such as hypoplasia, hemiagenesis or agenesis, and ectopy of the thyroid gland. Lateral to the thyroid are the carotid arteries and the internal jugular veins. The esophagus may be located dorsal to the trachea but may be often found dorsomedial to the left thyroid lobe. Normal parathyroid glands are usually not visible on ultrasound but in case of a parathyroid adenoma a hypoechogenic nodule may be found behind a thyroid lobe or elsewhere in the neck. The normal adult thyroid has a maximum volume of 18 mL for women and 25 mL for men. Thyroid function consists of synthesis, storage, and release of thyroid hormones (mainly thyroxine and to a lesser extent triiodthyronine) requiring adequate iodine supply with a recommended intake of 150–200 µg/day. In recent years, Germany has just achieved sufficient iodine supply as determined by a median iodine urine excretion of 132 µg/L [1]. Thyroid hormone synthesis consists of iodide trapping, organification, and coupling of iodotyrosine as well as release of thyroid hormones. Thyroid function is controlled by hypophyseal thyroid-stimulating hormone (TSH). Thyroxine is released from the thyroid as free hormone and bound to thyroxine-binding globuline while only a small fraction of less than 1% remains unbound. The major function of thyroid hormone is to regulate the body´s metabolism and heat

---

M. Schmidt
Department of Nuclear Medicine, University of Cologne,
Kerpener Str. 62, 50937 Köln, Germany
e-mail: Matthias.Schmidt@uni-koeln.de

J. Bucerius et al. (eds.), ^{99m}Tc-Sestamibi,
DOI 10.1007/978-3-642-04233-1_7, © Springer-Verlag Berlin Heidelberg 2012

production [2]. Thyroid hormones exhibit their main function in the cell nucleus where gene transcription is initiated. Thyroid hormones act on carbohydrate, lipid, and amino acid metabolism; influence bone development, and have influence on the central nervous system as well as on neuromuscular junctions and muscles.

7.1.1 Prevalence and Management of Thyroid Nodules

Due to the longstanding history of insufficient iodine supply in Germany thyroid nodules are very common. Reiners et al. published data on the prevalence of thyroid disorders in the working population of Germany: in a cross-sectional observational study on 96,278 unselected employees, ultrasound screening revealed goiter and/or thyroid nodules >0.5 cm in 32% of the men and 34.2% of the women [3]. Thus, thyroid nodules are frequent in Germany with an estimated prevalence of 15 million people being affected [4]. Thyroid evaluation consists of the combined evaluation of history, physical examination, laboratory tests including basal TSH, ultrasound, and – if indicated – thyroid scintigraphy. Thyroid ultrasound provides morphological information while thyroid scintigraphy is useful for global and regional functional assessment. Thyroid scintigraphy is valuable for nodule evaluation from a minimal diameter of 1 cm. Nowadays, mostly pertechnetate and rarely iodine-123 are used. Both scintigraphic techniques provide information on functional activity. A nodule with increased uptake is a so-called "hot nodule" being an almost exclusively benign finding ("autonomous adenoma") which does not require fine-needle aspiration biopsy holding the risk for false-positive findings. A nodule with decreased uptake is a so-called "cold nodule," raising the suspicion of malignancy. For further evaluation of cold thyroid nodules, fine-needle aspiration biopsy (FNAB) is indicated. However, there is a large regional variability in the percentage of nondiagnostic FNABs from less than 5% to more than 30%. For this reason, other radiopharmaceuticals have been evaluated for further characterization of thyroid nodules.

Tl-201-chloride and Tc-99m-Sestamibi are known to be unspecific tumor imaging agents [5] accumulating in malignant but also some benign thyroid nodules (e.g., follicular adenomas), but also in inflammatory lymphadenitis or parathyroid adenomas. The use of Tc-99m-MIBI as a tumor imaging radiopharmaceutical dates back to first reports from Müller et al. in 1987 [78]. In 1991, Briele et al. compared the diagnostic performance of Tl-201 and Tc-99m-MIBI in patients with recurrent differentiated thyroid carcinoma and concluded that Tc-99m-MIBI seems to be a promising alternative imaging agent in the follow-up of differentiated thyroid carcinomas [49]. In 1993, Szybiński et al. were among the first to use Tc-99m-MIBI for evaluation of cold thyroid nodules concluding that Tc-99m-labeled MIBI as used for scintigraphy of cold nodules of the thyroid is a useful marker of thyroid cancer in its early phase [6]. In the same year, Földes et al. compared pertechnetate and Tc-99m-MIBI scintigraphy but did not come to such a clear statement, probably because of the low number of only three follicular thyroid carcinomas in their series of 34 surgically removed thyroid nodules [7]. In sum, there are more than 20 years of experience with the use of Tc-99m-MIBI as a nonspecific tumor imaging agent for the evaluation of thyroid nodules.

7.2 Tc-99m-MIBI for Scintigraphy of Cold/Hypofunctioning Thyroid Nodules

Tc-99m-MIBI has become an important imaging technique for assessment of cold/hypofunctioning thyroid nodules because of its high negative predictive value excluding malignant thyroid tumors. The aim is to distinguish effectively between malignant and benign nodules in order to avoid expensive evaluation and treatment of patients with benign thyroid disease as well as to ensure appropriate and timely management of patients with thyroid cancer [8].

The strategy to evaluate thyroid nodules varies between countries. The main aim is to identify or exclude malignant thyroid nodules. In Germany, guidelines recommend thyroid scintigraphy (= scintigraphy with Tc-99m = pertechnetate scintigraphy) as standard procedure in thyroid nodules ≥1 cm for functional evaluation. Thyroid nodules which are cold (hypofunctional) in thyroid scintigraphy have a risk of malignancy of about 2–5% and require further evaluation with FNAB while hot nodules are almost exclusively of benign histopathology and do not require FNAB. Thus, standard thyroid scintigraphy using pertechnetate is established for risk stratification of thyroid nodules in Germany identifying nodules with an increased likelihood of malignancy, and thyroid scintigraphy guides the further diagnostic and therapeutic strategy.

European [9, 9a] and American [10, 10a] guidelines recommend the evaluation of thyroid nodules using FNAB: in case patients have normal thyroid function tests, FNAB of thyroid nodules is recommended and thyroid scintigraphy is reserved for patients with abnormal low TSH. These recommendations are repeated in the more recent international literature [11–13]. It would be erroneous to follow these recommendations in Germany because of the high incidence of autonomous adenomas in euthyroidism identified by thyroid scintigraphy. FNAB of autonomous adenomas is not indicated because this would increase the number of cytological findings of "follicular proliferation" which would increase the number of not-indicated surgical procedures.

There are several problems with FNAB in clinical practice related to

1. The high number of procedures to perform for diagnostic evaluation of the many thyroid nodules.
2. Inadequate material and/or inconclusive pathological results in 3–33% of cases.
3. Patient inacceptance of multiple and eventually repeated punctures, especially in multinodular goiter.

There is a large variability for FNA/ultrasound-guided fine-needle aspiration with sensitivities between 60% and 100%, specificity of 63–95%, a diagnostic accuracy of 80–95%, and an inadequacy rate of 3–33% [14–16]. Furthermore, the cytological result may not result in a clear definition of either benign or malignant category. There exists the possibility of "follicular proliferation" usually requiring definite operative evaluation of a thyroid nodule. The cytological finding of "follicular proliferation" raises the risk of malignancy to about 20%, meaning that this cytological finding leads to a benign finding in the majority of operated patients. Whether the Bethesda thyroid fine-needle aspiration classification system will improve this situation remains to be shown [17].

Ultrasound has been used to differentiate benign from malignant thyroid disease, looking at size, echogenicity, echo structure, border shape, and presence of calcifications in the thyroid nodules, as well as patterns of vascularity with power Doppler and vascular patterns, resistive index, and maximal systolic velocity with spectral Doppler ultrasound; however, none of these features are pathognomonic of thyroid cancer, even in patients with atypical cell cytology or follicular neoplasm cytology [8].

Therefore, the aim is to identify nodules with an increased likelihood of malignancy, to select nodules for FNAB, and decrease the number of unnecessary operations. In this clinical scenario, Tc-99m-MIBI has gained increasing interest as a noninvasive imaging tool to exclude thyroid malignancy with a very high negative predictive value.

7.2.1 Uptake Mechanism of Tc-99m-MIBI in Thyroid Nodules

Tc-99m-MIBI is a complex molecule of lipophilic cations. Although several hypotheses have been suggested regarding the accumulation of Tc-99m-MIBI in tumors, the exact uptake mechanism is still a matter of discussion. According to Földes et al., Tc-99m-MIBI uptake depends mainly on thyroid tissue viability [7]. The cationic charge and lipophilicity of Tc-99m-MIBI, the mitochondrial and plasma membrane potentials of the tumor cells and cellular mitochondrial content were considered to play a significant role in the mechanism of this agent's tumor uptake too [18]. However, other factors influencing uptake include blood flow, the number of mitochondria, and the size of the thyroid nodule. Sarikaya et al. investigated the ultrastructural cell type of thyroid tumors by electron microscopy and compared them with uptake of Tc-99m-MIBI. Thyroid cells were classified as A and B cells using electron microscopy. The cytoplasm of an A cell had the normal amount of mitochondria, whereas the cytoplasm of a B cell (mitochondria-rich oxyphilic cell) contained abundant mitochondria. According to the findings by Sarikaya et al., Tc-99m-MIBI accumulated in thyroid tumors with both A and B cells. Sarikaya et al. concluded that the mitochondrial content of tumors was not only responsible for Tc-99m-MIBI uptake and retention but other factors such as desmoplasia, cellular proliferation, plasma and mitochondrial membrane potentials, and active transport mechanisms may be responsible for Tc-99m-MIBI tumor uptake requiring further investigations [86].

7.2.2 Diagnostic/Therapeutic Indications for Thyroid Imaging with Tc-99m-MIBI

Tc-99m-MIBI is a
- Diagnostic agent to assist in the evaluation of cold/hypofunctioning thyroid nodules on pertechnetate scintigraphy after inconclusive FNAB or in case of difficulty to assess thyroid nodules by FNAB
- Diagnostic agent in multinodular disease ($\geq$3 nodules) with hot and cold nodules to select nodules requiring FNAB

7.2.3 Doses and Method of Administration

Tc-99m-MIBI is for intravenous use. The suggested dose for thyroid imaging ranges from 370 to 740 MBq injected intravenously to a patient of average weight (70 kg). Following the ALARA concept the dose used should in every case be as low as reasonably practical. It needs to be mentioned that, to the author's knowledge, at the time of writing of this manuscript, there has been no commercially available Tc-99m-MIBI having official approval for this indication.

7.2.4 Thyroid Imaging Technique with Tc-99m-MIBI and Image Interpretation

After injection of Tc-99m-MIBI, either a single-phase protocol with late planar and/or SPECT images about 1–2 h post injection or a double-phase protocol with early (about 15–30 min p.i.) and late images (about 2 h p.i.) can be used. Images are mostly interpreted visually and findings include a low, an isointense or an increased tracer accumulation in the thyroid nodule in comparison to the paranodular thyroid tissue and/or in comparison to pertechnetate thyroid scintigraphy. A "Match" between pertechnetate and Tc-99m-MIBI scintigraphy is a concordantly decreased uptake in the thyroid nodule in comparison to the normal thyroid gland. A definite "Mismatch" means a cold thyroid nodule on pertechnetate scintigraphy and an increased uptake of Tc-99m-MIBI in comparison to the MIBI-uptake of the paranodular thyroid tissue (Fig. 7.1). Apart from the fact that there are obvious "Match" (corresponding decreased uptake) and obvious "Mismatch" (decreased uptake in Tc-99m and increased uptake in Tc-99m-MIBI scintigraphy) images, there exists an "intermediate group" meaning that there is an increased uptake in Tc-99m-MIBI in comparison to the pertechnetate scan and this Tc-99m-MIBI uptake is isointense to the paranodular tissue in the Tc-99m-MIBI image. There is no unequivocal agreement whether this should be read as "Match" or "Mismatch" finding. To read these scans as "Mismatch" increases the negative predictive value, however it generates more false-positive findings and decreases the positive predictive value. Though standardization of image interpretation is important, this aim must be seen with respect to the prevalence of thyroid carcinomas in the patient population studied in the different publications. Hurtado-Lopez et al. read these intermediate category images as "Mismatch" while our group from Cologne reads this category as "Match." We did not find an increased risk of malignancy in our patients but our patient population had a much lower prevalence of thyroid carcinomas (11%) [27, 81] in comparison to the patient population in Mexico City (38%) [8].

Hurtado-Lopez et al. reported that Tc-99m-MIBI uptake within a hypofunctioning thyroid nodule should be visually read as either absent (no uptake, uptake similar to that of Tc-99m-pertechnetate) or present (uptake present and higher than Tc-99m-pertechnetate uptake). In the first case the Tc-99m-MIBI scan should be interpreted as a "negative MIBI study," while in the second case, when MIBI uptake

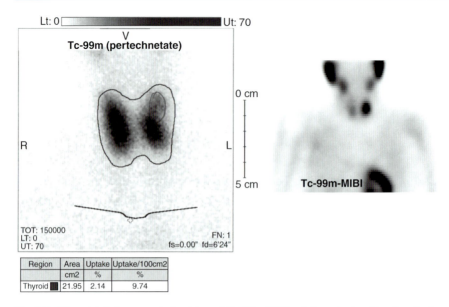

Fig. 7.1 Mismatch between pertechnetate and Tc-99m-MIBI-scintigraphy in a hypofunctioning thyroid nodule at the upper left thyroid lobe. Histology: follicular thyroid carcinoma, oxyphilic variant pT1 (UICC 6th edition). (Reproduction with permission from Lehmanns Media [81])

can be visually detected within the thyroid nodule, the scan should be interpreted as a "positive MIBI study." A "negative MIBI study" always indicated that the hypofunctioning thyroid nodule is benign, while a "positive MIBI study" is nonspecific, meaning that the hypofunctioning thyroid nodule may be benign or malignant and further nodule evaluation is mandatory [8].

Other authors introduced even more than three categories reading Tc-99m and Tc-99m-MIBI thyroid images and introduced a MIBI score from 0 to 3: MIBI-Score: 0 = cold, 1 = decreased, 2 = equal, 3 = hot [22]. Further image analysis included semiquantitative methods, that is, index calculation, washout rate calculation, and uptake differences between early and late images. Sharma et al. prospectively evaluated 77 patients with cold thyroid solitary nodules on Tc-99m pertechnetate scintigraphy by single injection, dual phase (30 and 120 min) thyroid scintigraphy using Tc-99m-MIBI. Using the 120/30-min thyroid lesion to background radiouptake ratio (RUR), malignant and benign thyroid nodules could be separated with a sensitivity of 84%, a specificity of 95%, and a positive predictive value of 93%. The mean RUR for malignant thyroid lesions was found to be 1.57 ± 0.32, whereas for benign lesions, the ratio was significantly lower, 0.32 ± 0.19. Sharma et al. concluded that fine needle aspiration cytology along with the 120/30 min Tc-99m MIBI scintigraphy ratio appeared to be useful in the preoperative assessment of solitary thyroid nodules [28]. Most investigators did not use a dual-phase protocol and the superiority of a dual phase protocol over late Tc-99m-MIBI images only has not been established.

7 Tc-99m-MIBI for Thyroid Imaging

Table 7.1 Tc-99m-MIBI for evaluation of hypofunctioning/cold thyroid nodules

First author, year	Pt. no	Papillary or follicular thyroid carcinomas (no)		Benign histology (no)		Negative predictive value (%)
		MIBI pos.	MIBI neg.	MIBI pos.	MIBI neg.	
1. Földes 1993 [7]	34*	3*	0	20*	10*	100
2. Sundram 1995 [19]	58	12	2	26	18	90
3. Nakahara 1996	25	13	0	8	4	100
4. Kresnik 1997 [20]	62	5	6	18	32	84
5. Alonso 1998 [30]	32	1	0	12	14	100
6. Mezosi 1999 [22]	56*	12*	0	39*	5*	100
7. Erdil 2000 [23]	40	21	0	14	5	100
8. Sarikaya 2001 [86]	25	6	0	13	6	100
9. Sathekge 2001 [24]	69**	20	1	11	37	97
10. Demirel 2003 [25]	43	8	0	31	3	100
11. Hurtado-L 2004 [26]	130	49	0	32	48	100
12. Theissen 2009 [27]	63	7	1	25	30	97
Sum	637					>97

The important clinical value is the negative predictive value of the technique, that is, thyroid nodules negative for MIBI uptake are almost always of benign histology and such a finding excludes thyroid malignancy. Sensitivity and specificity are of minor importance with this technique because it is not the aim to detect or exclude thyroid nodules with Tc-99m-MIBI scintigraphy but to assess their dignity.

MIBI pos. positive for MIBI uptake, *MIBI neg.* negative for MIBI uptake, *Pt. no* number of patients with either papillary or follicular thyroid carcinoma or benign histology after operation, except for these marked with an * denoting number of thyroid nodules

**Sathekge [24]: 71 patients – 1 medullary thyroid carcinoma – 1 anaplastic carcinoma=69 patients

It needs to be pointed out that uptake of Tc-99m-MIBI is not specific for thyroid nodules. Parathyroid adenomas usually accumulate Tc-99m-MIBI and must be considered as a differential diagnosis for Tc-99m-MIBI neck uptake [29].

7.2.5 Results for Thyroid Nodule Imaging with Tc-99m-MIBI

Papers reporting on the clinical value of Tc-99m-MIBI exist since 1993, that is, for more than 15 years now and since then included more than 600 patients. Table 7.1 compiles publications analyzing the results of Tc-99m-MIBI for thyroid nodule imaging against histology (table from [8], table modified by Schmidt M including further literature). The findings all point consistently in the same direction, that is, report on the very high negative predictive value. This means that a cold thyroid nodule not accumulating Tc-99m-MIBI 1–2 h after injection is a benign thyroid nodule with a very high degree of certainty and virtually excludes thyroid malignancy. Hurtado-Lopez et al. concluded that a negative MIBI thyroid scan excludes differentiated and medullary thyroid cancer in patients with hypofunctioning thyroid nodules. However, it needs to be admitted that the numbers of medullary cancer patients were small. In the papers (Tables 7.1 and 7.2), only four patients with

Table 7.2 Studies using Tc-99m-MIBI for evaluation of cold/hypofunctioning thyroid nodules: compilation of patient numbers, injected activity, start of acquisition, and use of planar and/or SPECT

First author, year	Patient number	Injected activity (MBq)	Start of acquisition after injection (min)	Planar/SPECT
1. Földes 1993 [7]	34*	370	4	Planar
2. Szybiński 1993 [6]	16	185	10	Planar
3. Sundram 1995 [19]	58	400	20	Planar
4. Nakahara 1996 [85]	25	185/740	10 and 120	Planar
5. Kresnik 1997 [20]	62	370	30 and 120	Planar
6. Alonso 1998 [21]	32	370	15	Planar
7. Mezosi 1999 [22]	56*	400	20–40	Planar
8. Erdil 2000 [23]	40	370	15 and 90	Planar
9. Sarikaya 2001 [86]	25	370	10 and 60	Planar
10. Sathekge 2001 [24]	69**	400	20 and 120	Planar
11. Demirel 2003 [25]	43	555	15 and 120	Planar
12. Hurtado-L 2004 [26]	130	296–370	15 and 120	Planar
13. Theissen 2009 [27]	63	740	60	Planar and SPECT

Pt. no number of patients with either papillary or follicular thyroid carcinoma or benign histology after operation, except for these marked with an * denoting number of thyroid nodules
**Sathekge [24]: 71 patients – 1 medullary thyroid carcinoma – 1 anaplastic carcinoma=69 patients

medullary cancer were reported and more patients with medullary thyroid cancer must be studied in order to draw more definitive conclusions.

There is only one study from Kresnik et al. reporting on a negative predictive value of Tc-99m-MIBI of 84% only due to seven MIBI-negative thyroid carcinomas. This figure is by far worse than in any other study. This may be most likely related to the author's individual interpretation of the scans of "intermediate category" and potential differences in imaging technique [20].

The main disadvantage of Tc-99m-MIBI is that an increased uptake does not differentiate between benign and malignant thyroid tissue. In our patient population the majority of patients with a positive Tc-99m-MIBI scan had a benign thyroid pathology. Thus, a second point of clinical interest is the positive predictive value, that is, the ability to predict a malignant thyroid tumor in case of a positive Tc-99m-MIBI result. This positive predictive value varies between studies, with values between <10% [21] and 60% [26]. The positive predictive value of a thyroid nodule accumulating Tc-99m-MIBI for thyroid cancer is dependent on the prevalence. In a study from Theissen et al., the positive predictive value was about 20% concerning patients from Germany [27]. This is a clinical relevant information too usually justifying surgery. The positive predictive value of 20% means that histopathological evaluation of these patients resulted in 20% malignant thyroid tumors while 80% had a benign histopathology in case of a positive Tc-99m-MIBI scan. For comparison, looking at the clinical value of FNAB the probability of 20% malignancy is in the same order as the cytological result of "follicular proliferation."

False-negative findings are rare: Kresnik et al. reported about a false-negative finding in a patient with an undifferentiated thyroid carcinoma [20] and Földes et al.

in a patient with an anaplastic thyroid carcinoma [7]. Sundram et al. did not detect two papillary and Sathekge one follicular thyroid carcinoma [19, 24]. In our patient population we did not detect a papillary microcarcinoma in the border zone between a cold and a hot thyroid nodule, that is, autonomous adenoma [27].

The results of the studies underscore the clinical usefulness of Tc-99m-MIBI for evaluation of thyroid nodules. Though these are all open, unblinded studies, the comparator is the histopathological "golden standard" which sets high clinical standards for a diagnostic study. The clinical usefulness of Tc-99m-Tetrofosmin in the evaluation of hypofunctioning thyroid nodules is less well investigated as only two studies were identified [77, 82]

7.2.6 Clinical Usefulness of Tc-99m-MIBI for Thyroid Nodule Imaging

The rationale for the use of Tc-99m-MIBI for evaluation of cold or suspicious thyroid nodules lies in the clinical usefulness of Tc-99m-MIBI to exclude thyroid malignancy in thyroid nodules because of its excellent negative predictive value.

According to German guidelines, thyroid nodules ≥1 cm are evaluated by thyroid scintigraphy and FNAB is recommended for further evaluation of cold thyroid nodules [73–75]. European and American guidelines are even more focused on the diagnostic evaluation by FNAB. However, guidelines are not consistent concerning the recommendation which nodules should be biopsied [9, 9a, 10, 10a, 12, 76, 79]. The European thyroid association recommends fine-needle aspiration of every thyroid nodule >1 cm and of every smaller suspicious nodule in ultrasound, and reserves thyroid scintigraphy for patients with low TSH or multinodular goiter. The American thyroid association [10] recommends FNAB of nodules >1–1.5 cm and reserves thyroid scintigraphy for patients with low TSH too. Other guidelines advocate the selection of nodules for biopsy on the basis of additional suspicious sonographic criteria [12]. In addition to these recommendations, one has to bear in mind that inconclusive results of FNAB occur in 3–33% and require repeat FNAB [14–16]. More recent literature expands the recommendation of fine-needle biopsy on nodules <1 cm [31]. In a country with long-standing iodine deficiency, FNAB to such an extent as recommended by guidelines would be impossible and not reasonable: under the hypothesis that all patients with such nodules would undergo FNAB and that sensitivity and specificity of cytology were 85%, the positive predictive value of a pathologic cytologic finding will reach 1.5% only according to the Bayes-theorem. This is clinically unacceptable and points towards the limited practicability of guidelines [4]. These conclusions are supported by an earlier publication of Raber et al.: under routine conditions of a teaching hospital in Austria, 2,071 cold thyroid nodules were diagnosed and evaluated by 49 doctors and 33 pathologists between 1975 and 1995. Only 47.3% of the fine-needle biopsies resulted in a conclusive diagnosis. The positive predictive value of a suspicious fine-needle biopsy for thyroid cancer was 35% only. A normal cytological result missed thyroid cancer in 15% [32]. Other support of the limited value of FNAB came from a literature review of Tee et al.: the authors analyzed the available literature and identified 12 studies with altogether 54,415 patients from 1966 until 2005 and concluded that FNAB missed one third of thyroid carcinomas [33]. As a consequence, preselection of thyroid nodules for FNAB is required to increase the pretest probability to at least 5–10%. A combination of sonographic criteria and scintigraphy, even in patients with normal TSH levels, is suited to select thyroid nodules for FNAB. In this scenario, Tc-99m-MIBI has gained increasing interest in the past years.

Tc-99m-MIBI has been used as a tumor imaging agent including the detection and localization of thyroid carcinomas for many years (e.g., papillary, follicular, Hürthle cell or medullary thyroid carcinomas, lymphoma) [34–36]. The clinical value of Tc-99m-MIBI as a tumor imaging agent lies in the fact that increased uptake in cold/hypofunctioning thyroid nodules (Mismatch between pertechnetate and Tc-99m-MIBI scan) increases the likelihood of malignancy while low uptake (Match between pertechnetate and Tc-99m-MIBI scan) excludes thyroid malignancies with a very high negative predictive value of >97% [8]. Hurtado-López summarized nine publications with 448 patients and reported on a negative predictive value of 100%. Further literature research identified additional publications [19, 24] with few false-negative results, that is, MIBI-negative in patients with differentiated thyroid cancer after operation. Our own data [27] included only one false-negative patient, in whom a papillary microcarcinoma was missed. Even in the light of the few false-negative patients in whom Tc-99m-MIBI was negative despite a thyroid carcinoma was identified after operation, the high negative-predictive value (>97%) of a negative Tc-99m-MIBI scan is clinically important and is an additional parameter to justify a conservative and nonsurgical management. In addition and in contrast, the positive predictive value of about 20% [27] of a pathological Tc-99m-MIBI scan for identification of a patient with a differentiated thyroid carcinoma is clinically helpful and relevant because it raises the likelihood of thyroid carcinoma to a level that surgery can be justified in analogy to the cytological diagnosis of follicular proliferation, having about the same positive predictive value for thyroid carcinoma as a positive Tc-99m-MIBI scan. However, the positive predictive value is dependent on the prevalence of thyroid malignancies of the patient population studied [37].

In conclusion, based on the available literature and our own institutional experience, Tc-99m-MIBI is a valuable method for further evaluation of (on pertechnetate scintigraphy) cold thyroid nodules, especially if the nodule is not easily amenable to fine needle aspiration biopsy (= FNAB) and/or FNAB is equivocal. There are at least 12 publications from 1993 to 2009 with more than 600 patients demonstrating the clinical usefulness for evaluation of thyroid nodules against the histopathological "golden standard" justifying the above-mentioned indications [8, 27]. The main finding is that a negative Tc-99m-MIBI excludes a malignant thyroid tumor. Apart from the evaluation of cold thyroid nodules, this technique is of special interest in nodules which are not easy to reach by FNAB and in multinodular goiter if patients do not want multiple or serial FNAB. It is the author´s opinion that the results of the publications and the many years of experience from different groups justify the use of Tc-99m-MIBI for thyroid imaging though to the author's knowledge no commercially available Tc-99m-MIBI kit has official approval for this indication at the time of writ

7 Tc-99m-MIBI for Thyroid Imaging

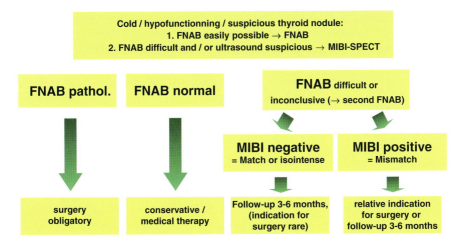

Fig. 7.2 Algorithm for management of cold/hypofunctioning thyroid nodule (reproduction with permission from Lehmanns Media [81])

ing this chapter. Figure 7.2 provides an algorithm on how to include Tc-99m-MIBI scintigraphy in the evaluation of cold thyroid nodules [81]. SPECT gave incremental diagnostic information in about 34% of examinations.

7.3 F-18-FDG-PET

7.3.1 F-18-FDG-PET for Thyroid Nodule Imaging

F-18-FDG-PET for oncological imaging has gained widespread use in recent years. The detection of iodine-131-negative but F-18-FDG-positive thyroid carcinoma metastases is just one example. In individual indications, F-18-FDG-PET has been used for evaluation of a nodular goiter. In case of nondiagnostic fine-needle aspiration, F-18-FDG-PET has been evaluated for assessment of the dignity of cytologically indeterminate thyroid nodules. European and American algorithms for evaluation of thyroid nodular goiter address the importance of fine-needle aspiration cytology. Though this is an established diagnostic method especially for cold thyroid nodules, there are about 3–33% nondiagnostic results. Repeated FNAB may not solve this problem too. De Geus-Oei et al. examined prospectively 44 consecutive patients with F-18-FDG-PET before hemithyroidectomy who had nondiagnostic fine-needle aspiration cytology. They found seven differentiated thyroid carcinomas in six patients which were all FDG-positive. The negative predictive value was 100%. However, FDG was also trapped in 13 of 38 benign thyroid nodules. The pre-PET likelihood was 14% (6/44 patients) and the post-PET likelihood raised this value to 32% (6/19 patients). Using a hypothetical algorithm, which would include FDG-PET as a diagnostic method before thyroid operation, the number of futile operations could be reduced by 66% (25/38 patients). De Geus-Oei et al. concluded that F-18-FDG-PET is a useful diagnostic tool for preoperative evaluation of thyroid patients with inconclusive results of FNAB. However, de Geus-Oei et al. did not answer the question as to how to handle the high number of benign thyroid nodules accumulating F-18-FDG [38]. Sebastianes et al. came to similar conclusions on the basis of his 42 consecutive patients with nondiagnostic FNAB. All 11 patients with a thyroid carcinoma were F-18-FDG-positive (sensitivity 100%). The negative predictive value was 100% too. 12/31 patients with a benign nodular goiter did not accumulate F-18-FDG [39]. The difficult situation in this publication is the high number of benign thyroid nodules accumulating F-18-FDG, which was the case for 19/31 patients. Specificity was low with 38.7%. A hypothetical algorithm including F-18-FDG-PET would lower the number of futile thyroid operations by 39%, and F-18-FDG-PET would raise the likelihood for thyroid malignancy from 26.2%, pre-FDG-PET to 36.7% post-FDG-PET. Finally, results from Hales et al. should be mentioned with less favorable results for FDG-PET. However, only 15 patients were examined [40].

7.3.2 PET-Associated Incidental Positive Thyroid (PAINs)

F-18-FDG-PET is not routinely used for evaluation of the many thyroid nodules. Usually, the situation is vice versa, that is, while performing an oncological F-18-FDG-PET, a focus of abnormal F-18-FDG uptake is incidentally found in the thyroid. In patients undergoing F-18-FDG-PET for tumor staging, secondary F-18-FDG-positive malignancies are found with an incidence of 4–6% ["PET-associated incidental neoplasms" (= PAINs)] and about 27–44% of these foci are found in the thyroid. Thus, incidental foci in the thyroid are not an infrequent clinical problem [41]. In a systematic review Shie et al. examined the incidence of malignant findings in case of incidental pathological FDG-foci in the thyroid while performing an oncological F-18-FDG-PET. Shie et al. identified 18 studies between 1998 and 2007 with a total of 55,160 patients of whom 571 patients (1%) had a pathological FDG foci in the thyroid. Further diagnostic evaluation was performed in 322 patients. In 200 patients (62.1%) a benign and in 107 patients (33.2%) a malignant result was confirmed while 15 patients (4.7%) had no final diagnosis. Papillary thyroid carcinomas were the leading malignant diagnosis with 82.2%. Shie et al. concluded that a pathological F-18-FDG foci requires further evaluation bearing in mind the high number of malignant findings [42]. The publication also confirmed that a pathological F-18-FDG accumulation in the thyroid does not necessarily mean a malignant finding because benign thyroid adenomas accumulate F-18-FDG too [42–44].

7.4 Tc-99m-MIBI and Multidrug Resistance

Saggiorato et al. reported on the use of Tc-99m-MIBI imaging in the presurgical characterization of thyroid follicular neoplasms and the relationship to multidrug resistance protein expression. The aim of their study was to investigate the usefulness of visual and semiquantitative analyses of Tc-99m-MIBI scintigraphy for preoperatively characterizing thyroid nodules with indeterminate cytologic diagnoses, segregating in advance nononcocytic variants from those that are oncocytic, which would help to increase the specificity of Tc-99m-MIBI for separating benign from malignant thyroid nodules. This study also aimed to analyze the relationship between Tc-99m-MIBI images and P-glycoprotein (P-gp)/multidrug resistance-associated protein-1 (MRP1) immunohistochemical expression. Fifty-one consecutive patients with cold thyroid nodules cytologically diagnosed as nononcocytic or oncocytic follicular neoplasm were prospectively studied. Visual and semiquantitative Tc-99m-MIBI scanning was performed and the diagnoses of the lesions were histologically proven by subsequent thyroidectomy. Immunohistochemical evaluation of P-gp and MRP1 was also performed on surgical samples. Visual and semiquantitative Tc-99m-MIBI scintiscans showed a low specificity in preoperatively discriminating malignant oncocytic lesions. In nononcocytic nodules, the semiquantitative method was more accurate than the visual (94.44% and 77.78%, respectively). P-gp protein expression was negative in all thyroid lesions, whereas apical plasma membrane MRP1 expression was found in 78% of the lesions with a negative Tc-99m-MIBI retention index, compared with 11% of lesions with a positive retention index, correlating most strongly with a negative Tc-99m-MIBI retention index in those cases with strong MRP1 apical expression. Saggiorato et al. concluded that semiquantitative Tc-99m-MIBI scintigraphy is an adjunctive method to predict preoperatively the malignant behavior of nononcocytic follicular thyroid nodules indeterminate at FNAB, with a potential impact on the definition of their clinical management. Moreover, the good correlation found between immunohistochemical apical expression of MRP1 and the scintigraphic findings supported the Tc-99m-MIBI results and provided tissue information on the molecular mechanisms responsible for Tc-99m-MIBI images in thyroid lesions. Furthermore, the authors provided an algorithm combining Tc-99m-MIBI scintigraphy with molecular markers (Galectin-3, Cytokeratin 19 and cell surface mesothelial antigen HBME-1) to decide between thyroidectomy and clinical follow-up [45]. Further prospective studies are needed to clarify the clinical usefulness of such an algorithm.

7.5 Tc-99m-MIBI and Amiodarone-Induced Thyrotoxicosis

In a review about Amiodarone-induced thyrotoxicosis by Piga and Serra et al., the authors summarized that Amiodarone, a potent class III antiarrhythmic drug, is an iodine-rich compound with a structural resemblance to thyroid hormones triiodothyronine (T3) and thyroxine (T4). At the commonly employed doses, Amiodarone causes iodine overload up to 50–100 times the optimal daily intake, which may be responsible for a spectrum of effects on thyroid function often counterbalancing its heart benefits. Although most patients on chronic AM treatment remain euthyroid, a consistent proportion may develop thyrotoxicosis (Amiodarone-induced thyrotoxicosis, AIT) or hypothyroidism. Amiodarone-induced thyrotoxicosis is more prevalent in iodine-deficient areas and is currently subdivided in two different clinicopathological forms (AIT I and AIT II). Amiodarone-induced thyrotoxicosis type I (AIT I) develops in subjects with underlying thyroid disease, and is caused by an exacerbation by iodine load of thyroid autonomous function while Amiodarone-induced thyrotoxicosis type II (AIT II) occurs in patients with no underlying thyroid disease and is probably consequent to a drug-induced destructive thyroiditis. Mixed or indeterminate forms of Amiodarone-induced thyrotoxicosis encompassing several features of both AIT I and AIT II may be also observed. The differential diagnosis between AIT I and AIT II (which is important for the choice of the appropriate therapy) is currently made on radioiodine uptake, which may be high, normal, or low but detectable in AIT I, while it is consistently very low or undetectable in AIT II and on color-flow Doppler sonography showing normal or increased vascularity in AIT I and absent vascularity in AIT II. Quite recently, studies carried out at the University of Cagliari, Italy, showed that Tc-99m-MIBI thyroid scintigraphy may represent the best single test to differentiate AIT I (showing increased MIBI retention) from AIT II (displaying no significant uptake) [46]. Piga et al. examined 20 patients and found that a positive Tc-99m-MIBI uptake was detected in all patients with a final diagnosis of Amiodarone-induced thyrotoxicosis type I (AIT I, $n=6$) or an indefinite form of AIT (AIT Ind, $n=4$), while it was absent in all patients affected by Amiodarone-induced thyrotoxicosis type II (AIT II, $n=10$). Patients with an indefinite form of AIT showed low, patchy, and persistent uptake in two cases and in the other two evident MIBI uptake followed by a rapid washout. Tc-99m-MIBI scintigraphy was superior to all other diagnostic tools, including thyroid color-flow Doppler sonography or thyroid radioiodine uptake, which was measurable in all patients with AIT I, and also in 4 out of the 10 patients with AIT II. Piga et al. concluded that thyroid Tc-99m-MIBI scintigraphy may be proposed as an easy and highly effective tool for the differential diagnosis of different forms of Amiodarone-induced thyrotoxicosis [47].

7.6 Thyroid Carcinoma

In Germany, there is an estimated prevalence of 15 million thyroid nodules [3, 4] with an estimated risk of malignancy of about 1:1,000 nodules [3, 80]. About 6,000 patients are diagnosed with thyroid cancer each year in Germany with about 3,500 women and 1,500 men being affected [72]. In the United States approximately 44670 new cases of thyroid cancer were diagnosed in 2010 [83]. Clinical risk factors for thyroid cancer include age <20 or age >60 years, previous head and neck irradiation, male gender and a positive family history (for multiple endocrine neoplasia type II or Cowden syndrome). Early clinical signs do not exist and rapid thyroid nodule growth, fixed thyroid node, lymph node involvement, vocal cord paralysis or the presence of distant metastases indicate advanced disease. There is a broad spectrum of biological behavior in thyroid cancer ranging from very slow growth over years in differentiated thyroid carcinoma to rapid progressive disease in anaplastic thyroid cancer usually being fatal within a few months after diagnosis. Except for papillary thyroid carcinomas pT1 <1 cm in diameter, for whom operation alone is considered as adequate treatment, patients with differentiated

7 Tc-99m-MIBI for Thyroid Imaging

thyroid carcinoma usually undergo thyroidectomy followed by radioiodine ablation. Most patients with a diagnosis of differentiated thyroid carcinoma can be cured and long-term prognosis is usually excellent [48] with 10-year survival rates above 90%. Surveillance includes neck ultrasound and thyroglobuline measurements. Less than 10% of patients with a diagnosis of thyroid carcinoma develop recurrent disease during follow-up. Most metastases are located in cervical or upper mediastinal lymph nodes. Pulmonary or osteomedullary metastases are the most frequent distant metastatic sites while liver or brain metastases are rare. Usually, the earliest suspicion of recurrent disease comes from an elevated thyroglobuline level. Further diagnostic work-up usually includes I-131-whole body scintigraphy under either rhTSH stimulation or in hypothyroidism to detect iodine-131-positive metastases. Patients with elevated thyroglobuline levels but negative iodine-131-whole body scintigraphy require further evaluation in order to detect iodine-negative metastases. Nowadays, usually F-18-FDG-PET is used for this purpose. Thus, iodine-131 whole body scintigraphy and F-18-FDG-PET in combination aim to detect thyroid carcinoma metastases with different degrees of differentiation – named "flip-flop-phenomenon." However, this is not a strict separation as metastases may accumulate either radiopharmaceutical.

7.6.1 Tc-99m-MIBI for Detection of Radioiodine-Negative Metastases

There exist a number of publications reporting on the use of either planar or SPECT imaging with Tc-99m-MIBI for detection of recurrent disease after a diagnosis of differentiated thyroid cancer and rising thyroglobuline levels. It was the aim to detect iodine-131-negative thyroid carcinoma metastases. Briele et al. were among the first to compare the diagnostic performance of Tl-201 and Tc-99m-MIBI in patients with suspected recurrence of differentiated thyroid carcinoma. Except in one case, the findings concerning tumor localization and extension were identical in the 12 patients examined. In all cases, locoregional lymph node metastases as well as osseous metastases were imaged by Tl-201 and Tc-99m-MIBI scintigraphy. However, the sensitivity of the two methods was relatively low in the detection of pulmonary metastases which were imaged in 1 out of 3 patients only. Discrepancies between Tl-201 and Tc-99m-MIBI were observed in a case of axillary lymph node metastasis. Although tumor-/background ratios were slightly higher for Tl-201, Tc-99m-MIBI SPECT showed a higher imaging quality compared to Tl-201 SPECT, especially in deeply situated tumor lesions. Briele et al. concluded that Tc-99m-MIBI seems to be a promising alternative imaging agent in the follow-up of differentiated thyroid carcinomas [49]. Tc-99m-MIBI does not replace radioiodine whole-body scintigraphy but is used for detection of radioiodine-negative recurrences or metastases [50]. Table 7.3 compiles publications providing information about the ability of Tc-99m-MIBI to detect thyroid carcinoma metastases. One advantage over F-18-FDG-PET lies in the fact that patients need not have hypothyroidism or under rhTSH stimulation using Tc-99m-MIBI while it has been documented that F-18-FDG-PET

Table 7.3 Tc-99m-MIBI for detection of iodine-negative (recurrent) thyroid carcinoma

First author, year	Patient number	Sensitivity (%)	Specificity (%)	Accuracy (%)
Dadparvar 1995 [51]	34	36[a]	89[a]	69[a]
Uğur 1996 [84]	36	50[b]	88[b]	67[b]
Němec 1996 [52]	200	81–100[c]	71–99[b]	78–99[c]
Grünwald 1997 [53]	44	100[d]	71[d]	85[d]
Alam 1998 [30]	68	78–94[e]	91–100[e]	–/–
Seabold 1999 [54]	54	53	100	69
Rubello 2000 [55]	122	86–100[f]	100[f]	–/–
Iwata 2004 [56]	19	63	–/–	–/–
Fujie 2005 [57]	36	44[g]	99[g]	85[g]
Küçük 2006 [61]	19	63	–/–	–/–
Ronga 2007 [58]	84	76(–100)[h]	–/–	–/–

[a]Dadparvar [51]: Sensitivity, specificity, and diagnostic accuracy for post-^{131}I-Na ablation patients

[b]Uğur 1996 [84]: Sensitivity, specificity, and diagnostic accuracy for 18 post-^{131}I-Na ablation patients

[c]Němec [52]: Range due to differences between tumor recurrence in the neck, pulmonary, and bone metastases

[d]Grünwald [53]: Data extracted from Table 7.2: TP 12, TN 10, FP 4, FN 0

[e]Alam [30]: Sensitivity and specificity on a lesion basis for neck, lung, and bone

[f]Rubello [55]: Group 1 comprising 122 patients with high thyroglobuline levels and negative iodine-131 scintigraphy provided data for calculation of sensitivity (94% for cervical metastases, 100% for mediastinal metastases, 100% for pulmonary metastases and 86% for bone metastases) and Group 2 with 27 disease-free patient were taken for calculation of specificity

[g]Fujie [57]: Results of diagnostic studies after iodine-131 ablation for patients with thyroid carcinoma

[h]Ronga [58]: Group A ($n=50$) with iodine-131 positive metastases and Group B ($n=34$) with iodine-131-negative metastases. Iodine-131-negative metastases had sensitivities of 82% for local recurrence, 100% for cervical and mediastinal nodes and bone metastases, and 75% for nodular lung metastases, while all miliaric lung metastases were missed

is more sensitive in hypothyroidism or under rhTSH stimulation in comparison to TSH suppression. However, Tc-99m-MIBI is less sensitive than F-18-FDG-PET for detection of thyroid carcinoma metastases [53, 59]. As a rare phenomenon there exists a case report about a patient with recurrent poorly differentiated insular carcinoma being iodine-131- and Tc-99m-MIBI positive but FDG-negative [60]. There exists a wide range for sensitivity and specificity for Tc-99m-MIBI to detect metastatic thyroid carcinoma tissue, which depends on the location and size of the metastases. While Tc-99m-MIBI has fairly high sensitivities for the detection of local cervical recurrence and bone metastases, pulmonary metastases may be missed by Tc-99m-MIBI [61]. Němec et al. reported on sensitivities for detecting tumor tissue in the neck of 81%, pulmonary metastases of 95% and bone metastases of 100% [52]. Alam et al. found a higher sensitivity for neck lesions of 94% but lower for lung lesions with 78% [30], and Fujie reported about a sensitivity for detecting pulmonary metastases of 30% only [57]. Ronga et al. were able to detect nodular lung metastases but missed all cases with miliary lung involvement using Tc-99m-MIBI [58]. Therefore, lung computed tomography may be used for identification

7 Tc-99m-MIBI for Thyroid Imaging

of iodine-negative pulmonary metastases. Comparing Tc-99m-MIBI with Tl-201-chloride as another nonspecific tumor imaging radiopharmaceutical, the overall diagnostic results were about the same [54] while Tl-201 has the higher patient radiation exposure. Dadparvar et al. found 97% concordance between Tl-201 and Tc-99m-MIBI studies for postablation patients and both methods were especially valuable when iodine-131 whole body examinations were negative [51]. Dadparvar et al. concluded that the results of iodine-131 scintigraphy were significantly better than those of Tc-99m-MIBI imaging in the detection of thyroid carcinoma in pre- and post-iodine-131-ablation patients and recommended that iodine-131 scintigraphy and serum thyroglobulin estimation be the primary studies performed on both pre- and postablation patients. If the iodine-131 study is negative and the quantitative thyroglobulin level is elevated, and/or there is a high clinical suspicion for the presence of thyroid cancer, Tc-99m-MIBI or Tl-201 chloride scintigraphy could be used as an alternative diagnostic tool. The combination of ^{131}I-Na scintigraphy with serum thyroglobulin and Tc-99m-MIBI or a Tl-201 scintigraphy offered the highest diagnostic yield [51]. From the present point of view, Tl-201 is a historical radiopharmaceutical for tumor imaging. As F-18-FDG-PET is superior for detection of iodine-131-negative thyroid carcinoma, metastases Tc-99m-MIBI may be reserved for situations when F-18-FDG-PET is unavailable.

7.6.2 Head to Head Comparison Tc-99m-MIBI Versus FDG-PET

As early as in 1999, Grünwald et al. summarized the clinical impact of functional imaging with tracers besides radioiodine. In direct comparison, FDG-PET had the highest sensitivity exceeding 80% in cases with negative whole body scintigraphy. Thus, FDG-PET should be considered in all patients suffering from differentiated thyroid cancer with suspected recurrence and/or metastases, particularly in cases with elevated thyroglobulin values and negative whole body scintigraphy [62].

Wu et al. compared FDG-PET and Tc-99m-MIBI for their ability to detect metastatic cervical lymph nodes in 15 patients with a diagnosis of well-differentiated thyroid carcinoma after total thyroidectomy and I-131 treatment. Patients had elevated serum human thyroglobulin levels, but negative I-131 whole body scan under TSH stimulation FDG-PET could detect all of the 15 (100%) patients with metastatic cervical lymph nodes, but Tc-99m MIBI-SPECT revealed lesions in only 9 out of 15 (60%) patients (p value <0.05) demonstrating that FDG-PET was more sensitive than Tc-99m MIBI SPECT in detecting metastatic cervical lymph nodes in radioiodine negative patients with elevated thyroglobulin levels [59].

Iwata et al. reported about the comparison of whole-body FDG-PET, Tc-99m-MIBI SPECT, and post-therapeutic I-131 scintigraphy under TSH stimulation for the detection of metastatic thyroid cancer in 19 patients with a total of 22 iodine-positive and ten iodine-negative lesions. FDG-PET was positive in 17 (78.3%) iodine-positive and in 9 (90.0%) iodine-negative lesions while Tc-99m-MIBI SPECT was only positive in 14 (63.6%) iodine-positive and in 6 (60.0%) iodine negative lesions. Comparison of FDG-PET with Tc-99m-MIBI SPECT revealed

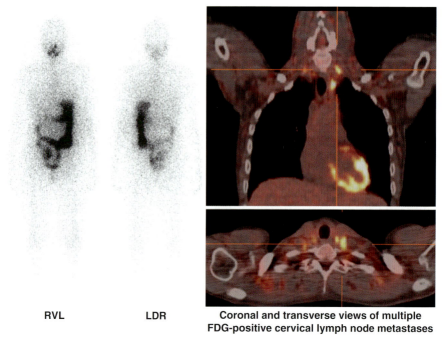

Fig. 7.3 A 33-year-old female patient with papillary thyroid cancer pT3 pN1 after operation and ablative radioiodine therapy [3.7 GBq I-131] with radioiodine negative whole-body scintigraphy and FDG-positive recurrent left cervical lymph node metastases histologically confirmed after subsequent surgery

concordant results in 24 lesions and discordant results in eight lesions (seven with positive FDG-PET alone and one with positive Tc-99m-MIBI SPECT alone). Thus, even using whole-body SPECT, FDG-PET was superior to Tc-99m-MIBI in terms of ability to detect metastases of differentiated thyroid cancer [56].

Figures 7.3–7.5 provide clinical examples of patients with radioiodine negative, FDG-PET positive cervical lymph node (Fig. 7.3), pulmonary and soft tissue (Fig. 7.4), and osteomedullary metastases (Fig. 7.5) visualizing the excellent combined metabolic and morphological information provided by FDG-PET-CT.

7.7 Tc-99m-MIBI for Imaging Medullary Thyroid Carcinoma

Kloos et al. (The American Thyroid Association Guidelines Task Force) published management guidelines for medullary thyroid cancer recently [63]. A number of diagnostic test are available for initial staging and from a nuclear medicine perspective more importantly in the search for metastatic disease in case of persistent or increasing calcitonin levels after operation [63, 64]. Thus, imaging methods include Penta-DMSA-SPECT, somatostatin receptor imaging including SPECT and PET somatostatin analogs, F-18-FDG PET and – if available – gastrin receptor imaging. Due to the rarity of a medullary thyroid carcinoma, tumor imaging methods are difficult to

7 Tc-99m-MIBI for Thyroid Imaging

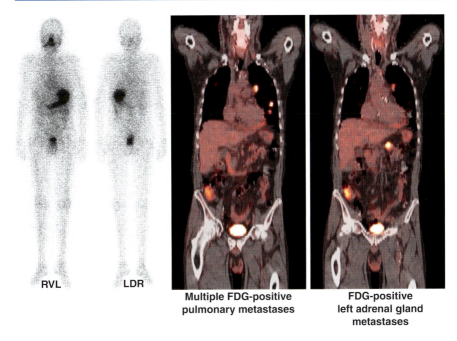

Fig. 7.4 A 62-year-old male patient with follicular thyroid cancer pT3 pN1 after operation, ablative radioiodine therapy and several high-dose radioiodine therapies [Σ 21,2 GBq I-131] with radioiodine negative whole-body scintigraphy and FDG-positive pulmonary metastases and right adrenal gland and pancreatic metastases – the latter two locations histologically confirmed by biopsy

compare and none of the methods provided brilliant results. Tc-99m-MIBI has been reported to have only a low sensitivity of about 25–47% for the detection of metastatic medullary thyroid carcinoma [65, 66]. Therefore, Tc-99m-MIBI SPECT can only be recommended in selected clinical situations. Tc-99m-MIBI SPECT is usually not useful for staging patients with medullary thyroid carcinoma and has limited success to detect recurrent metastatic disease in medullary thyroid carcinoma patients with raising calcitonin levels. The use of Tc-99m-MIBI to detect medullary thyroid carcinoma metastases is mainly based on case reports or small patient series [34, 67–71]. Roelants et al. reported the case of a MEN 2a patient with a history of medullary thyroid cancer treated by total thyroidectomy, who presented an increasing calcitonin level, suggesting tumor recurrence. Conventional radiographic and radionuclide imaging failed to localize the responsible lesions. A planar and tomographic (SPECT) Tc-99m-MIBI scan, performed in order to investigate a recent hyperparathyroidism, localized a parathyroid adenoma and revealed an abnormal uptake in the left lateral neck region, corresponding to apparently banal lymph nodes on magnetic resonance imaging. This abnormal uptake was also observed on a F-18-FDG positron emission tomography study and was proven to be an uptake in MTC lymph nodes metastases as confirmed by histopathologic analysis. Thus, Tc-99m-MIBI scintigraphy is potentially able to localize both parathyroid adenoma and recurrent medullary thyroid carcinoma at one and the same time, particularly in case of nondiagnostic conventional imaging

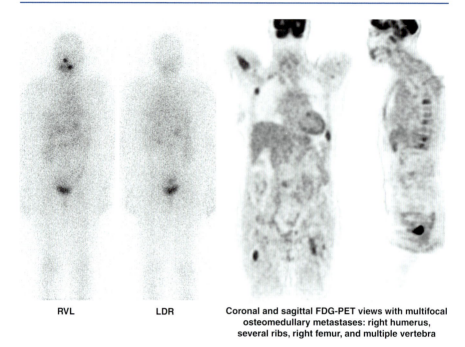

RVL LDR Coronal and sagittal FDG-PET views with multifocal osteomedullary metastases: right humerus, several ribs, right femur, and multiple vertebra

Fig. 7.5 A 68-year-old female patient with follicular thyroid cancer pT4 pN0 after operation, ablative radioiodine therapy, and subsequent high-dose radioiodine therapies [Σ 18,5 GBq I-131] with radioiodine negative whole-body scintigraphy and FDG-positive predominantly osteomedullary metastases

techniques [70]. Sato et al. reported on the detection of a hepatic metastasis from medullary thyroid cancer with Tc-99m-MIBI scintigraphy, negative in I-131-mIBG scintigraphy, in a 28-year-old male patient with Sipple's syndrome [71]. In a series of 14 patients, Adalet et al. reported on average sensitivities of 73% for Tl-201, 82% for Tc-99m(V)DMSA and 81% for Tc-99m-MIBI. Three patients were scanned with Tc-99m-tetrofosmin and two of four pathological foci as well as residual thyroid tissue were identified. The sensitivities of Tl-201, Tc-99m(V)DMSA, and Tc-99m-MIBI were 100%, 100%, and 85% in identifying lymphadenopathies; 40%, 50%, and 71% for soft tissue foci; 100% and 100% for foci in pulmonary parenchyma; and 100%, 66%, and 100% for recurrences in thyroid gland. Although Tc-99m(V)DMSA identified all bony metastases in three patients (100%), Tc-99m-MIBI detected only two of three foci (66%) and Tl-201 none. Tl-201, Tc-99m-MIBI, and Tc-99m-tetrofosmin accumulated in residual thyroid tissue, but Tc-99m(V)DMSA did not. Adalet et al. concluded that these agents were complementary, since they had different sensitivities in different tissues [67]. Learoyd et al. reported on the use of Tc-99m-MIBI for scanning ten patients with recurrent medullary thyroid carcinoma with 7/10 patients having at least one site of abnormal Tc-99m-MIBI uptake, however all of these patients had extremely high basal serum calcitonin values >6,000 ng/L [68].

7.8 Summary

The clinical usefulness of Tc-99m-MIBI in benign and malignant thyroid conditions is presented. Tc-99m-MIBI is a complex molecule of lipophilic cations and a nonspecific radiopharmaceutical for tumor imaging. It has become a clinically useful imaging technique for the assessment of cold/hypofunctioning thyroid nodules because of its high negative predictive value excluding malignant thyroid tumors. After injection of Tc-99m-MIBI, either a single-phase protocol with late planar and/or SPECT images about 1–2 h post injection or a double-phase protocol with early (about 15–30 min p.i.) and late images (about 2 h p.i.) can be used. Findings include a low, an isointense or an increased tracer accumulation in the thyroid nodule on late images in comparison to the paranodular thyroid tissue and in comparison to pertechnetate thyroid scintigraphy. A "Match" between pertechnetate and Tc-99m-MIBI scintigraphy is a concordantly decreased uptake in the thyroid nodule in comparison to the normal thyroid gland. This finding has a negative predictive value of >97% to exclude thyroid nodule malignancy. A definite "Mismatch" means a cold thyroid nodule on pertechnetate scintigraphy and an increased uptake of Tc-99m-MIBI in comparison to the MIBI-uptake of the paranodular thyroid tissue. The positive predictive value of this finding for malignancy varies between studies and is in the range of <10–65% depending on the prevalence of malignant thyroid tumors in the patient population studied. Another indication for Tc-99m-MIBI thyroid scintigraphy in benign thyroid conditions is the differentiation of Amiodarone-induced thyrotoxicosis type I from type II.

Concerning differentiated thyroid carcinomas, an indication of Tc-99m-MIBI scintigraphy is the search for recurrent tumor tissue in patients with iodine-negative differentiated thyroid carcinomas and usually positive thyroglobuline levels. However, this technique is inferior to FDG-PET and should be restricted to situations in which FDG-PET is unavailable. Case reports and small patient series exist about the clinical value of Tc-99m-MIBI to detect medullary thyroid carcinoma metastases with mostly reporting about low sensitivities so that this technique is only rarely indicated.

References

1. Hampel R, Bennöhr G, Gordalla A, Below H (2009) Jodidurie bei Erwachsenen in Deutschland 2005 im WHO-Zielbereich. Med Klin 104:425–428
2. Park HM (2006) The thyroid gland. In: Henkin RE, Bova D, Dillehay GL, Halama JR, Karesh SM, Wagner RH, Zimmer AM (eds) Nuclear medicine, 2nd edn. Mosby, Philadelphia, pp 790–819
3. Reiners C, Wegscheider K, Schicha H, Theissen P, Vaupel R, Wrbitzky R, Schumm-Draeger PM (2004) Prevalence of thyroid disorders in the working population of Germany: ultrasonography screening in 96,278 unselected employees. Thyroid 14:926–932
4. Schicha H, Hellmich M, Lehmacher W, Eschner W, Schmidt M, Kobe C, Schober O, Dietlein M (2009) Should all patients with thyroid nodules ≥1 cm undergo fine-needle aspiration biopsy? Nuklearmedizin 48:79–83

5. Dillehay GL (2006) Non-FDG tumor imaging. In: Henkin RE, Bova D, Dillehay GL, Halama JR, Karesh SM, Wagner RH, Zimmer AM (eds) Nuclear medicine, 2nd edn. Mosby, Philadelphia, pp 1443–1479
6. Szybiński Z, Huszno B, Gołkowski F, Atneisha A (1993) Technetium-99 m-methoxyisobutylisonitrile in early diagnosis of thyroid cancer. Endokrynol Pol 44:427–433
7. Földes I, Lévay A, Stotz G (1993) Comparative scanning of thyroid nodules with technetium-99 m pertechnetate and technetium-99 m methoxyisobutylisonitrile. Eur J Nucl Med 20:330–333
8. Hurtado-López LM, Martínez-Duncker C (2007) Negative MIBI thyroid scans exclude differentiated and medullary thyroid cancer in 100% of patients with hypofunctioning thyroid nodules. Eur J Nucl Med Mol Imaging 34:1701–1703
9. Pacini F, Schlumberger M, Dralle H, Elisei R, Smit JW, Wiersinga W, European Thyroid Cancer Taskforce (2006) European consensus for the management of patients with differentiated thyroid carcinoma of the follicular epithelium. Eur J Endocrinol 154:787–803
9a. Pacini F, Castagna MG, Brilli L, Pentheroudakis G (2009) ESMO Guidelines Working Group Differentiated thyroid cancer: ESMO clinical recommendations for diagnosis, treatment and follow-up. Ann Oncol 20 (Suppl 4): 143–146 http://www.ncbi.nlm.nih.gov/pubmed
10. Cooper DS, Doherty GM, Haugen BR, Kloos RT, Lee SL, Mandel SJ, Mazzaferri EL, McIver B, Sherman SI, Tuttle RM (2006) The American Thyroid Association Guidelines Taskforce Management guidelines for patients with thyroid nodules and differentiated thyroid cancer. Thyroid 16:109–142
10a. Cooper DS, Doherty GM, Haugen BR, Kloos RT, Lee SL, Mandel SJ, Mazzaferri EL, McIver B, Pacini F, Schlumberger M, Sherman SI, Steward DL, Tuttle RM (2009) American Thyroid Association (ATA) Guidelines Taskforce on Thyroid Nodules and Differentiated Thyroid Cancer Revised American Thyroid Association management guidelines for patients with thyroid nodules and differentiated thyroid cancer. Thyroid 19: 1167–1214 http://www.ncbi.nlm.nih.gov/pubmed/19860577
11. Rosen JE, Stone MD (2006) Contemporary diagnostic approach to the thyroid nodule. J Surg Oncol 94:649–661
12. Shirodkar M, Jabbour SA (2008) Endocrine incidentalomas. Int J Clin Pract 62:1423–1431
13. Yeung MJ, Serpell JW (2008) Management of the solitary thyroid nodule. Oncologist 13:105–112
14. Oertel YC, Miyahara-Felipe L, Mendoza MG, Yu K (2007) Value of repeated fine needle aspirations of the thyroid: an analysis of over ten thousand FNAs. Thyroid 17:1061–1066
15. Orija IB, Piñeyro M, Biscotti C, Reddy SS, Hamrahian AH (2007) Value of repeating a nondiagnostic thyroid fine-needle aspiration biopsy. Endocr Pract 13:735–742
16. Izquierdo R, Shankar R, Kort K, Khurana K (2009) Ultrasound-guided fine-needle aspiration in the management of thyroid nodules in children and adolescents. Thyroid 19:703–705
17. Theoharis CGA, Schofield KM, Hammers L, Udelsman R, Chhieng DC (2009) The Bethesda thyroid fine-needle aspiration classification system: year 1 at an academic institution. Thyroid 19:1215–1223
18. Chiu ML, Kronauge JF, Worms DP (1990) Effect of mitochondrial and plasma membrane potentials on accumulation of hexakis (2-methoxyisobutylisonitrile) technetium(I) in cultured mouse fibroblast. J Nucl Med 31:1646–1653
19. Sundram FX, Mack P (1995) Evaluation of thyroid nodules for malignancy using ^{99m}Tc-sestamibi. Nucl Med Commun 16:687–693
20. Kresnik E, Gallowitsch HJ, Mikosch P, Gomez I, Lind P (1997) Technetium-99 m-MIBI scintigraphy of thyroid nodules in an endemic goiter area. J Nucl Med 38:62–65
21. Alonso O, Mut F, Lago G, Aznarez A, Nunez M, Canepa J et al (1998) Tc-99 m-MIBI scanning of the thyroid gland in patients with markedly decreased pertechnetate uptake. Nucl Med Commun 19:257–261
22. Mezosi E, Bajnok L, Gyory F, Varga J, Sztojka I, Szabo J, Galuska L, Leovey A, Kakuk G, Nagy E (1999) The role of technetium-99 m methoxyisobutylisonitrile scintigraphy in the differential diagnosis of cold thyroid nodules. Eur J Nucl Med 26:798–803

7 Tc-99m-MIBI for Thyroid Imaging

23. Erdil TY, Ozker K, Kabasakal L, Kanmaz B, Sönmezoglu K, Atasoy KC, Turoglu HT, Uslu I, Isitman AT, Onsel C (2000) Correlation of technetium-99 m MIBI and thallium-201 retention in solitary cold thyroid nodules with postoperative histopathology. Eur J Nucl Med 27:713–720

24. Sathekge MM, Mageza RB, Muthuphei MN, Modiba MC, Clauss RC (2001) Evaluation of thyroid nodules with technetium-99 m MIBI and technetium-99 m pertechnetate. Head Neck 23:305–310

25. Demirel K, Kapucu O, Yücel C, Ozdemir H, Ayvaz G, Taneri F (2003) A comparison of radionuclide thyroid angiography, (99 m)Tc-MIBI scintigraphy and power Doppler ultrasonography in the differential diagnosis of solitary cold thyroid nodules. Eur J Nucl Med Mol Imaging 30:642–650

26. Hurtado-López LM, Arellano-Montaño S, Torres-Acosta EM, Zaldivar-Ramirez FR, Duarte-Torres RM, Alonso-De-Ruiz P, Martínez-Duncker I, Martínez-Duncker C (2004) Combined use of fine-needle aspiration biopsy, MIBI scans and frozen section biopsy offers the best diagnostic accuracy in the assessment of the hypofunctioning solitary thyroid nodule. Eur J Nucl Med Mol Imaging 31:1273–1279

27. Theissen P, Schmidt M, Ivanova T, Dietlein M, Schicha H (2009) MIBI scintigraphy in hypofunctioning thyroid nodules – Can it predict the dignity of the lesion? Nuklearmedizin 48:144–152

28. Sharma R, Mondal A, Shankar LR, Sahoo M, Bhatnagar P, Sawroop K, Chopra MK, Kashyap R (2004) Differentiation of malignant and benign solitary thyroid nodules using 30- and 120-minute Tc-99 m MIBI scans. Clin Nucl Med 29:534–537

29. Schmidt M, Thoma N, Dietlein M, Moka D, Eschner W, Faust M, Schröder W, von Hülst-Schlabrendorff M, Ehses W, Schicha H (2008) ^{99m}Tc-MIBI SPECT in primary hyperparathyroidism – Influence of concomitant vitamin D deficiency for visualization of parathyroid adenomas. Nuklearmedizin 47:1–7

30. Alam MDS, Kasagi K, Misaki T, Miyamoto S, Iwata M, Iida Y, Konishi J (1998) Diagnostic value of technetium-99 m methoxyisobutyl I sonitrile (^{99m}Tc-MIBI) scintigraphy in detecting thyroid cancer metastases: a critical evaluation. Thyroid 8:1091–1100

31. Berker D, Aydin Y, Ustun I, Gul K, Tutuncu Y, Işik S, Delibasi T, Guler S (2008) The value of fine-needle aspiration biopsy in subcentimeter thyroid nodules. Thyroid 18:603–608

32. Raber W, Kmen E, Kaserer K, Waldhäusl W, Vierhapper H (1997) Der kalte knoten der Schilddrüse: 20jährige Erfahrungen mit 2071 Patienten und diagnostische Grenzen der Feinnadelbiopsie. Wien Klein Wochenschr 109/4:116–122

33. Tee YY, Lowe AJ, Brand CA, Judson RT (2007) Fine-needle aspiration may miss a third of all malignancy in palpable thyroid nodules: a comprehensive literature review. Ann Surg 246:714–720

34. O'Driscoll CM, Baker F, Casey MJ et al (1991) Localization of recurrent medullary thyroid carcinoma with technetium-99 m-methoxyisobutylnitrile scintigraphy: a case report. J Nucl Med 32:2281–2283

35. Balon HR, Fink-Bennett D, Stoffer SS (1992) Technetium-99 m-sestamibi uptake by recurrent Hurthle cell carcinoma of the thyroid. J Nucl Med 33:1393–1395

36. Scott AM, Kostakoglu L, O'Brien JP et al (1992) Comparison of technetium-99 m-MIBI and thallium-201-chloride uptake in primary thyroid lymphoma. J Nucl Med 33:1396–1398

37. Schmidt M, Schicha H (2010) MIBI-SPECT in hypofunctioning thyroid nodules for detection of thyroid carcinoma [MIBI-SPECT bei kalten Knoten zur Schilddrüsenkarzinomdetektion]. Nuklearmediziner 33:214–221

38. De Geus-Oei LF, Pieters GF, Bonenkamp JJ, Mudde AH, Bleeker-Rovers CP, Corstens FH, Oyen WJ (2006) 18F-FDG PET reduces unnecessary hemithyroidectomies for thyroid nodules with inconclusive cytologic results. J Nucl Med 47:770–775

39. Sebastianes FM, Cerci JJ, Zanoni PH, Soares J Jr, Chibana LK, Tomimori EK, de Camargo RY, Izaki M, Giorgi MC, Eluf-Neto J, Meneghetti JC, Pereira MA (2007) Role of 18 F-fluorodeoxyglucose positron emission tomography in preoperative assessment of cytologically indeterminate thyroid nodules. J Clin Endocrinol Metab 92:4485–4488

40. Hales NW, Krempl GA, Medina JE (2008) Is there a role for fluorodeoxyglucose positron emission tomography/computed tomography in cytologically indeterminate thyroid nodules? Am J Otolaryngol 29:113–118

41. Katz SC, Shaha A (2008) PET-associated incidental neoplasms of the thyroid. J Am Coll Surg 207:259–264
42. Shie P, Cardarelli R, Sprawls K, Fulda KG, Taur A (2009) Systematic review: prevalence of malignant incidental thyroid nodules identified on fluorine-18 fluorodeoxyglucose positron emission tomography. Nucl Med Commun 30:742–748
43. Börner AR, Voth E, Theissen P, Wienhard K, Wagner R, Schicha H (2000) Glucose metabolism of the thyroid in autonomous goiter measured by F-18-FDG-PET. Exp Clin Endocrinol Diabetes 108:191–196
44. Gianoukakis AG, Karam M, Cheema A, Cooper JA (2003) Autonomous thyroid nodules visualized by positron emission tomography with 18 F-fluorodeoxyglucose: a case report and review of the literature. Thyroid 13:395–399
45. Saggiorato E, Angusti T, Rosas R, Martinese M, Finessi M, Arecco F, Trevisiol E, Bergero N, Puligheddu B, Volante M, Podio V, Papotti M, Orlandi F (2009) ^{99m}Tc-MIBI imaging in the presurgical characterization of thyroid follicular neoplasms: relationship to multidrug resistance protein expression. J Nucl Med 50:1785–1793
46. Piga M, Serra A, Boi F, Tanda ML, Martino E, Mariotti S (2008) Amiodarone-induced thyrotoxicosis. A review. Minerva Endocrinol 33:213–228
47. Piga M, Cocco MC, Serra A, Boi F, Loy M, Mariotti S (2008) The usefulness of 99mTc-sestaMIBI thyroid scan in the differential diagnosis and management of amiodarone-induced thyrotoxicosis. Eur J Endocrinol 159:423–429
48. Verburg FA, Stokkel MP, Düren C, Verkooijen RB, Mäder U, van Isselt JW, Marlowe RJ, Smit JW, Reiners C, Luster M (2010) No survival difference after successful (131)I ablation between patients with initially low-risk and high-risk differentiated thyroid cancer. Eur J Nucl Med Mol Imaging 37:276–283
49. Briele B, Hotze A, Kropp J, Bockisch A, Overbeck B, Grünwald F, Kaiser W, Biersack HJ (1991) Vergleich von 201Tl und 99mTc-MIBI in der Nachsorge des differenzierten Schilddrüsenkarzinoms [A comparison of 201Tl and 99mTc-MIBI in the follow-up of differentiated thyroid carcinomas]. Nuklearmedizin 30:115–124
50. Dietlein M, Scheidhauer K, Voth E, Theissen P, Schicha H (1998) Follow-up of differentiated thyroid cancer: What is the value of FDG and sestamibi in the diagnostic algorithm? Nuklearmedizin 37:12–17
51. Dadparvar S, Chevres A, Tulchinsky M, Krishna-Badrinath L, Khan AS, Slizofski WJ (1995) Clinical utility of technetium-99 m methoxyisobutylisonitrile imaging in differentiated thyroid carcinoma: comparison with thallium-201 and iodine-131 Na scintigraphy, and serum thyroglobulin quantitation. Eur J Nucl Med 22:1330–1338
52. Němec J, Nývltová O, Blazek T, Vlcek P, Racek P, Novák Z, Preiningerová M, Hubáčková M, Krízo M, Zimák J, Bílek R (1996) Positive thyroid cancer scintigraphy using technetium-99 m methoxyisobutylisonitrile. Eur J Nucl Med 23:69–71
53. Grünwald F, Menzel C, Bender H, Palmedo H, Willkomm P, Ruhlmann J, Franckson T, Biersack HJ (1997) Comparison of ^{18}FDG-PET with ^{131}iodine and ^{99m}Tc-sestamibi scintigraphy in differentiated thyroid cancer. Thyroid 7:327–335
54. Seabold JE, Gurll N, Schurrer ME, Aktay R, Kirchner PT (1999) Comparison of ^{99m}Tc-methoxy-isobutylisonitrile and ^{201}Tl-scintigraphy for detection of residual thyroid cancer after ^{131}I ablative therapy. J Nucl Med 40:1434–1440
55. Rubello D, Mazzarotto R, Casara D (2000) The role of technetium-99 m methoxyisobutylisonitrile scintigraphy in the planning of therapy and follow-up of patients with differentiated thyroid carcinoma after surgery. Eur J Nucl Med 27:431–440
56. Iwata M, Kasagi K, Misaki T, Matsumoto K, Iida Y, Ishimori T, Nakamoto Y, Higashi T, Saga T, Konishi J (2004) Comparison of whole-body ^{18}F-FDG PET, ^{99m}Tc-MIBI SPET, and post-therapeutic ^{131}I-Na scintigraphy in the detection of metastatic thyroid cancer. Eur J Nucl Med Mol Imaging 31:491–498
57. Fujie S, Okumura Y, Sato S, Akaki S, Katsui K, Himei K, Takemoto M, Kanazawa S (2005) Diagnostic capabilities of I-131, TI-201, and Tc-99 m-MIBI scintigraphy for metastatic differentiated thyroid carcinoma after total thyroidectomy. Acta Med Okayama 59:99–107

58. Ronga G, Ventroni G, Montesano T, Filesi M, Ciancamerla M, Di Nicola AD, Travascio L, Vestri AR, Signore A (2007) Sensitivity of [99mTc]methoxyisobutylisonitrile scan in patients with metastatic differentiated thyroid cancer. Q J Nucl Med Mol Imaging 51:364–371

59. Wu HS, Huang WS, Liu YC, Yen RF, Shen YY, Kao CH (2003) Comparison of FDG-PET and technetium-99 m MIBI SPECT to detect metastatic cervical lymph nodes in well-differentiated thyroid carcinoma with elevated serum HTG but negative I-131 whole body scan. Anticancer Res 23:4235–4238

60. Zetting G, Leitha T, Niederle B, Kaserer K, Becherer A, Kletter K, Dudczak R (2001) FDG positron emission tomographic, radioiodine, and MIBI imaging in a patient with poorly differentiated insular thyroid carcinoma. Clin Nucl Med 26:599–601

61. Küçük ON, Gültekin SS, Aras G, Ibiş E (2006) Radioiodine whole-body scans, thyroglobulin levels, 99mTc-MIBI scans and computed tomography: results in patients with lung metastases from differentiated thyroid cancer. Nucl Med Commun 27:261–266

62. Grünwald F, Briele B, Biersack HJ (1999) Non-131I-scintigraphy in the treatment and follow-up of thyroid cancer. Single-photon-emitters or FDG-PET? Q J Nucl Med 43:195–206

63. Kloos RT, Eng C, Evans DB, Francis GL, Gagel RF, Gharib H, Moley JF, Pacini F, Ringel MD, Schlumberger M, Wells SA, The American Thyroid Association Guidelines Task Force (2009) Medullary thyroid cancer: management guidelines of the American Thyroid Association. Thyroid 19:565–612

64. Schmidt M, Eschner W, Dietlein M, Theissen P, Schicha H (2005) Konventionelle nuklearmedizinische Tumordiagnostik (Tumor-SPECT): Was ist angesichts von 18F-FDG-PT noch aktuell? [Established nuclear medicine techniques for tumour diagnosis (tumour SPECT): Can they still compete with 18F-FDG-PET?]. Nuklearmedizin 44:37–48

65. Ugur O, Kostakğlu L, Güler N, Caner B, Uysal U, Elahi N, Haliloğlu M, Yüksel D, Aras T, Bayhan H, Bekdik C (1996) Comparison of 99mTc(V)-DMSA, 201Tl and 99mTc-MIBI imaging in the follow-up of patients with medullary carcinoma of the thyroid. Eur J Nucl Med 23:1367–1371

66. Diehl M, Risse JH, Brandt-Mainz K, Dietlein M, Bohuslavizki KH, Matheja P, Lange H, Bredow J, Körber C, Grünwald F (2001) Fluorine-18 fluorodeoxyglucose positron emission tomography in medullary thyroid cancer: results of a multicentre study. Eur J Nucl Med 28:1671–1676

67. Adalet I, Koçak M, Oğüz H, Alagöl F, Cantez S (1999) Determination of medullary thyroid carcinoma metastases by 201Tl, 99mTc(V)DMSA, 99mTc-MIBI and 99mTc-tetrofosmin. Nucl Med Commun 20:353–359

68. Learoyd DL, Roach PJ, Briggs GM, Delbridge LW, Wilmshurst EG, Robinson BG (1997) Technetium-99 m-sestamibi scanning in recurrent medullary thyroid carcinoma. J Nucl Med 38:227–230

69. Lebouthillier G, Morais J, Picard M, Picard D, Chartrand R, D'Amour P (1993) Tc-99 m sestamibi and other agents in the detection of metastatic medullary carcinoma of the thyroid. Clin Nucl Med 18:657–661

70. Roelants V, Michel L, Lonneux M, Lacrosse M, Delgrange E, Donckier JE (2001) Usefulness of [99mTc]MIBI and [18F]fluorodeoxyglucose for imaging recurrent medullary thyroid cancer and hyperparathyroidism in MEN 2a syndrome. Acta Clin Belg 56:373–377

71. Sato S, Okumura Y, Tamizu A, Maki K, Akaki S, Takeda Y, Kanazawa S, Hiraki Y (2001) Detection of hepatic metastasis from medullary thyroid cancer with Tc-99 m-MIBI scintigraphy in a patient with Sipple's syndrome. Ann Nucl Med 15:443–446

72. Bertz J, Kraywinkel K (Robert Koch-Institut - Hrsg.) (2010) Verbreitung von Krebserkrankungen in Deutschland. Entwicklung der Prävalenzen zwischen 1990 und 2010. Beiträge zur Gesundheitsberichterstattung des Bundes. [Incidence and prevalence of cancer in Germany between 1990 and 2010. Federal health reports] Robert Koch-Institut, Berlin, pp 124–131

73. Dietlein M, Dressler J, Grünwald F, Joseph K, Leisner B, Moser E, Reiners C, Rendl J, Schicha H, Schneider P, Schober O (2003) Deutsche Gesellschaft für Nuklearmedizin. Leitlinie zur Schilddrüsendiagnostik (Version 2) [Guideline for in vivo- and in vitro procedures for thyroid diseases (version 2)]. Nuklearmedizin 42:109–115

74. Dietlein M, Kobe C, Schmidt M, Schicha H (2005) Das Inzidentalom der Schilddrüse: Über- oder Unterdiagnostik eines epidemiologischen Befundes? Nuklearmedizin 44:213–224

75. Führer D, Holzapfel HP, Ruschenburg I, Paschke R (2001) Diagnostik des Schilddrüsenknotens. Deutsches Ärzteblatt 98:A2427–A2437
76. Hurtado-López LM, Monroy-Lozano BE, Martínez-Duncker C (2008) TSH alone is not sufficient to exclude all patients with a functioning thyroid nodule from undergoing testing to exclude thyroid cancer. Eur J Nucl Med Mol Imaging 35:1173–1178
77. Klain M, Maurea S, Cuocolo A, Colao A, Marzano L, Lombardi G, Salvatore M (1996) Technetium-99 m tetrofosmin imaging in thyroid diseases: comparison with Tc-99 m-pertechnetate, thallium-201 and Tc-99 m-methoxyisobutylisonitrile scans. Eur J Nucl Med 23: 1568–1574
78. Müller S, Guth-Tougelides B, Creutzig H (1987) Imaging of malignant tumors with ^{99m}Tc-MIBI SPECT [Abstract]. J Nucl Med 28:562
79. Reiners C (2008) Scintigraphy or fine-needle aspiration biopsy to exclude thyroid malignancy: What should be done first in iodine deficiency? Eur J Nucl Med Mol Imaging 35:1171–1172
80. Reiners C, Schumm-Draeger PM, Geling M, Mastbaum C, Schönberger J, Laue-Savic A, Hackethal K, Hampel R, Heinken U, Kullak W, Linke R, Uhde W (2003) [Thyroid gland ultrasound screening (Papillon Initiative). Report of 15 incidentally detected thyroid cancers]. Internist 44:412–419
81. Schmidt M (2010) Risk stratification in suspicious thyroid nodules by nuclear medicine techniques: PET or SPECT? In: Dralle H (ed) Thyroid 2009, 19th conference on the human thyroid – Heidelberg. [Nuklearmedizinische Risikostratifizierung bei suspekten Schilddrüsenknoten: PET oder SPECT? In: Schilddrüse 2009, 19. Konferenz über die menschliche Schilddrüse – Heidelberg.]. Lehmanns Media, Berlin, pp 179–189
82. Sharma R, Chakravarty KL, Tripathi M, Kaushik A, Bharti P, Sahoo M, Chopra MK, Rawat H, Misra A, Mondal A, Kashyap R (2007) Role of 99mTc-Tetrofosmin delayed scintigraphy and color Doppler sonography in characterization of solitary thyroid nodules. Nucl Med Commun 28:847–851
83. Jemal A, Siegel R, Xu J, Ward E (2010) Cancer statistics, 2010. CA Cancer J Clin 60: 277–300
84. Uğur O, Kostakoğlu L, Caner B, Güler N, Gülaldi NC, Ozmen M, Uysal U, Elahi N, Erbengi G, Bejdik C (1996) Comparison of ^{201}Tl, ^{99m}Tc-MIBI and ^{131}I imaging in the follow-up of patients with well-differentiated thyroid carcinoma. Nucl Med Commun 17:373–377
85. Nakahara H, Noguchi S, Murakami N, Hoshi H, Jinnouchi S, Nagamachi S, Ohnishi T, Futami S, Flores LG 2nd, Watanabe K (1996) Technetium-99m-sestamibi scintigraphy compared with thallium-201 in evaluation of thyroid tumors. J Nucl Med. 37:901–904 http://www.ncbi.nlm.nih.gov/sites/entrez
86. Sarikaya A, Huseyinova G, Irfanoglu ME, Erkmen N, Cermik TF, Berkarda S (2001) The relationship between ^{99m}Tc-sestamibi uptake and ultrastructural cell types of thyroid tumours. Nucl Med Commun 22:39–44

Tc-99m Sestamibi in Miscellaneous Tumors

8

Amir Sabet

8.1 Lung Cancer

Lung cancer is the leading cause of cancer-related mortality. The single most important cause of lung cancer is smoking. The other risk factors include radiation therapy to the breast or chest and exposure to second-hand smoke, radon, arsenic, asbestos, and chromates [1]. The 5-year relative survival rate varies markedly depending on the stage at diagnosis. To facilitate treatment and prognostic decisions, lung cancer is broadly classified into two types: small cell lung cancers (SCLC) and non-small cell lung cancers (NSCLC).

NSCLC are the most common lung cancers, accounting for about 80% of all cases. The major histologic classes of NSCLC are adenocarcinoma, squamous cell carcinoma, small cell carcinoma, and large cell carcinoma. SCLC is the most aggressive and rapidly growing of all lung cancers. Histologic diagnosis may be obtained with sputum cytology, thoracentesis, accessible lymph node biopsy, bronchoscopy, transthoracic needle aspiration, video-assisted thoracoscopy, or thoracotomy. Treatment and prognosis of lung cancer are closely tied to the type and stage of the identified tumor. For the patients with low stages of non-small cell carcinoma, surgical resection is preferred. Advanced non-small cell carcinoma is treated with a multimodality approach that may include radiotherapy, chemotherapy, and palliative care. Chemotherapy (combined with radiotherapy for limited disease) is the mainstay of treatment for small cell carcinoma.

Imaging is a common way to diagnose lung cancer. In addition to the common chest x-ray procedure, other conventional imaging techniques such as CT scans and magnetic resonance imaging (MRI) are regularly used for this purpose. However, pulmonary nodules and masses frequently present a diagnostic dilemma especially when they are solitary, surrounded by normal lung tissue, and not greater than

---

A. Sabet
Klinik und Poliklinik für Nuklearmedizin, Universität Bonn,
Sigmund-Freud-Straße 25, 53127 Bonn, Germany
e-mail: amir.sabet@ukb.uni-bonn.de

J. Bucerius et al. (eds.), ^{99m}Tc-Sestamibi,
DOI 10.1007/978-3-642-04233-1_8, © Springer-Verlag Berlin Heidelberg 2012

3.0 cm in their largest diameter without radiographic evidence of hilar or mediastinal adenopathy (solitary pulmonary nodules). Conventional imaging techniques have a limited diagnostic accuracy since interpretation relies principally on lesion size and other nonspecific findings [2]. Radiological findings suggestive of malignancy are thickening of the cavity wall and presence of speculated or nodular edge, whereas central, laminated, or diffuse calcifications are more likely to be related to a benign etiology. Definitive diagnoses have traditionally depended on invasive techniques as mentioned before. However, even invasive procedures such as bronchoscopy and transbronchial or transthoracic biopsy have sensitivities of <80% in certain settings and may be associated with significant complications [3].

There is thus an increased interest in the functional noninvasive radioisotopic methods to reduce the number of invasive diagnostic procedures. In this setting, F-18-2-fluoro-2-deoxyglucose (FDG) positron emission tomography (PET) is a useful modality which takes advantage of increased glucose utilization by tumor cells [4, 5]. However, FDG-PET has some limits not only because a variety of inflammatory lesions (tuberculosis, sarcoidosis, inflammatory pseudotumor, fungal infection, pneumonia, and abscess) have all been associated with FDG-PET uptake [6] but also some tumors such as adenocarcinoma and bronchioloalveolar lung carcinoma may not be visualized by FDG-PET, probably because they are less aggressive and slow-growing [7]. Consequently, despite the growing applications of PET, single photon emission computed tomography (SPECT) studies are still of benefit in numerous conditions in pulmonary neoplasms [8, 9] and various radionuclides, such as 67Ga, 201Tl, and Tc-99m sestamibi have been utilized in lung cancer for staging [10, 11] follow-up, and monitoring the therapy response [12].

The ability of sestamibi to detect lung malignancies has been evaluated in a number of studies. In the largest patient series assessed to date, Tc-99m sestamibi SPECT demonstrated 100% specificity and positive predictive values, while sensitivity, accuracy, and negative predictive values were 90%, 91%, and 63%, respectively. The correlation between the pathologic data and the scintigraphic results was high (k:0.72), but age, sex, histological type and grade of lung cancer, as well as the type of benign lesion did not appear to affect this correlation. No relationship was found between lesion size and scintigraphic results [13]. Similar findings were obtained in a more recent study in a small series of patients, all with a single nodule <6 cm in diameter completely surrounded by lung tissue, which was considered indeterminate by clinical and radiographic criteria. The overall sensitivity, specificity, positive predictive value, and negative predictive value Tc-99m sestamibi SPECT for malignancy were 86%, 100%, 100%, and 57%, respectively. The correlation between sestamibi uptake and nodule diameter was statistically significant [14].

However, Tc-99m sestamibi SPECT was reported to have a low specificity in differentiating malignant from benign lung lesions in another study [15] apparently due to misinterpreted areas of radiotracer accumulation by visual evaluation. This may be specially the case when an increase of radiotracer is low or in the presence of lung lesions characterized by a focal uptake with a central hypoactive focus as well as a ring-like appearance of increased uptake. In these cases, interobserver variability could be extremely high, and should not be resolved by a consensus of readers. The authors concluded that, in a clinical setting, if the lung mass has a small tumor/contralateral normal lung (T/N) ratio value in patients with a lesion that is estimated to have a low likelihood of being malignant (age < 30 years, no history of previous malignancy, no smoking history, no features of malignancy at radiological evaluation) lung cancer can be ruled out with a reasonable degree of reliability and invasive diagnostic procedures like thoracotomy may be avoided with the potential for significant cost savings [16].

Evaluation of mediastinal lymph node metastases is a crucial part of preoperative staging in patients with NSCLC and computed tomography (CT) is the most commonly used noninvasive staging method, despite its well-known limitations [17]. These shortcomings have led to a fast growing role of functional imaging in assessing mediastinal lymph nodes. While FDG-PET is widely used in this setting, Tc-99m sestamibi and SPECT can also play a role.

The diagnostic efficacy of Tc-99m sestamibi SPECT in detecting mediastinal lymph node involvement in NSCLC was first investigated in a series of patients who also underwent other staging procedures such as conventional radiography, CT, and fiberoptic bronchoscopy. Lymph node involvement was demonstrated by histology. SPECT and CT had a diagnostic sensitivity and specificity of 91% versus 84% and 84% versus 60%, respectively. Scintigraphic results were also better than those of CT with regard to positive and negative predictive values and accuracy [18]. Other studies have confirmed these findings [13, 19].

Moreover, whole body imaging with Tc-99m sestamibi can detect distant metastases in patients with advanced NSCLC, such as in brain, bones, and soft tissues [20, 21]. It can also distinguish between viable and necrotic tumor tissue, which may have important implications for clinical management and follow-up of patients with NSCLC.

Tc-99m sestamibi SPECT has also proven useful as a noninvasive imaging method to monitor therapy response in lung cancer. It has showed a sensitivity of 90% and a specificity of 100%, using a T/N ratio decrease >10% as a threshold value for monitoring the treatment response after 3 cycles of chemotherapy [22].

Another interesting aspect of sestamibi imaging is its involvement in multidrug resistance. An inverse correlation was reported between the ability of cancers to accumulate Tc-99m sestamibi and the density of P-glycoprotein (P-gp) expression [23, 24]. In another study the increased levels of P-gp expression correlated with a high washout rate. Neither multidrug resistance-associated protein (MRP), resistance protein (LRP) expression at the protein level nor mRNA correlated significantly with tumor accumulation or efflux of Tc-99m sestamibi [25]. In a group of patients with NSCLC pre-therapeutic tracer uptake was significantly higher in responders than in nonresponders and there was a significant positive correlation between survival rate and both early and delayed ratios [26].

There have been clinical studies in patients with SCLC demonstrating that negative Tc-99m sestamibi uptake at the time of diagnosis correlates with poor prognosis [12, 27] and retention Index of Tc-99m sestamibi SPECT appears even as the only useful parameter in predicting the survival of patients with SCLC [28].

Physiological uptake of Tc-99m sestamibi, 201Tl, and 99mTc- HMFG1-MoAb in the liver, spleen, and other splenic areas limit their utility for tumor localization in these organs and in their neighboring areas [29, 30]. Fused images can aid in the correct characterization of pulmonary lesions located near sites of physiologic radiopharmaceutical uptake such as the liver, the myocardium, and vascular structures. Hybrid images may facilitate SPECT interpretation in some cases [31].

A positive Tc-99m sestamibi SPECT study may suggest a malignant lesion and may help to detect the extent of its spread and, consequently, its resectability. Negative SPECT imaging, conversely, may indicate a benign lesion, a vascular tumor, a tumor with extensive necrosis, or a tumor with P-gp overexpression leading to rapid MIBI efflux. This suggests the value of MIBI as a tumor imaging agent not only in demonstrating malignant intrathoracic tumor masses, but potentially also in evaluating their resectability and their chemotherapeutic responsiveness.

8.2 Myeloma

Multiple myeloma (MM) is a malignant hematologic disorder characterized by proliferation of clonal plasma cells and overproduction of monoclonal immunoglobulins [32]. It accounts for 10% of all hematological malignancies [33]. Although the median survival time is 3–4 years, overall survival ranges from less than 6 months to more than 10 years. This variability derives from the heterogeneity in both myeloma cell biology and multiple host factors. In the recent years, cumulative and event-free survival rates and quality of life improved with high dose chemotherapy protocols and autologous stem cell transplantation [34].

The clinical staging is important to establish the treatment modality. The estimation of the tumor mass in multiple myeloma still follows the staging system described by Durie and Salmon in 1975 [35] which includes biochemical parameters of the disease activity and bone lesions (punched-out lesions and/or fractures) on skeletal X-ray survey. However, radiographs can significantly underestimate the extent of bone and bone marrow involvement, especially in the early phases of the disease [36]. Therefore, more advanced imaging modalities – including whole-body 18F-FDG-PET/CT, whole-body Tc-99m sestamibi scintigraphy, and magnet resonance imaging (MRI) – have been proposed in the effort to improve the management of MM patients in a noninvasive manner.

Various radionuclides such as gallium-67 [37] and 99mTc-diphosphonate [38] have been suggested in the past to predict neoplastic bone marrow infiltration in MM. The ability of Tc-99m sestamibi scanning to detect bone marrow involvement in MM has also been known for decades [39–42]. Whole body Tc-99m sestamibi scan reveals the presence of infiltrating myeloma cells rather than its consequence, neoplastic bone destruction [41–47].

Compared to Tc-99m sestamibi images, radiographic changes are not reliable indicators of prognosis often showing only occasional punched out lesions or diffuse osteopenia, which is difficult to quantitate. In a large study, Tc-99m sestamibi was able to detect a positive pattern in 40% of the cases with a negative X-ray, possibly enabling the therapeutic approaches to be modified. Conventional X-ray shows lytic lesions only when the cortical bone damage is more than 40%. In addition, X-ray is not able to distinguish active from nonactive bone osteolytic lesions and accordingly yields a confounding pattern in the monitoring of the response to treatment. Therefore, Tc-99m sestamibi could be very useful in this setting.

Basically, three patterns may be observed by whole body Tc-99m sestamibi scintigraphy in plasma cell proliferations [48]: (i) normal, with physiologic uptake in salivary glands, thyroid, heart, liver, spleen, small intestine, bladder; (ii) diffuse bone uptake, designing bone profiles with variable extension and intensity; (iii) focal, in bones or in soft tissues. A mixed diffuse and focal pattern can also be seen.

Tc-99m sestamibi scans with diffuse patterns correlate with a diffuse and high percentage of plasma cell infiltration and a lower clinical response rate. Therefore, a diffuse sestamibi pattern could be interpreted as a potentially negative prognostic factor for myeloma [43].

The positive scan was found to correlate with disease activity and tumor burden represented by high levels of CRP, b2M, IL-6, and sIL-6r and bone marrow infiltration. A significant association has also been observed between the baseline scintigraphic pattern and clinical status at follow-up in the group of patients evaluated after chemotherapy as well as in those not undergoing chemotherapy [39, 40, 46, 49].

It has also been observed that combined use of Tc-99m sestamibi and 99mTc-V-DMSA scanning during chemotherapy allows evaluation of the effectiveness of the administered chemotherapy. The high-dose chemotherapy eliminated uptake of Tc-99m sestamibi by the lesions, whereas 99mTc-V-DMSA uptake was increased in lesions presenting significant initial Tc-99m sestamibi uptake [50].

However, Tc-99m sestamibi could produce false-negative results in patients with refractory myeloma due to the presence of the multidrug resistance P-gp, which is responsible for the elimination of Tc-99m sestamibi from malignant cells [51, 52]. Tc-99m sestamibi has a high specificity to identify the absence of disease (patients in complete remission) but is less sensitive for the identification of residual disease when response is not complete.

A new staging system was announced more recently called the Durie and Salmon PLUS staging system that integrates MRI and 18F-FDG-PET scanning into the former system.

It has also been suggested that the washout of Tc-99m sestamibi may be used as a sensitive tool for whole-body imaging of P-gp expression in multiple myeloma patients providing functional and quantitative characterization of the multidrug resistance (MDR) phenotype – before, during, or after chemotherapy [44, 52].

In whole-body analysis, 18F-FDG-PET/CT performed better than Tc-99m sestamibi in the detection of focal lesions, whereas Tc-99m sestamibi was superior in the visualization of diffuse disease. In the spine and pelvis, MRI was comparable to 18F-FDG-PET/CT and Tc-99m sestamibi in the detection of focal and diffuse disease, respectively [48]. Thus, whole-body Tc-99m sestamibi, despite its limited capacity in detecting focal lesions, may be an alternative option when a PET facility is not available.

8.3 Brain Tumors

Primary brain tumors are classified by light microscopy according to their predominant cell type and graded based upon the presence or absence of standard pathologic features in too different types and subtypes: Tumors of Glial Cells (astrocytic tumors, astrocytoma, glioblastoma multiforme, oligodendroglioma, and ependymoma), neuronal tumors (ganglioglioma, gangliocytoma, central neurocytoma), embryonal tumors (medulloblastoma), tumor of cranial and spinal nerves (schwannoma and neurofibroma), meningeal tumors (meningioma), mesenchymal tumors (sarcoma and hemangioblastoma), cerebral lymphomas, germ cell tumors (teratoma and craniopharyngioma), tumors of the pituitary gland (pituitary adenoma) and metastatic tumors.

Primary brain tumors are commonly located in the posterior cranial fossa in children and in the anterior two thirds of the cerebral hemispheres in adults. Survival rates in primary brain tumors depend on the type of tumor, age, functional status of the patient, and the extent of surgical tumor removal [53]. Medulloblastoma has a good prognosis while glioblastoma multiforme, the most common form of malignant brain tumor, has a median survival of only 12 months. Brainstem gliomas have the poorest prognosis of any form of brain cancer, with most patients dying within 1 year. Although there is no generally accepted therapeutic management for primary brain tumors, a surgical attempt at tumor removal or at least cytoreduction is considered in most cases. Postoperative radiotherapy and chemotherapy are integral parts of the therapeutic standard for malignant tumors [54].

Brain perfusion scintigraphy was used in the past to confirm the presence of cerebral masses suspicious of cancer at clinical examination. CT and MRI are now considered the most sensitive imaging methods in detecting neoplastic lesions, differentiating benign from malignant lesions and determining lesion size and extension in surrounding structures [55].

In patients with supratentorial expanding brain lesions, Tc-99m sestamibi brain SPECT showed a significant higher uptake and a more elevated T/N ratio in high-grade than in low-grade gliomas, thus providing information for the differential diagnosis of these two different forms [56]. A relationship between sestamibi uptake and tumor grade was also determined in cases of astrocytoma but not in glioblastoma, where Tc-99m sestamibi uptake was variable, probably because of the solid to cystic ratio observed in these patients. Furthermore, tracer uptake has been shown to be elevated in meningiomas according to their vascular supply, while it is absent in normal parenchyma [57].

With respect to the histological type, a higher Tc-99m sestamibi retention index has been noted in glioblastoma multiforme compared with metastatic tumor. In addition, while sestamibi SPECT shows high uptake and retention in malignant gliomas, washout from metastatic brain tumors is better than from glioblastomas [58].

In a study on patients in the presurgical phase for intraparenchymal brain tumors, Tc-99m sestamibi SPECT identified tumors in the frontotemporal regions more easily than in the temporal regions or in the posterior fossa [57]. It could identify tumor tissue also in hemorrhage areas [59].

Tc-99m sestamibi delayed imaging is thought to reflect the presence of P-gp [60] and hence delayed images might be false-negative (with absence of sestamibi uptake) despite tumor progression [61]. Early imaging on the other hand offers the highest diagnostic yield and is not affected by the multidrug resistant phenotype [62].

In brain tumors, response to chemotherapy is generally evaluated on CT or MRI. Response assessment is based on major changes in tumor size on enhanced CT or MRI scans. There are, however, several limitations to these criteria: they are not applicable to non-enhancing malignant tumors, it may be difficult to measure the size of a nonhomogeneous or multifocal tumor, and nonpathological changes induced by surgery, radiotherapy, or corticosteroid treatment can hinder image interpretation. Therefore, functional imaging techniques, such as Tc-99m sestamibi SPECT, thallium-201 [63, 64], or PET with carbon-11 methionine or FDG [65] can be a useful complement to morphological studies, providing information on tumor metabolism. Tc-99m sestamibi SPECT is able to detect early response or resistance to chemotherapy in high-grade gliomas, providing information on treatment efficacy and primary or secondary resistance. In cases of tumor progression, Tc-99m sestamibi SPECT is shown to be an earlier indicator of escape from chemotherapy, an average of 4 months before MRI changes [66].

Tc-99m sestamibi has also been successfully used in high-grade gliomas to distinguish recurrent tumor from radionecrosis after radiotherapy [67] where the results of both CT and MRI are difficult to interpret because of the inflammation resulting from surgery or the radiation, and offer only an imperfect indication of tumor viability [68]. Tc-99m sestamibi concentrates in mitochondria by active diffusion because of an increased negative transmembrane potential [69] – an advantage over 18F-FDG, which can be found in the inflamed area.

The physiological distribution of Tc-99m sestamibi in the choroid plexus could be a disadvantage for the evaluation of lesions lying close to the ventricule in the deep paraventricular regions [70] although it offers a useful landmark for lesion localization. This and the other major drawback of sestamibi, that is, poor morphological resolution could be overcome by dual-modality, integrated systems (SPECT/CT). SPECT/CT can distinguish tumor from the skull and other sites of physiological uptake. Thus, it may permit exact localization of viable tumor tissue after surgery and/or radiotherapy within areas of anatomical changes, as well as differentiating tumor from gliosis, or other regions such as the infratentorial posterior fossa, where SPECT has proven to be a poor sensitive diagnostic modality [71].

Tc-99m sestamibi SPECT seems to be less accurate than 18F-FDG-PET and PET/CT [72] in delineating tumor metabolism, and it has a lower resolution. An increasing number of studies have also shown that 11 C-methionine [73] or 3-deoxy-3-18F-fluorothymidine [74] are more accurate and correlate better with proliferation indexes (such as Ki-67) than SPECT tracers (including sestamibi) or even 18F-FDG-PET. SPECT/CT thus seems a useful additional tool in brain tumor management, especially when MRI is not feasible or PET/CT is not available.

8.4 Lymphoma

Typically, lymphomas present as a solid tumor of lymphoid cells. It can also affect other organs in which case it is referred to as extranodal lymphoma. Extranodal sites include the skin, brain, bowels, and bone. The WHO Classification, updated in 2008, is the latest classification of lymphoma and is based upon the foundations laid within the "Revised European-American Lymphoma classification" (REAL). This system attempts to group lymphomas by cell type (i.e., the normal cell type that most resembles the tumor) and defining phenotypic, molecular, or cytogenetic characteristics. There are three large groups: the B cell, T cell, and natural killer cell tumors. Hodgkin's lymphoma, although considered separately within the World Health Organization (and preceding) classifications, is now recognized as being a tumor of lymphocytes of mature B cell lineage. Non-Hodgkin's lymphoma on the other hand refers to any type of lymphoma that does not have the distinctive Reed-Sternberg cell present in Hodgkin's lymphoma. Non-Hodgkin's lymphoma is the most common type of lymphoma classified broadly in to high-grade or aggressive non-Hodgkin's lymphoma and low-grade or indolent non-Hodgkin's lymphoma.

18F-FDG-PET is now considered the most accurate imaging procedure in the diagnosis, staging and follow-up of Lymphoma. A wide range of gamma radiopharmaceuticals has also been employed for this purpose in the past. In particular, 67Ga [75–79] has been extensively used with good results and still maintains its usefulness, especially when FDG-PET is not available.

Both Tc-99m sestamibi and Tc-tetrofosmin have also been used, but because they are eliminated by the biliary-intestinal route, investigation of the infradiaphragmatic regions is very difficult, as it occurs in 67Ga scintigraphy. In a comparative study with Tc-99m sestamibi versus 67Ga SPECT on both Hodgkin's and non-Hodgkin's lymphoma patients, the overall sensitivity and specificity of Tc-99m sestamibi were superior (71% and 76%, versus 68% and 44) [80]. The sensitivity for residual masses was 44% for both tracers, and the specificity was 80% for Tc-99m sestamibi and 53% for 67Ga.

In another study, the diagnostic accuracy of Tc-99m sestamibi imaging for lesion detection in Lymphoma (Hodgkin's or non-Hodgkin's) was 85% without any false positive results [81]. However, its accuracy was higher (94%) in non-Hodgkin's patients than in those with Hodgkin's lymphomas (72%). The difference was probably related to lesion size rather than the specific histologic type of the lymphoma, since the Hodgkin's lymphoma lesions were smaller than the non-Hodgkin's lesions.

Tc-99m sestamibi brain SPECT has proved to be valuable in detecting intracranial lymphomas in AIDS patients, with sensitivity and specificity of 100% and 69%, respectively [82]. The false-positive results were due to toxoplasmosis, which showed a pattern of healing after medical treatment.

Tc-99m sestamibi was also evaluated with respect to therapy outcome [82] and showed a high uptake in patients who went on to improve after therapy or transformed into stable disease.

The usefulness of Tc-99m sestamibi in predicting response to chemotherapy in malignant lymphoma patients has also been reported in children irrespective of the lymphoma type [83]. In adults, the role of Tc-99m sestamibi imaging as a predictor of chemotherapy has been also investigated, comparing with P-gp expression, MRP expression, and other prognostic factors. Negative P-gp and MRP expression, positive Tc-99m sestamibi scan, or a slow tumor clearance in double-phase Tc-99m sestamibi scintigraphy [83–87] before treatment were predictors of a good chemotherapy response, whereas patients with a poor response had negative Tc-99m sestamibi scans and positive P-gp or MRP expression.

However, because of the diagnostic limitations of Tc-99m sestamibi scans for detecting nodal lesions in the lower chest and abdomen as well as extranodal lesions in the liver, spleen, and gastrointestinal wall and the lesions with small tumor size due to biliary and intestinal excretion of Tc-99m sestamibi, the precise prediction of chemotherapy response in these lesions is difficult [80, 81].

Therefore, employment of hybrid devices (SPECT/CT) may be advisable in clinical conditions requiring highly accurate functional characterization and disease staging at diagnosis, post-treatment localization of active tumor tissue inside a residual mass, or an early diagnosis of relapse that may not be easily interpretable because of inconclusive anatomic studies.

8.5 Bone Tumors

While primary bone tumors occur most commonly in children and adolescents, older adults develop more often metastatic bone tumors. The most common primary bone tumors include osteosarcoma, Ewing's sarcoma, chondrosarcoma, malignant fibrous histiocytoma, fibrosarcoma, and chordoma. Osteosarcoma is the most common primary malignant bone cancer. It often occurs in the long bones of the arms and legs at areas of rapid growth around the knees and shoulders of children. On the other hand, Ewing's sarcoma occurs in the middle of the long bones of the arms and legs. It is the most aggressive bone tumor and affects younger people between 4 and 15 years of age. Chondrosarcoma is the second most common bone tumor and accounts for about 25% of all malignant bone tumors. These tumors arise from the cartilage cells and can either be very aggressive or relatively slow growing. Unlike many other bone tumors, chondrosarcoma is most common in people over 40 years of age. An accurate diagnosis of bone tumors relies on a cooperative clinical and imaging effort. The patient's age, sex, history, clinical findings, and presentation, in addition to the radiographic features, allow for proper diagnosis. Aside from a biopsy, the radiograph is clearly the most important single approach to the diagnosis of bone tumors.

The introduction of aggressive chemotherapy before surgical intervention has resulted in dramatic improvement of the prognosis of the patients with malignant bone and soft tissue tumors, may make limb-sparing surgery possible, and permits excellent quality of life [88]. Therefore, a good response to preoperative chemotherapy is crucial and an accurate evaluation of chemotherapeutic effects is essential for proper treatment strategy [89, 90].

Several studies have suggested that the change of Tc-99m sestamibi uptake from pre- to postchemotherapy might reflect the chemotherapeutic effect in patients with bone sarcomas [91–93]. Moreover, Tc-99m sestamibi scintigraphy performed in the middle of chemotherapy in patients with bone and soft tissue tumors has been suggested as an accurate predictor of the final response to chemotherapy with high positive and negative predictive values, 93% and 85% respectively. Separate analysis showed relatively better values for bone tumors versus soft tissue tumors, 100% and 82% versus 86% and 88%, respectively. Thus, this method might be worthy as one of the gatekeepers for the decision-making process in the middle of chemotherapy, namely, in determining whether the chemotherapy should be continued or changed [94].

Some studies [95, 96] showed a significant correlation between the washout rate of Tc-99m sestamibi and both P-gp and MRP1 expression in patients with osteosarcoma whereas others [97] could not identify this correlation.

Possible drawbacks of Tc-99m sestamibi include its high uptake by the liver and excretion via the intestines and urinary system, which interfere with abdominal and pelvic evaluation. However, lesions of the extremities, where most bone and soft tissue tumors are found, are unaffected by these issues.

8.6 Gastrointestinal Tumors

Prognosis of gastrointestinal tumors depends almost entirely on the specific type of cancer. Esophageal cancer has a dismal prognosis, largely because it is often detected late, while colon cancer has an excellent prognosis, when detected early.

Gastrointestinal endoscopy is the method of choice for diagnosis and follow-up of gastrointestinal malignancies [98]. Several alternative methods, including virtual endoscopy with CT [99, 100] or MRI [101], 18F-FDG-PET imaging – alone or in combination with CT imaging [102] are also being utilized.

It is well known, that tracer Tc-99m sestamibi has a negligible role in subdiaphragmatic tumor detection because of its rapid passage in the intestine by immediate biliary secretion of the tracer, thus causing high background activity, which makes the interpretation of images rather impossible [103]. In addition, high liver biliary tract and bladder uptake of the tracer further complicate image analysis.

In a study to overcome biliary secretion of the tracer, morphine hydrochloride was intravenously administered before the administration of Tc-99m sestamibi and early and delayed images were acquired at 30 and 120 min after iv injection of the tracer. Prescintigraphic morphine administration could inhibit background activity coming from biliary secretion, and enables better intraabdominal Tc-99m sestamibi imaging but with limited sensitivity and poor specificity [104].

Studies reported that an increased expression of P-gp, but not of MRP, correlates with low accumulation of Tc-99m sestamibi in gastric cancers [105] as some other types of malignancy [25, 106].

References

1. Wingo PA et al (1999) Annual report to the nation on the status of cancer, 1973–1996, with a special section on lung cancer and tobacco smoking. J Natl Cancer Inst 91(8):675–690
2. Webb WR et al (1991) CT and MR imaging in staging non-small cell bronchogenic carcinoma: report of the Radiologic Diagnostic Oncology Group. Radiology 178(3):705–713

3. Salathe M et al (1992) Transbronchial needle aspiration in routine fiberoptic bronchoscopy. Respiration 59(1):5–8
4. Gould MK et al (2001) Accuracy of positron emission tomography for diagnosis of pulmonary nodules and mass lesions: a meta-analysis. JAMA 285(7):914–924
5. van Tinteren H et al (2002) Effectiveness of positron emission tomography in the preoperative assessment of patients with suspected non-small-cell lung cancer: the PLUS multicentre randomised trial. Lancet 359(9315):1388–1393
6. Kapucu LO et al (1998) Fluorine-18-fluorodeoxyglucose uptake in pneumonia. J Nucl Med 39(7):1267–1269
7. Higashi K et al (1998) Fluorine-18-FDG PET imaging is negative in bronchioloalveolar lung carcinoma. J Nucl Med 39(6):1016–1020
8. Beller GA, Watson DD (1991) Physiological basis of myocardial perfusion imaging with the technetium 99m agents. Semin Nucl Med 21(3):173–181
9. Schomacker K, Schicha H (2000) Use of myocardial imaging agents for tumour diagnosis–A success story? Eur J Nucl Med 27(12):1845–1863
10. Yokoi K et al (1994) Mediastinal lymph node metastasis from lung cancer: evaluation with Tl-201 SPECT–comparison with CT. Radiology 192(3):813–817
11. Tonami N et al (1991) 201Tl SPECT in the detection of mediastinal lymph node metastases from lung cancer. Nucl Med Commun 12(9):779–792
12. Piwnica-Worms D et al (1993) Functional imaging of multidrug-resistant P-glycoprotein with an organotechnetium complex. Cancer Res 53(5):977–984
13. Nosotti M et al (2002) Role of (99m)tc-hexakis-2-methoxy-isobutylisonitrile in the diagnosis and staging of lung cancer. Chest 122(4):1361–1364
14. Minai OA et al (2000) Role of Tc-99m MIBI in the evaluation of single pulmonary nodules: a preliminary report. Thorax 55(1):60–62
15. Kao CH et al (1993) Differentiation of single solid lesions in the lungs by means of single-photon emission tomography with technetium-99m methoxyisobutylisonitrile. Eur J Nucl Med 20(3):249–254
16. Mountain CF (2000) The international system for staging lung cancer. Semin Surg Oncol 18(2):106–115
17. Friedman PJ (1992) Lung cancer staging: efficacy of CT. Radiology 182(2):307–309
18. Chiti A et al (1996) Assessment of mediastinal involvement in lung cancer with technetium-99m-sestamibi SPECT. J Nucl Med 37(6):938–942
19. Spanu A et al (2003) The usefulness of 99mTc-tetrofosmin SPECT in the detection of intrathoracic malignant lesions. Int J Oncol 22(3):639–649
20. Cermik TF et al (2003) Thallium-201 SPECT in advanced non-small cell lung cancer: in relation with chemotherapeutic response, survival, distant metastasis and p53 status. Ann Nucl Med 17(5):369–374
21. Sobic-Saranovic D et al (2008) Assessment of non-small cell lung cancer viability and necrosis with three radiopharmaceuticals. Hell J Nucl Med 11(1):16–20
22. Yuksel M et al (2001) Monitoring the chemotherapeutic response in primary lung cancer using 99mTc-MIBI SPET. Eur J Nucl Med 28(7):799–806
23. Maublant JC et al (1993) *In vitro* uptake of technetium-99m-teboroxime in carcinoma cell lines and normal cells: comparison with technetium-99m-sestamibi and thallium-201. J Nucl Med 34(11):1949–1952
24. Kostakoglu L et al (1998) Association of tumor washout rates and accumulation of technetium-99m-MIBI with expression of P-glycoprotein in lung cancer. J Nucl Med 39(2):228–234
25. Zhou J et al (2001) Expression of multidrug resistance protein and messenger RNA correlate with (99m)Tc-MIBI imaging in patients with lung cancer. J Nucl Med 42(10):1476–1483
26. Yuksel M et al (2002) 99mTc-MIBI SPET in non-small cell lung cancer in relationship with Pgp and prognosis. Eur J Nucl Med Mol Imaging 29(7):876–881
27. Hassan IM et al (1989) Uptake and kinetics of Tc-99m hexakis 2-methoxy isobutyl isonitrile in benign and malignant lesions in the lungs. Clin Nucl Med 14(5):333–340

28. Mohan HK, Miles KA (2009) Cost-effectiveness of 99mTc-sestamibi in predicting response to chemotherapy in patients with lung cancer: systematic review and meta-analysis. J Nucl Med 50(3):376–381
29. Abdel-Dayem HM et al (1994) Tracer imaging in lung cancer. Eur J Nucl Med 21(1):57–81
30. Pauwels EK et al (1998) The mechanism of accumulation of tumour-localising radiopharmaceuticals. Eur J Nucl Med 25(3):277–305
31. Schillaci O et al (2004) Is SPECT/CT with a hybrid camera useful to improve scintigraphic imaging interpretation? Nucl Med Commun 25(7):705–710
32. Malpas JS et al (1995) Myeloma during a decade: clinical experience in a single centre. Ann Oncol 6(1):11–18
33. Baur-Melnyk A et al (2005) Role of MRI for the diagnosis and prognosis of multiple myeloma. Eur J Radiol 55(1):56–63
34. Attal M et al (1996) A prospective, randomized trial of autologous bone marrow transplantation and chemotherapy in multiple myeloma Intergroupe Francais du Myelome. N Engl J Med 335(2):91–97
35. Durie BG, Salmon SE (1975) A clinical staging system for multiple myeloma. Correlation of measured myeloma cell mass with presenting clinical features, response to treatment, and survival. Cancer 36(3):842–854
36. Durie BG et al (2002) Whole-body (18)F-FDG PET identifies high-risk myeloma. J Nucl Med 43(11):1457–1463
37. Otsuka N et al (1993) Bone and 67 Ga scintigraphy in the evaluation of rib lesions in patients with multiple myeloma. Radiat Med 11(3):75–80
38. Lindstrom E, Lindstrom FD (1980) Skeletal scintigraphy with technetium diphosphonate in multiple myeloma–a comparison with skeletal x-ray. Acta Med Scand 208(4):289–291
39. Ak I et al (2003) Tc-99m methoxyisobutylisonitrile bone marrow imaging for predicting the levels of myeloma cells in bone marrow in multiple myeloma: correlation with CD38/CD138 expressing myeloma cells. Ann Hematol 82(2):88–92
40. Alexandrakis MG et al (2002) Correlation between the uptake of Tc-99m-sestaMIBI and prognostic factors in patients with multiple myeloma. Clin Lab Haematol 24(3):155–159
41. Catalano L et al (1999) Detection of focal myeloma lesions by technetium-99m-sestaMIBI scintigraphy. Haematologica 84(2):119–124
42. Durie BG (1986) Staging and kinetics of multiple myeloma. Semin Oncol 13(3):300–309
43. Pace L et al (1998) Different patterns of technetium-99m sestamibi uptake in multiple myeloma. Eur J Nucl Med 25(7):714–720
44. Fonti R et al (2001) Bone marrow uptake of 99mTc-MIBI in patients with multiple myeloma. Eur J Nucl Med 28(2):214–220
45. Tirovola EB et al (1996) The use of 99mTc-MIBI scanning in multiple myeloma. Br J Cancer 74(11):1815–1820
46. Adams BK, Fataar A, Nizami MA (1996) Technetium-99m-sestamibi uptake in myeloma. J Nucl Med 37(6):1001–1002
47. el Shirbiny AM et al (1997) Technetium-99m-MIBI versus fluorine-18-FDG in diffuse multiple myeloma. J Nucl Med 38(8):1208–1210
48. Mele A et al (2007) Technetium-99m sestamibi scintigraphy is sensitive and specific for the staging and the follow-up of patients with multiple myeloma: a multicentre study on 397 scans. Br J Haematol 136(5):729–735
49. Bacovsky J et al (2005) Scintigraphy using (99m)Tc-MIBI (sestamibi), a sensitive parameter of activity of multiple myeloma. Neoplasma 52(4):302–306
50. Koutsikos J et al (2006) Scintigraphy with technetium-99m methoxyisobutylisonitrile in multiple myeloma patients: correlation with the International Staging System. Hell J Nucl Med 9(3):177–180
51. Koutsikos J et al (2005) Combined use of 99mTc-sestamibi and 99mTc-V-DMSA in the assessment of chemotherapy effectiveness in patients with multiple myeloma. J Nucl Med 46(6):978–982

8 Tc-99m Sestamibi in Miscellaneous Tumors

52. Fonti R et al (2004) Functional imaging of multidrug resistant phenotype by 99mTc-MIBI scan in patients with multiple myeloma. Cancer Biother Radiopharm 19(2):165–170
53. Nicolato A et al (1995) Prognostic factors in low-grade supratentorial astrocytomas: a uni-multivariate statistical analysis in 76 surgically treated adult patients. Surg Neurol 44(3):208–221, discussion 221–223
54. Nakamura M et al (2000) Analysis of prognostic and survival factors related to treatment of low-grade astrocytomas in adults. Oncology 58(2):108–116
55. Del Sole A et al (2004) Position of nuclear medicine techniques in the diagnostic work-up of brain tumors. Q J Nucl Med Mol Imaging 48(2):76–81
56. Baillet G et al (1994) Evaluation of single-photon emission tomography imaging of supratentorial brain gliomas with technetium-99m sestamibi. Eur J Nucl Med 21(10):1061–1066
57. Bagni B et al (1995) SPET imaging of intracranial tumours with 99Tcm-sestamibi. Nucl Med Commun 16(4):258–264
58. Nishiyama Y et al (2001) Comparison of 99Tcm-MIBI with 201Tl chloride SPET in patients with malignant brain tumours. Nucl Med Commun 22(6):631–639
59. Minutoli F et al (2003) 99mTc-MIBI SPECT in distinguishing neoplastic from nonneoplastic intracerebral hematoma. J Nucl Med 44(10):1566–1573
60. Yokogami K et al (1998) Application of SPET using technetium-99m sestamibi in brain tumours and comparison with expression of the MDR-1 gene: Is it possible to predict the response to chemotherapy in patients with gliomas by means of 99mTc-sestamibi SPET? Eur J Nucl Med 25(4):401–409
61. Beauchesne P, Soler C (2002) Correlation of 99mTc-MIBI brain spect (functional index ratios) and survival after treatment failure in malignant glioma patients. Anticancer Res 22(5):3081–3085
62. Leitha T, Glaser C, Lang S (1998) Is early sestamibi imaging in head and neck cancer affected by MDR status, p53 expression, or cell proliferation? Nucl Med Biol 25(6):539–541
63. Kallen K et al (2000) Quantitative 201Tl SPET imaging in the follow-up of treatment for brain tumour: A sensitive tool for the early identification of response to chemotherapy? Nucl Med Commun 21(3):259–267
64. Roesdi MF et al (1998) Thallium-201 SPECT as response parameter for PCV chemotherapy in recurrent glioma. J Neurooncol 40(3):251–255
65. Brock CS et al (2000) Early evaluation of tumour metabolic response using [18F]fluorodeoxyglucose and positron emission tomography: a pilot study following the phase II chemotherapy schedule for temozolomide in recurrent high-grade gliomas. Br J Cancer 82(3):608–615
66. Prigent-Le Jeune F et al (2004) Technetium-99m sestamibi brain SPECT in the follow-up of glioma for evaluation of response to chemotherapy: first results. Eur J Nucl Med Mol Imaging 31(5):714–719
67. Le Jeune FP et al (2006) Sestamibi technetium-99m brain single-photon emission computed tomography to identify recurrent glioma in adults: 201 studies. J Neurooncol 77(2):177–183
68. O'Tuama LA et al (1993) Thallium-201 versus technetium-99m-MIBI SPECT in evaluation of childhood brain tumors: a within-subject comparison. J Nucl Med 34(7):1045–1051
69. Delmon-Moingeon LI et al (1990) Uptake of the cation hexakis(2-methoxyisobutylisonitrile)-technetium-99m by human carcinoma cell lines *in vitro*. Cancer Res 50(7):2198–2202
70. Louis DN et al (2007) The 2007 WHO classification of tumours of the central nervous system. Acta Neuropathol 114(2):97–109
71. Barai S et al (2003) Evaluation of single photon emission computerised tomography (SPECT) using Tc99m-tetrofosmin as a diagnostic modality for recurrent posterior fossa tumours. J Postgrad Med 49(4):316–320, discussion 320–321
72. Henze M et al (2006) Comparison of diagnostic accuracy of (18)F-FDG PET, (123)I-IMT- and (99m)Tc-MIBI SPECT: evaluation of tumour progression in irradiated low grade astrocytomas. Nuklearmedizin 45(1):49–56
73. Kim S et al (2005) 11 C-methionine PET as a prognostic marker in patients with glioma: comparison with 18F-FDG PET. Eur J Nucl Med Mol Imaging 32(1):52–59

74. Chen W et al (2005) Imaging proliferation in brain tumors with 18F-FLT PET: comparison with 18F-FDG. J Nucl Med 46(6):945–952
75. Turner DA et al (1972) The use of 67 Ga scanning in the staging of Hodgkin's disease. Radiology 104(1):97–101
76. Iosilevsky G et al (1985) Uptake of gallium-67 citrate and [2-3 H]deoxyglucose in the tumor model, following chemotherapy and radiotherapy. J Nucl Med 26(3):278–282
77. Kostakoglu L et al (1992) Validation of gallium-67-citrate single-photon emission computed tomography in biopsy-confirmed residual Hodgkin's disease in the mediastinum. J Nucl Med 33(3):345–350
78. Schuster DM, Alazraki N (2002) Gallium and other agents in diseases of the lung. Semin Nucl Med 32(3):193–211
79. Even-Sapir E, Israel O (2003) Gallium-67 scintigraphy: a cornerstone in functional imaging of lymphoma. Eur J Nucl Med Mol Imaging 30(Suppl 1):S65–S81
80. Ziegels P et al (1995) Comparison of technetium-99m methoxyisobutylisonitrile and gallium-67 citrate scanning in the assessment of lymphomas. Eur J Nucl Med 22(2):126–131
81. Maurea S et al (1998) Tc-99m sestamibi imaging in the diagnostic assessment of patients with lymphomas: comparison with clinical and radiological evaluation. Clin Nucl Med 23(5):283–290
82. Naddaf SY et al (1998) Comparison between 201Tl-chloride and 99Tc(m)-sestamibi SPET brain imaging for differentiating intracranial lymphoma from non-malignant lesions in AIDS patients. Nucl Med Commun 19(1):47–53
83. Kapucu LO et al (1997) Evaluation of therapy response in children with untreated malignant lymphomas using technetium-99m-sestamibi. J Nucl Med 38(2):243–247
84. Shih WJ et al (1998) Functional retention of Tc-99m MIBI in mediastinal lymphomas as a predictor of chemotherapeutic response demonstrated by consecutive thoracic SPECT imaging. Clin Nucl Med 23(8):505–508
85. Kao CH et al (2001) Evaluation of chemotherapy response using technetium-99M-sestamibi scintigraphy in untreated adult malignant lymphomas and comparison with other prognosis factors: a preliminary report. Int J Cancer 95(4):228–231
86. Kao CH et al (2001) Technetium-99m-sestamethoxyisobutylisonitrile scan as a predictor of chemotherapy response in malignant lymphomas compared with P-glycoprotein expression, multidrug resistance-related protein expression and other prognosis factors. Br J Haematol 113(2):369–374
87. Matsui R et al (1995) Tc-99m sestamibi uptake by malignant lymphoma and slow washout. Clin Nucl Med 20(4):352–356
88. Tsuchiya H et al (1997) Limb salvage using distraction osteogenesis. A classification of the technique. J Bone Joint Surg Br 79(3):403–411
89. Jaffe N, Patel SR, Benjamin RS (1995) Chemotherapy in osteosarcoma. Basis for application and antagonism to implementation; early controversies surrounding its implementation. Hematol Oncol Clin North Am 9(4):825–840
90. Tsuchiya H et al (1999) Marginal excision for osteosarcoma with caffeine assisted chemotherapy. Clin Orthop Relat Res 358:27–35
91. Taki J et al (1997) Evaluating benign and malignant bone and soft-tissue lesions with technetium-99m-MIBI scintigraphy. J Nucl Med 38(4):501–506
92. Moustafa H et al (2003) 99mTc-MIBI in the assessment of response to chemotherapy and detection of recurrences in bone and soft tissue tumours of the extremities. Q J Nucl Med 47(1):51–57
93. Soderlund V et al (1997) Use of 99mTc-MIBI scintigraphy in the evaluation of the response of osteosarcoma to chemotherapy. Eur J Nucl Med 24(5):511–515
94. Taki J et al (2008) Prediction of final tumor response to preoperative chemotherapy by Tc-99m MIBI imaging at the middle of chemotherapy in malignant bone and soft tissue tumors: comparison with Tl-201 imaging. J Orthop Res 26(3):411–418
95. Burak Z et al (2003) 99mTc-MIBI imaging as a predictor of therapy response in osteosarcoma compared with multidrug resistance-associated protein and P-glycoprotein expression. J Nucl Med 44(9):1394–1401

96. Burak Z et al (2001) The role of 99mTc-MIBI scintigraphy in the assessment of MDR1 over-expression in patients with musculoskeletal sarcomas: comparison with therapy response. Eur J Nucl Med 28(9):1341–1350
97. Gorlick R et al (2001) Lack of correlation of functional scintigraphy with (99m)technetium-methoxyisobutylisonitrile with histological necrosis following induction chemotherapy or measures of P-glycoprotein expression in high-grade osteosarcoma. Clin Cancer Res 7(10): 3065–3070
98. Bond JH (2003) Update on colorectal polyps: management and follow-up surveillance. Endoscopy 35(8):S35–S40
99. Pickhardt PJ et al (2003) Computed tomographic virtual colonoscopy to screen for colorectal neoplasia in asymptomatic adults. N Engl J Med 349(23):2191–2200
100. Ajaj W et al (2005) MR colonography in patients with incomplete conventional colonoscopy. Radiology 234(2):452–459
101. Jadvar H, Fischman AJ (2001) Evaluation of pancreatic carcinoma with FDG PET. Abdom Imaging 26(3):254–259
102. Stahl A et al (2004) PET/CT molecular imaging in abdominal oncology. Abdom Imaging 29(3):388–397
103. Krolicki L et al (2002) Technetium-99m MIBI imaging in diagnosis of pelvic and abdominal masses in patients with suspected gynaecological malignancy. Nucl Med Rev Cent East Eur 5(2):131–137
104. Ferlitsch A et al (2007) Prescintigraphic morphine application for abdominal adenocarci-noma imaging, with technetium-99m methoxy isobutyl isonitrile. Hell J Nucl Med 10(1): 14–18
105. Kawata K et al (2004) Usefulness of 99mTc-sestamibi scintigraphy in suggesting the thera-peutic effect of chemotherapy against gastric cancer. Clin Cancer Res 10(11):3788–3793
106. Chang CS et al (2003) Effect of P-glycoprotein and multidrug resistance associated protein gene expression on Tc-99m MIBI imaging in hepatocellular carcinoma. Nucl Med Biol 30(2):111–117

Oncologic Applications of Sestamibi: *In Vivo* Imaging of Multi-Drug Resistance

9

Ali Gholamrezanezhad

Each year millions of new cancers are diagnosed, and chemotherapy remains the principal mode of treatment for many of them. Development of chemoresistance, first described in 1970, is a challenging obstacle during the treatment of local and disseminated malignancies and has been described as the single most common reason for discontinuation of a chemotherapeutic agent. The phenomenon of multi-drug resistance (MDR), as one of the major causes of chemotherapy failure, has been defined as the insensitivity of various tumors to a variety of chemically related or unrelated anti-neoplastic or cytotoxic agents, mediated by a process of inactivating the drug or removing it from the target tumor cells [1]. Numerous etiologies have been identified in studies of patients suffering from MDR, among which are the following: enhanced drug degradation due to augmented expression of metabolizing enzymes, altered target enzyme (e.g. mutation of topoisomerase II), decreased drug activation, increased drug inactivation, subcellular redistribution, drug interaction, metabolic effects and growth factors, enhanced DNA repair and failure to apoptosis (as a result of mutated cell cycle proteins such as p53) [1].

In this context, probably one of the most significant forms of chemoresistance against the variety of currently used anti-neoplastic agents may include drug efflux involving the multi-drug transporter P-glycoprotein (P-gp), product of the MDR gene, as well as other associated proteins [1]. In fact, altered membrane transport of chemotherapy agents induced by the approximately 170 kDa integral membrane P-gp, a protein of 1,280 amino acids, has been considered as a significant contributor for MDR in many malignancies. Relative resistance to different drugs depends on the specific P-gp isoforms that alter the substrate specificity of P-gp [2]. Belonging to a superfamily of adenosine triphosphate (ATP) binding cassette transporters, P-gp consists of two analogous halves and contains 12 potential transmembrane

---

A. Gholamrezanezhad
Research Institute for Nuclear Medicine, Tehran University of Medical Sciences,
Shariati Hospital, 14114 Tehran, Iran
e-mail: gholamrezanejhad@razi.tums.ac.ir

domains with two putative cytoplasmic sites, which utilize ATP and serves as an energy-dependent drug efflux pump [3].

Logically, the ability to predict or *in vivo* detection of MDR is of paramount importance for oncologic applications and is likely to improve patients' outcome: Several studies have confirmed that drug efflux mediated by P-gp can be blocked by methods such as *in vivo* RNA interference-mediated ablation of MDR1 P-glycoprotein [4] or many non-cytotoxic agents, including nifedipine, verapamil, quinine, amiodarone, WK-X-34, etc [5]. Circumventing MDR using these potent, non-toxic modulators of P-gp combined with conventional chemotherapy has been reported to improve the treatment efficacy [5]. Application of such an approach is, however, dependent upon precise *in vivo* diagnosis of P-gp-induced MDR or *in vitro* confirming of the existence of P-gp isoforms on tumoral cells.

On the other hand, in the current cost-conscious environment, increasing costs of management coupled with increasing drug resistance are important concerns of health care providers, which can be overcome with the adoption of techniques to predict or diagnose the MDR, before or during chemotherapy of patients with cancer [6]. This will result in a significant financial commitment from the health care system through the reduction of unnecessary and futile chemotherapies and also significant decrease in the number of side effects produced by ineffective chemotherapy in patients with MDR [6].

Numerous techniques are available to detect the existence of P-gp in tumoral tissues [3]. Immunocytochemical studies using the P-gp monoclonal antibodies, application of nucleic acid probes in northern blot and slot blot analyses, studies using monoclonal antibodies against P-gp by western immunoblot analysis, flow cytometry of fluorescent substrates and in situ RNA hybridization with nucleic acid probes have been described [3]. Although the level of P-gp can be easily investigated on tissue biopsies, detection of MDR in tumor cells during and following treatment with cytotoxic agents is not systematically performed and "the usefulness of these approaches has been limited by the labor intensity of current protocols, the invasiveness of biopsies, sampling errors from heterogeneous tumors, and the sensitivity and specificity required of RNA and antibody probes" [7]. More importantly, *in vitro* tests cannot provide any reliable information about the *in vivo* functionality of these drug efflux pumps. Hence, clinically, it would be very invaluable to be able to detect and monitor the status of tumors' chemoresistance by means of *in vivo* non-invasive tools [8] and ultimately provide a means to direct patients to specific cancer therapies [7].

9.1 ^{99m}Tc-Sestamibi, an *In Vivo* Imaging Indicator of MDR

The first study to test the hypothesis that ^{99m}Tc-Sestamibi may interact with P-gp as a novel organometallic substrate was reported by Piwnica-Worms et al. in 1993. In this way, they characterized the accumulation and inhibition profile of ^{99m}Tc-Sestamibi in MDR cell lines [7]. Their results indicated that ^{99m}Tc-Sestamibi is a transport substrate recognized by P-gp and further demonstrate the feasibility of *in vivo*

9 Oncologic Applications of Sestamibi: *In Vivo* Imaging of Multi-Drug Resistance

imaging P-gp function using a nude mouse tumor model [7]. Finally, the authors concluded that functional imaging using ^{99m}Tc-Sestamibi may provide a novel approach to rapidly detect P-gp expression in neoplastic cells *in vivo* and introduced it as a sensitive assay to evaluate functional expression of P-gp and for the quantitative investigation of the transporter modulation and regulation.

It was the beginning of the long journey to confirm that ^{99m}Tc-Sestamibi can be used as a non-invasive marker for *in vivo* diagnosis of MDR-related P-gp expression in cancer patients and their chemoresistance status. Subsequent *in vitro* and animal studies supported the potential application of ^{99m}Tc-Sestamibi for functional imaging of P-gp activity [9–15]. Using ^{99m}Tc-Sestamibi as the P-gp scintigraphic imaging agent, rapid cell accumulation (t1/2 approximately 6 min) of the agent to a steady state is observed, which is inversely proportional to P-gp levels [16, 17]. These data suggest that ^{99m}Tc-Sestamibi imaging is useful as a non-invasive technique to diagnose MDR in a variety of tumors *in vivo* [18].

On the other hand, ^{99m}Tc-Sestamibi is extruded from resistant tumoral cells by the action of P-gp and therefore ^{99m}Tc-Sestamibi scintigraphy may be less useful for tumor detection, when the tumoral cells highly express P-gp [19, 20]. In other words, expression of P-gp has negative effect on the diagnostic accuracy of ^{99m}Tc-Sestamibi imaging.

More recently, computer-aided diagnosis model has been generated, which predicts the probability of drug resistance. Using quantified ^{99m}Tc-Sestamibi efflux on tumor tissues, the model has the potential to non-invasively assign P-gp-mediated efflux correlated with MDR proteins' expression on tumoral cells to predict the therapeutic impact of a P-gp inhibitor or modulator, and to non-invasively assess the likelihood of MDR phenomenon [21].

9.2 Image Acquisition for Clinical Purposes

Different approaches have been used based on the institutions' policies. Routinely, 10–20 mCi (370–740 MBq) of ^{99m}Tc-Sestamibi is injected, intravenously. Image acquisition can be done just once (namely Single Phase Imaging Protocol), within 20 min following radiotracer injection, in order to calculate tumor-to-background (T/B) ratio. However, we strongly recommend not to use Single Phase Protocol. Passive influx of ^{99m}Tc-Sestamibi is consistently related to large plasma membrane and mitochondrial inner membrane negative potentials, as well as a reversible mitochondrial accumulation with rapid intake, allowing to achieve a maximum tumor uptake in 10–20 min. Hence, single time point ^{99m}Tc-Sestamibi imaging to assess the net temporal content of ^{99m}Tc-Sestamibi is just an indicator of tumor avidity for ^{99m}Tc-Sestamibi and a function of passive potential-dependent influx, not the function of MDR1 P-gp-mediated active extrusion of ^{99m}Tc-Sestamibi. Overexpression of P-gp, in contrast, causes an enhanced P-gp dependent outward transport or clearance (washout) of the already absorbed tracer and may not affect the early stages of ^{99m}Tc-Sestamibi uptake. For example, tissue perfusion will impact pharmacokinetics of ^{99m}Tc-Sestamibi *in vivo* in a manner that will tend to diminish P-gp-mediated phenotypic differences between tissues, when they are perfusion-limited [22]. To better understand the overall fidelity of ^{99m}Tc-Sestamibi to report MDR activity *in vivo*, dynamic imaging to extract efflux rate is strongly advised. Efflux rate indices are independent of tissue perfusion or some other confounding factors and may represent the highest quality methodology for collecting the desired information regarding activity of the efflux transposter [22]. In fact, sequential or dynamic imaging is, logically, a more effective approach to reflect the physiologic sequence of P-gp-mediated functions and to make an image of the quantity of the radiotracer expelled out from the cell: Following injection of radiotracer, the images are acquired 15 min (early imaging: ER, which show passive uptake of ^{99m}Tc-Sestamibi) and 2–3 h later (delayed imaging: DR, which reveal the remaining percentage of radiotracer in the temporal tissue after the function of P-gp). Retention index (RI) is calculated using the following formula: (DR-ER)/ER × 100%. Also data from the region of interest analysis on sequential images can be fitted with a mono-exponential function to calculate the efflux rates of ^{99m}Tc-Sestamibi from decay-corrected time-activity curves [23] or to calculate the time to half-clearance of the tracer [24]. It should be emphasized that in highly resistant tumors with high levels of P-gp expression, the process of radiotracer washout can be completed so rapidly that even the early images are negative and are unable to delineate the tumor. For example, a negative ^{99m}Tc-Sestamibi scintimammography predicts chemoresistance of breast cancers with a specificity of 100% [25]. Hence, as usual, all studies using ^{99m}Tc-Sestamibi must be interpreted in the clinical context.

SPECT acquisition is recommended and its superiority has been confirmed [26–29]. ^{99m}Tc-Sestamibi indices are calculated from the ratio of tumor ROI to a normal reference tissue (for example, contra-lateral normal ROI).

9.3 Clinical Evidences

Following *in vitro* evidences suggesting the potential of ^{99m}Tc-Sestamibi to predict the outcome in response to chemotherapy, numerous clinical evidences from different human cancers were reported, validating and emphasizing on the importance and feasibility of functional imaging with this readily available radiopharmaceutical [30]. The consistency of the results from different institutions and trials strongly support the clinical application of this scintigraphic imaging for individual tailoring of chemotherapeutic regimens and to administer P-gp modulators [31]. Also, the results were so encouraging which lead to attempts for the application of the related compounds or the design of further radiotracers with more specificity to P-gp [27, 32–39]. Subsequently, for better quantification of P-gp-mediated transport with positron emission tomography (PET) *in vivo*, a number of agents, such as [^{11}C]Colchicine, [^{11}C]Verapamil and [^{11}C]Daunorubicin or ^{124}I and [40]Br radiolabeled Doxorubicin analogues were examined. *In vivo* results suggest that these radiopharmaceuticals are useful to image P-gp function in tumors [41] and provide the possibility for separation of MDR from other variables affecting tracer uptake in tumors [42].

9.4 Breast Cancer

[99m]Tc-Sestamibi is the paradigm of new class of compounds suitable for breast imaging [24]. Early *in vitro* studies on breast cancer cell lines were discouraging, as they just relied on ^{99m}Tc-Sestamibi uptake (T/B ratio) calculation in a single time point. They reached the conclusion that ^{99m}Tc-Sestamibi uptake does not necessarily indicate that a cancer is sensitive to chemotherapeutic agents [43]. Based on the description of the function of P-gp (see the section on Image acquisition for clinical purposes), such a conclusion is expected. However, further investigations made more promising conclusions, particularly when kinetic indices such as RI were applied. In fact, these reports stated that determination of ^{99m}Tc-Sestamibi RI by sequential or dynamic imaging has the potential to be used clinically as a simple, non-invasive, and functional test to assess P-gp expression in untreated breast cancers and to identify patients with high probability to develop MDR [28, 44, 45]. We generally believe that it is better not to rely on a single phase imaging in these settings. The major advantage of ^{99m}Tc-Sestamibi scan is to make an image of the dynamic physiology of P-gp function using ^{99m}Tc-Sestamibi kinetics.

Based on these observations, human trials with promising results were published. Most of the studies confirm that the values for the T/B ratio on single static view ^{99m}Tc-Sestamibi scintimammography are significantly lower for those tumors expressing P-gp at high levels than those with scattered or no expression, showing an inverse correlation between T/B ratio and P-gp levels [25, 46–51]. However, reviewing all available reports, generally it can be concluded that on pre-chemotherapy scan, a simple ^{99m}Tc-Sestamibi T/B ratio, although very invaluable, but does not correlate with *in vitro* results of P-gp overexpression on patients' tissue specimens, constantly. Both false-positives (mastopathy) and false-negatives (wide tumor necrosis and deep location in the breast) have been described [26, 52].

On the other hand, calculating ^{99m}Tc-Sestamibi efflux rates using dynamic or sequential imaging (at least two sets of image acquisition) has an additional value on simple T/B ratios, increasing the diagnostic accuracy and reliability of the test [23, 53, 54]. ^{99m}Tc-Sestamibi efflux from breast carcinomas with high levels of P-gp expression is 2.7 times higher than that observed in benign breast lesions or carcinomas with low levels of P-gp expression, showing a sensitivity of 80% and a specificity of 95% for the *in vivo* identification of MDR [23]. In fact, ^{99m}Tc-Sestamibi RI is closely correlated to tumor chemosensitivity, suggesting that double-phase scintimammography allows preoperative prediction of chemosensitivity of breast cancer [53, 55]. A rapid tumor washout of ^{99m}Tc-Sestamibi (time to half-clearance of less than 205 min) can predict the lack of tumor response to neoadjuvant chemotherapy with drugs affected by MDR phenotype, while slower tracer clearance (> or = 205 min) does not guarantee an objective tumor response to chemotherapy in all patients, as several P-gp-independent mechanisms of MDR also exist [24]. In the other words, the presence of other factors contributing to drug sensitivity in tumor response, such as apoptosis-related genes, should be considered, when the results of [99mTc]-Sestamibi imaging are interpreted [51]. At the end, it should be noted that few reports that reject the added value of RI calculation exist, claiming on the adequacy of T/B ratios. Hence, larger patient cohorts are needed to enable a better validation of the imaging and interpretation method and to determine optimal early and delayed T/B ratios [56]. Generally, [99mTc]-Sestamibi radionuclide breast scanning is an invaluable tool to select the appropriate treatment regimen for each patient as a guide to subsequent chemotherapy [50].

9.5   Lung Cancers

A recent review of the available literature on the use of [99mTc]-Sestamibi in predicting the clinical response to chemotherapy in lung cancer has found a total of 235 patients included in 8 studies [6]. The overall sensitivity of [99mTc]-Sestamibi in identifying responders to chemotherapy is 94% with the specificity of 90%, and the accuracy of 92% [57–64]. Although the number of published studies examining the effectiveness of [99mTc]-Sestamibi in preselecting lung cancer patients before chemotherapy is limited, it can be concluded that when [99mTc]-Sestamibi is used, it is very effective in differentiating responders from non-responder patients [6]. The best scintigraphic index for predicting the response to chemotherapy is the degree of initial [99mTc]-Sestamibi uptake by the tumor, better than delayed retention, percentage washout, and RI [65]. Generally, patients who had less [99mTc]-Sestamibi uptake are less likely to respond to chemotherapy than those with more uptake [66–68]. However, some overlap in initial T/B ratio between responders and non-responders reduces the accuracy of the test [6]. Interestingly, tumor [99mTc]-Sestamibi washout rates are not very reliable in identifying non-responders. In some cases, responders show [99mTc]-Sestamibi washout as early as non-responders, although some reports emphasize on the fact that increased tumor clearance of [99mTc]-Sestamibi significantly correlates with resistance to chemotherapy as well as the existence of distant metastasis [69, 70], even better than early T/B ratios [71]. Regarding these discrepancies, we again recommend not to rely on a single scintigraphic parameter, and calculating both early and kinetic indices seems to be more helpful.

More importantly, cost-effectiveness analysis has revealed an incremental cost-effectiveness ratio of greater than £30,000 (approximately $42,900) for the strategy of treating all patients to recover the small loss of life expectancy (7.5 d) associated with the bring into play of [99mTc]-Sestamibi scintigraphy to preselect candidates for chemotherapy [6]. It has the potential to yield significant cost savings in the health care system without a significant reduction of life expectancy for patients.

Dipyridamole, the widely used drug in the pharmacologic stress protocols of cardiac imaging, is a P-gp modulator, which is able to improve the accuracy of identifying responders by nearly twofold [64]. A reduction in the initial uptake of [99mTc]-Sestamibi followed by a subsequent increase after Dipyridamole infusion is a strong negative predictor of the response to chemotherapy.

9 Oncologic Applications of Sestamibi: *In Vivo* Imaging of Multi-Drug Resistance

9.6 Brain Tumors

In vitro studies have shown that ^{99m}Tc-Sestamibi uptake is significantly (almost 50%) lower in resistant glioma cell lines [8, 72]. However, there is no agreement on the correlation between ^{99m}Tc-Sestamibi findings and MDR-1 gene expression in glioma patients, clinically. Some studies have found significant associations and support the bring into play of ^{99m}Tc-Sestamibi imaging as a non-invasive method for *in vivo* detection of MDR [73], while others have rejected this hypothesis [40, 74, 75]. Although *in vitro* studies had confirmed that P-gp expression is related to ^{99m}Tc-Sestamibi retention in brain tumors, discordant clinical results illustrated the difficulty to go from bench to bed. In the *in vivo* situation, many factors affect the imaging of a tumor, other than membrane P-gp levels, including vascular endothelium, tumor viability, etc.

Non-glioma brain tumors: RI of ^{99m}Tc-Sestamibi is significantly lower in P-gp positive meningiomas as compared to P-gp positive intracranial meningiomas and hence it can be used as a marker of P-gp-related MDR [76]. Also based on a small number of patients, it has been concluded that ^{99m}Tc-Sestamibi has the potential to predict P-gp-related MDR in pituitary adenomas [77]. Further investigations on both intracranial meningiomas and pituitary adenomas are still needed.

9.7 Lymphomas and Multiple Myeloma

^{99m}Tc-Sestamibi scan represents P-gp expression more accurately than other prognostic factors and is able to predict the chemotherapy response in malignant lymphomas [14, 78–82]. In fact, ^{99m}Tc-Sestamibi scan would be beneficial to malignant lymphoma patients. As stated earlier, we recommend measuring all scintigraphic variables, including T/B ratios of both early and late images and the washout rate, as different studies have not reached a common conclusion as to which one of the scintigraphic markers is the most reliable predictor of response to treatment.

^{99m}Tc-Sestamibi has been extensively used to study patients with multiple myeloma [83, 84]. Although ^{99m}Tc-Sestamibi scan is a useful indicator of activity of multiple myeloma, based on the discordant results obtained from different groups, further large studies are needed to evaluate the usefulness of this agent as a potential predictor of MDR in multiple myeloma. One of the major disadvantages is the fact that a partial overlap of washout values is present in different classes of P-gp expression, thus preventing the discrimination of individual patients [85].

9.8 Other Tumors

In all other tumors, the number of the reported studies and studied patients are too low that reaching a definite conclusion is problematic and further investigations are strongly needed. ^{99m}Tc-Sestamibi scintigraphy has shown no promising results to detect MDR in patients with different types of head and neck cancers [86]. Also

^{99m}Tc-Sestamibi has no role in the staging of neuroblastoma, and its value to provide prognostic information on the responsiveness to chemotherapy has not confirmed in all studies [87, 88]. False negative cases have been reported (no accumulation of ^{99m}Tc-Sestamibi in primary and metastatic foci in a patient with good response to chemotherapy) [89].

There are limited encouraging *in vitro* or *in vivo* experiences concerning the hepatic neoplasms and advanced gastric cancer [90–92]. The association of enhanced ^{99m}Tc-Sestamibi efflux in ^{99m}Tc-Sestamibi SPECT with overexpression of P-gp in hepatocellular carcinoma has been observed to be strong [93]. P-gp expression is detected in tumor tissues of all patients without ^{99m}Tc-Sestamibi uptake, whereas among patients with ^{99m}Tc-Sestamibi uptake, no P-gp expression is seen in tumor lesions. Although it seems that ^{99m}Tc-Sestamibi SPECT is useful for non-invasively forecasting the existence of MDR1 gene-encoded P-gp in patients with hepatocellular carcinoma, due to limited reported experiences, further studies in larger number of patients are advised.

^{99m}Tc-Sestamibi scintigraphy in malignant musculoskeletal sarcomas has shown discordant results in different studies. While some investigators have reported a positive correlation between the washout rate and P-gp status or therapy response [the percentage of washout of ^{99m}Tc-Sestamibi is significantly higher in patients with high P-gp expression than in those with a low Pgp score (33% vs 17%) [94–96], others have found no significant association [97]. As discussed earlier, the initial uptake of ^{99m}Tc-Sestamibi (early T/B ratio) in bone and soft tissue sarcomas and Ewing's sarcoma does not correlate with Pgp expression [94], consistently.

9.9 Monitoring or Planning of the Treatment

It seems clear that ^{99m}Tc-Sestamibi can be used before treatment to detect MDR and to predict treatment efficacy [98]. However, after initiation of the treatment, it may lose its applicability: Although it has been suggested that ^{99m}Tc-Sestamibi might be used to monitor tumor response to chemotherapy, it is unable to differentiate tumors with ongoing apoptosis from those developing MDR [98]. At early stages of tumoral cell apoptosis, the electrical driving forces of ^{99m}Tc-Sestamibi uptake are impaired, which lead to reduced influx and accumulation of the radiotracer, a finding which is seen similarly in those developing MDR. Interpreting in the clinical context decreases the shortcoming.

However, functional imaging of the malignant tumors with ^{99m}Tc-Sestamibi scintigraphy or related radiopharmaceuticals before and after administration of P-gp modulators/inhibitors or MDR gene therapy is useful to identify those patients who could benefit from P-gp manipulation [8, 32, 33, 99–103]. The modulators or inhibitors are potent enhancing agents of ^{99m}Tc-Sestamibi net uptake, and known MDR-reversing agents (such as Verapamil and cyclosporine A) enhance ^{99m}Tc-Sestamibi levels [7, 19, 104]. Unidirectional efflux of ^{99m}Tc-Sestamibi can be blocked using the P-gp inhibitors such as Verapamil [7]. In the presence of Verapamil, ^{99m}Tc-Sestamibi uptake increases by a factor of 2 in cells expressing no detectable levels of

9 Oncologic Applications of Sestamibi: *In Vivo* Imaging of Multi-Drug Resistance

P-gP, but by a factor of 12 in cells with high P-gP levels [18]. Although ^{99m}Tc-Sestamibi is useful *in vivo* as a means of monitoring the effects of MDR reversal agents on various tumors and normal tissues that express Pgp [105], in clinical practice, however, discordant therapeutic benefits for solid tumors that have accrued from use of agents that reverse the effects of P-gp have been observed, which may be explained, partly, by the fact that these agents increase the sensitivity of perivascular tumoral cells, but decrease the penetration of P-gp substrates to more distal cells [106]. Moreover, in the MDR biological diagnosis, other chemoresistant mechanisms (topoisomerases, glutathione system, etc.) could be present simultaneously or successively during tumor spreading or during successive antineoplastic treatments. Similarly, unexpected effects of MDR reversing agents on ^{99m}Tc-Sestamibi uptake are also observed [107]. Hence, although the results support the feasibility of this approach, the alteration of tracer pharmacokinetics induced by numerous confounding factors certainly constitutes a challenge in the development of a simple functional test suitable in clinical practice [108].

9.10 Conclusion

[99m]Tc-Sestamibi provides the opportunity and makes it feasible to study the functionality of MDR transporters *in vivo*, particularly in breast, lung and lymphoma cancers. This imaging technique possesses the potential to become an important tool for treatment planning. However, additional clinicopathological studies are strongly required to confirm whether ^{99m}Tc-Sestamibi uptake kinetics correlates with clinical MDR, P-gp expression, intratumoral angiogenesis, or other mechanisms.

References

1. Luqmani YA (2005) Mechanisms of drug resistance in cancer chemotherapy. Med Princ Pract 14(Suppl 1):35–48
2. Georges E, Bradley G, Gariepy J, Ling V (1990) Detection of P-glycoprotein isoforms by gene-specific monoclonal antibodies. Proc Natl Acad Sci USA 87:152–156
3. Rothenberg M, Ling V (1989) Multidrug resistance: molecular biology and clinical relevance. J Natl Cancer Inst 81:907–910
4. Pichler A, Zelcer N, Prior JL, Kuil AJ, Piwnica-Worms D (2005) *In vivo* RNA interference-mediated ablation of MDR1 P-glycoprotein. Clin Cancer Res 11:4487–4494
5. Ferry DR, Kerr DJ (1994) Multidrug resistance in cancer. BMJ 308:148–149
6. Mohan HK, Miles KA (2009) Cost-effectiveness of 99mTc-sestamibi in predicting response to chemotherapy in patients with lung cancer: systematic review and meta-analysis. J Nucl Med 50:376–381
7. Piwnica-Worms D, Chiu ML, Budding M, Kronauge JF, Kramer RA, Croop JM (1993) Functional imaging of multidrug-resistant P-glycoprotein with an organotechnetium complex. Cancer Res 53:977–984
8. Perek N, Le Jeune N, Denoyer D, Dubois F (2005) MRP-1 protein expression and glutathione content of *in vitro* tumor cell lines derived from human glioma carcinoma U-87-MG do not interact with 99mTc-glucarate uptake. Cancer Biother Radiopharm 20:391–400

9. Lorke DE, Kruger M, Buchert R, Bohuslavizki KH, Clausen M, Schumacher U (2001) *In vitro* and *in vivo* tracer characteristics of an established multidrug-resistant human colon cancer cell line. J Nucl Med 42:646–654

10. Ballinger JR, Hua HA, Berry BW, Firby P, Boxen I (1995) 99Tcm-sestamibi as an agent for imaging P-glycoprotein-mediated multi-drug resistance: *in vitro* and *in vivo* studies in a rat breast tumour cell line and its doxorubicin-resistant variant. Nucl Med Commun 16:253–257

11. Moretti JL, Duran Cordobes M, Starzec A et al (1998) Involvement of glutathione in loss of technetium-99m-MIBI accumulation related to membrane MDR protein expression in tumor cells. J Nucl Med 39:1214–1218

12. Yamaguchi S, Yachiku S, Hashimoto H et al (2002) Relation between technetium 99m-methoxyisobutylisonitrile accumulation and multidrug resistance protein in the parathyroid glands. World J Surg 26:29–34

13. Utsunomiya K, Ballinger JR, Piquette-Miller M et al (2000) Comparison of the accumulation and efflux kinetics of technetium-99m sestamibi and technetium-99m tetrofosmin in an MRP-expressing tumour cell line. Eur J Nucl Med 27:1786–1792

14. Tsai SC, Shiau YC, Wang JJ, Ho YJ, Kao CH (2001) Comparison of the uptake and clearance of Tc-99m MIBI, Tl-201 and Ga-67 in drug-resistant lymphoma cell lines. Cancer Lett 171:147–152

15. Marian T, Szabo G, Goda K et al (2003) *In vivo* and *in vitro* multitracer analyses of P-glycoprotein expression-related multidrug resistance. Eur J Nucl Med Mol Imaging 30:1147–1154

16. Ballinger JR, Bannerman J, Boxen I, Firby P, Hartman NG, Moore MJ (1996) Technetium-99m-tetrofosmin as a substrate for P-glycoprotein: *in vitro* studies in multidrug-resistant breast tumor cells. J Nucl Med 37:1578–1582

17. Piwnica-Worms D, Rao VV, Kronauge JF, Croop JM (1995) Characterization of multidrug resistance P-glycoprotein transport function with an organotechnetium cation. Biochemistry 34:12210–12220

18. Cordobes MD, Starzec A, Delmon-Moingeon L et al (1996) Technetium-99m-sestamibi uptake by human benign and malignant breast tumor cells: correlation with mdr gene expression. J Nucl Med 37:286–289

19. Ballinger JR, Sheldon KM, Boxen I, Erlichman C, Ling V (1995) Differences between accumulation of 99mTc-MIBI and 201Tl-thallous chloride in tumour cells: role of P-glycoprotein. Q J Nucl Med 39:122–128

20. Gomes CM, Abrunhosa AJ, Pauwels EK, Botelho MF (2009) P-glycoprotein versus MRP1 on transport kinetics of cationic lipophilic substrates: a comparative study using [99mTc]sestamibi and [99mTc]tetrofosmin. Cancer Biother Radiopharm 24:215–227

21. van Leeuwen FW, Buckle T, Kersbergen A, Rottenberg S, Gilhuijs KG (2009) Noninvasive functional imaging of P-glycoprotein-mediated doxorubicin resistance in a mouse model of hereditary breast cancer to predict response, and assign P-gp inhibitor sensitivity. Eur J Nucl Med Mol Imaging 36:406–412

22. Bae KT, Piwnica-Worms D (1997) Pharmacokinetic modeling of multidrug resistance P-glycoprotein transport of gamma-emitting substrates. Q J Nucl Med 41:101–110

23. Vecchio SD, Ciarmiello A, Potena MI et al (1997) *In vivo* detection of multidrug-resistant (MDR1) phenotype by technetium-99m sestamibi scan in untreated breast cancer patients. Eur J Nucl Med 24:150–159

24. Salvatore M, Del Vecchio S (1998) Dynamic imaging: scintimammography. Eur J Radiol 27(Suppl 2):S259–S264

25. Cayre A, Cachin F, Maublant J et al (2002) Single static view 99mTc-sestamibi scintimammography predicts response to neoadjuvant chemotherapy and is related to MDR expression. Int J Oncol 20:1049–1055

26. Sergieva SB, Timcheva KV, Hadjiolov ND (2006) 99mTc-MIBI scintigraphy as a functional method for the evaluation of multidrug resistance in breast cancer patients. J BUON 11:61–68

27. Liu Z, Stevenson GD, Barrett HH et al (2005) Imaging recognition of inhibition of multidrug resistance in human breast cancer xenografts using 99mTc-labeled sestamibi and tetrofosmin. Nucl Med Biol 32:573–583

28. Liu Z, Stevenson GD, Barrett HH et al (2004) Imaging recognition of multidrug resistance in human breast tumors using 99mTc-labeled monocationic agents and a high-resolution stationary SPECT system. Nucl Med Biol 31:53–65
29. Dirlik A, Burak Z, Goksel T et al (2002) The role of Tc-99m sestamibi imaging in predicting clinical response to chemotherapy in lung cancer. Ann Nucl Med 16:103–108
30. Moretti JL, Caglar M, Boaziz C, Caillat-Vigneron N, Morere JF (1995) Sequential functional imaging with technetium-99m hexakis-2-methoxyisobutylisonitrile and indium-111 octreotide: Can we predict the response to chemotherapy in small cell lung cancer? Eur J Nucl Med 22:177–180
31. Del Vecchio S, Ciarmiello A, Salvatore M (2000) Scintigraphic detection of multidrug resistance in cancer. Cancer Biother Radiopharm 15:327–337
32. Chen WS, Luker KE, Dahlheimer JL, Pica CM, Luker GD, Piwnica-Worms D (2000) Effects of MDR1 and MDR3 P-glycoproteins, MRP1, and BCRP/MXR/ABCP on the transport of (99m)Tc-tetrofosmin. Biochem Pharmacol 60:413–426
33. Muzzammil T, Moore MJ, Ballinger JR (2000) In vitro comparison of sestamibi, tetrofosmin, and furifosmin as agents for functional imaging of multidrug resistance in tumors. Cancer Biother Radiopharm 15:339–346
34. Dyszlewski M, Blake HM, Dahlheimer JL, Pica CM, Piwnica-Worms D (2002) Characterization of a novel 99mTc-carbonyl complex as a functional probe of MDR1 P-glycoprotein transport activity. Mol Imaging 1:24–35
35. Ballinger JR, Muzzammil T, Moore MJ (1997) Technetium-99m-furifosmin as an agent for functional imaging of multidrug resistance in tumors. J Nucl Med 38:1915–1919
36. Rao VV, Herman LW, Kronauge JF, Piwnica-Worms D (1998) A novel areneisonitrile Tc complex inhibits the transport activity of MDR P-glycoprotein. Nucl Med Biol 25:225–232
37. Crankshaw CL, Marmion M, Luker GD et al (1998) Novel technetium (III)-Q complexes for functional imaging of multidrug resistance (MDR1) P-glycoprotein. J Nucl Med 39:77–86
38. Bergmann R, Brust P, Scheunemann M et al (2000) Assessment of the in vitro and in vivo properties of a (99m)Tc-labeled inhibitor of the multidrug resistant gene product P-glycoprotein. Nucl Med Biol 27:135–141
39. Ballinger JR (2001) 99mTc-tetrofosmin for functional imaging of P-glycoprotein modulation in vivo. J Clin Pharmacol 41(Suppl):39S–47S
40. Yokogami K, Kawano H, Moriyama T et al (1998) Application of SPET using technetium 99m sestamibi in brain tumours and comparison with expression of the MDR-1 gene: Is it possible to predict the response to chemotherapy in patients with gliomas by means of 99mTc-sestamibi SPET? Eur J Nucl Med 25:401–409
41. Hendrikse NH (2000) Monitoring interactions at ATP-dependent drug efflux pumps. Curr Pharm Des 6:1653–1668
42. Lewis JS, Dearling JL, Sosabowski JK et al (2000) Copper bis(diphosphine) complexes: radiopharmaceuticals for the detection of multi-drug resistance in tumours by PET. Eur J Nucl Med 27:638–646
43. Kabasakal L, Ozker K, Hayward M et al (1996) Technetium-99m sestamibi uptake in human breast carcinoma cell lines displaying glutathione-associated drug-resistance. Eur J Nucl Med 23:568–570
44. Del Vecchio S, Ciarmiello A, Pace L et al (1997) Fractional retention of technetium-99m-sestamibi as an index of P-glycoprotein expression in untreated breast cancer patients. J Nucl Med 38:1348–1351
45. Muzzammil T, Ballinger JR, Moore MJ (1999) 99Tcm-sestamibi imaging of inhibition of the multidrug resistance transporter in a mouse xenograft model of human breast cancer. Nucl Med Commun 20:115–122
46. Kostakoglu L, Elahi N, Kiratli P et al (1997) Clinical validation of the influence of P-glycoprotein on technetium-99m-sestamibi uptake in malignant tumors. J Nucl Med 38:1003–1008
47. Sun SS, Hsieh JF, Tsai SC, Ho YJ, Kao CH (2000) Expression of drug resistance protein related to Tc-99m MIBI breast imaging. Anticancer Res 20:2021–2025

48. Sun SS, Hsieh JF, Tsai SC, Ho YJ, Lee JK, Kao CH (2000) Expression of mediated P-glycoprotein multidrug resistance related to Tc-99m MIBI scintimammography results. Cancer Lett 153:95–100

49. Kao CH, Tsai SC, Liu TJ et al (2001) P-Glycoprotein and multidrug resistance-related protein expressions in relation to technetium-99m methoxyisobutylisonitrile scintimammography findings. Cancer Res 61:1412–1414

50. Alonso O, Delgado L, Nunez M et al (2002) Predictive value of (99m)Tc sestamibi scintigraphy in the evaluation of doxorubicin based chemotherapy response in patients with advanced breast cancer. Nucl Med Commun 23:765–771

51. Kim R, Osaki A, Hirai T, Toge T (2002) Utility of technetium-99m methoxyisobutyl isonitrile uptake analysis for prediction of the response to chemotherapy in advanced and relapsed breast cancer. Breast Cancer 9:240–247

52. Baena-Canada JM, Partida-Palma F, Palomo-Gonzalez MJ, Benitez E, Rueda-Ramos A, Garcia-Curiel A (2005) Evaluation of response to neoadjuvant chemotherapy using breast scintigraphy in breast cancer. Med Clin Barc 125:601–605

53. Fujii H, Nakamura K, Kubo A et al (1998) Preoperative evaluation of the chemosensitivity of breast cancer by means of double phase 99mTc-MIBI scintimammography. Ann Nucl Med 12:307–312

54. Cui SD, Liu ZZ, Liu H, Li LF, Yang H, Li WL (2005) The relationship between 99mTc-MIBI scintimammography of breast cancer and multidrug-resistant proteins. Zhonghua Zhong Liu Za Zhi 27:606–608

55. Mubashar M, Harrington KJ, Chaudhary KS et al (2002) 99mTc-sestamibi imaging in the assessment of toremifene as a modulator of multidrug resistance in patients with breast cancer. J Nucl Med 43:519–525

56. Kim IJ, Bae YT, Kim SJ, Kim YK, Kim DS, Lee JS (2006) Determination and prediction of P-glycoprotein and multidrug-resistance-related protein expression in breast cancer with double-phase technetium-99m sestamibi scintimammography. Visual and quantitative analyses. Oncology 70:403–410

57. Yamamoto Y, Nishiyama Y, Fukunaga K, Satoh K, Fujita J, Ohkawa M (2001) 99mTc-MIBI SPECT in small cell lung cancer patients before chemotherapy and after unresponsive chemotherapy. Ann Nucl Med 15:329–335

58. Yüksel M, Cermik TF, Karlikaya C et al (2001) Monitoring the chemotherapeutic response in primary lung cancer using 99mTc-MIBI SPET. Eur J Nucl Med Mol Imaging 28:799–806

59. Yüksel M, Cermik TF, Do anay L et al (2002) 99mTc-MIBI SPET in non-small cell lung cancer in relationship with Pgp and prognosis. Eur J Nucl Med Mol Imaging 29:876–881

60. Kao A, Shiun SC, Hsu NY, Sun SS, Lee CC, Lin CC (2001) Technetium-99m methoxyisobutylisonitrile chest imaging for small-cell lung cancer: relationship to chemotherapy response (six courses of combination of cisplatin and etoposide) and p-glycoprotein or multidrug resistance related protein expression. Ann Oncol 12:1561–1566

61. Nishiyama Y, Yamamoto Y, Satoh K et al (2000) Comparative study of Tc-99m MIBI and Tl-201 SPECT in predicting chemotherapeutic response in non-small-cell lung cancer. Clin Nucl Med 25:364–369

62. Kao CH, Hsieh JF, Tsai SC, Ho YJ, Lee JK (2000) Quickly predicting chemotherapy response to paclitaxel-based therapy in non-small cell lung cancer by early technetium-99m methoxyisobutylisonitrile chest single-photon-emission computed tomography. Clin Cancer Res 6:820–824

63. Ceriani L, Giovanella L, Bandera M, Beghe B, Ortelli M, Roncari G (1997) Semiquantitative assessment of 99Tcm-sestamibi uptake in lung cancer: relationship with clinical response to chemotherapy. Nucl Med Commun 18:1087–1097

64. Bom HS, Lim SC, Kim YC et al (1999) Dipyridamole modulated Tc-99m sestamibi lung SPECT in small cell lung cancer. Clin Nucl Med 24:97–101

65. Kostakoglu L, Kiratli P, Ruacan S et al (1998) Association of tumor washout rates and accumulation of technetium-99m-MIBI with expression of P-glycoprotein in lung cancer. J Nucl Med 39:228–234

9 Oncologic Applications of Sestamibi: *In Vivo* Imaging of Multi-Drug Resistance

66. Bom HS, Kim YC, Song HC, Min JJ, Kim JY, Park KO (1998) Technetium-99m-MIBI uptake in small cell lung cancer. J Nucl Med 39:91–94
67. Kao CH, ChangLai SP, Chieng PU, Yen TC (1998) Technetium-99m methoxyisobutylisonitrile chest imaging of small cell lung carcinoma: relation to patient prognosis and chemotherapy response–a preliminary report. Cancer 83:64–68
68. Shih CM, Hsu WH, Huang WT, Wang JJ, Ho ST, Kao A (2003) Usefulness of chest single photon emission computed tomography with technetium-99m methoxyisobutylisonitrile to predict taxol based chemotherapy response in advanced non-small cell lung cancer. Cancer Lett 199:99–105
69. Koukourakis MI, Koukouraki S, Giatromanolaki A, Skarlatos J, Georgoulias V, Karkavitsas N (1997) Non-small cell lung cancer functional imaging: increased hexakis-2-methoxy-isobutyl-isonitrile tumor clearance correlates with resistance to cytotoxic treatment. Clin Cancer Res 3:749–754
70. Zhou J, Higashi K, Ueda Y et al (2001) Expression of multidrug resistance protein and messenger RNA correlate with (99m)Tc-MIBI imaging in patients with lung cancer. J Nucl Med 42:1476–1483
71. Ak I, Gulbas Z, Ocak S et al (2007) TC-99m MIBI SPECT imaging in patients with lung carcinoma: Is it a functional probe of multidrug resistance genes? J Comput Assist Tomogr 31:795–799
72. Sasajima T, Shimada N, Naitoh Y et al (2007) (99m)Tc-MIBI imaging for prediction of therapeutic effects of second-generation MDR1 inhibitors in malignant brain tumors. Int J Cancer 121:2637–2645
73. Andrews DW, Das R, Kim S, Zhang J, Curtis M (1997) Technetium-MIBI as a glioma imaging agent for the assessment of multi-drug resistance. Neurosurgery 40:1323–1332, discussion 33–34
74. Shibata Y, Matsumura A, Nose T (2002) Effect of expression of P-glycoprotein on technetium-99m methoxyisobutylisonitrile single photon emission computed tomography of brain tumors. Neurol Med Chir Tokyo 42:325–330, discussion 30–31
75. Hau P, Fabel K, Baumgart U et al (2004) Pegylated liposomal doxorubicin-efficacy in patients with recurrent high-grade glioma. Cancer 100:1199–1207
76. Kunishio K, Morisaki K, Matsumoto Y, Nagao S, Nishiyama Y (2003) Technetium-99m sestamibi single photon emission computed tomography findings correlated with P-glycoprotein expression, encoded by the multidrug resistance gene-1 messenger ribonucleic acid, in intracranial meningiomas. Neurol Med Chir Tokyo 43:573–580, discussion 81
77. Kunishio K, Okada M, Matsumoto Y, Nagao S, Nishiyama Y (2006) Technetium 99m sesta mibi single photon emission computed tomography findings correlated with P-glycoprotein expression in pituitary adenoma. J Med Invest 53:285–291
78. Kao CH, Tsai SC, Wang JJ, Ho YJ, Ho ST, Changlai SP (2001) Technetium-99m-sestamethoxyisobutylisonitrile scan as a predictor of chemotherapy response in malignant lymphomas compared with P-glycoprotein expression, multidrug resistance-related protein expression and other prognosis factors. Br J Haematol 113:369–374
79. Qiao SK, Guo XN, Wang Y, Xu SR (2007) The clinical value of the 99Tcm-MIBI imaging in predicting the prognosis of malignant lymphoma. Zhonghua Yi Xue Za Zhi 87:2003–2006
80. Shih WJ, Rastogi A, Stipp V, Magoun S, Coupal J (1998) Functional retention of Tc-99m MIBI in mediastinal lymphomas as a predictor of chemotherapeutic response demonstrated by consecutive thoracic SPECT imaging. Clin Nucl Med 23:505–508
81. Kostakoglu L (2002) Noninvasive detection of multidrug resistance in patients with hematological malignancies: Are we there yet? Clin Lymphoma 2:242–248
82. Ak I, Aslan V, Vardareli E, Gulbas Z (2003) Assessment of the P-glycoprotein expression by 99mTc-MIBI bone marrow imaging in patients with untreated leukaemia. Nucl Med Commun 24:397–402
83. Pace L, Catalano L, Del Vecchio S et al (2005) Washout of [99mTc] sestamibi in predicting response to chemotherapy in patients with multiple myeloma. Q J Nucl Med Mol Imaging 49:281–285
84. Fallahi B, Beiki D, Mousavi SA et al (2009) 99mTc-MIBI whole body scintigraphy and P-glycoprotein for the prediction of multiple drug resistance in multiple myeloma patients. Hell J Nucl Med 12:255–259

85. Fonti R, Del Vecchio S, Zannetti A et al (2004) Functional imaging of multidrug resistant phenotype by 99mTc-MIBI scan in patients with multiple myeloma. Cancer Biother Radiopharm 19:165–170
86. Leitha T, Glaser C, Lang S (1998) Is early sestamibi imaging in head and neck cancer affected by MDR status, p53 expression, or cell proliferation? Nucl Med Biol 25:539–541
87. Burak Z, Yuksel DA, Cetingul N, Kantar M, Ozkilic H, Moretti JL (1999) The role of 99Tcm-sestamibi scintigraphy in the staging and prediction of the therapeutic response of stage IV neuroblastoma: comparison with 131I-MIBG and 99Tcm-MDP scintigraphy. Nucl Med Commun 20:991–1000
88. De Moerloose B (2005) The prognostic significance of P-glycoprotein in children with acute lymphoblastic leukemia and neuroblastoma. Verh K Acad Geneeskd Belg 67:45–54
89. Ozcan Z, Erenel G, Aksoylar S, Kansoy S, Burak Z, Ozkilic H (1999) False-negative scintigraphy with Tc-99m sestamibi in stage IV neuroblastoma. Clin Nucl Med 24:267–270
90. Han Y, Chen XP, Huang ZY, Zhu H (2005) Nude mice multi-drug resistance model of orthotopic transplantation of liver neoplasm and Tc-99m MIBI SPECT on p-glycoprotein. World J Gastroenterol 11:3335–3338
91. Chang CS, Yang SS, Yeh HZ, Kao CH, Chen GH (2004) Tc-99m MIBI liver imaging for hepatocellular carcinoma: correlation with P-glycoprotein-multidrug-resistance gene expression. Hepatogastroenterology 51:211–214
92. Kawata K, Kanai M, Sasada T, Iwata S, Yamamoto N, Takabayashi A (2004) Usefulness of 99mTc-sestamibi scintigraphy in suggesting the therapeutic effect of chemotherapy against gastric cancer. Clin Cancer Res 10:3788–3793
93. Kim YS, Cho SW, Lee KJ et al (1999) Tc-99m MIBI SPECT is useful for noninvasively predicting the presence of MDR1 gene-encoded P-glycoprotein in patients with hepatocellular carcinoma. Clin Nucl Med 24:874–879
94. Burak Z, Ersoy O, Moretti JL et al (2001) The role of 99mTc-MIBI scintigraphy in the assessment of MDR1 overexpression in patients with musculoskeletal sarcomas: comparison with therapy response. Eur J Nucl Med 28:1341–1350
95. Burak Z, Moretti JL, Ersoy O et al (2003) 99mTc-MIBI imaging as a predictor of therapy response in osteosarcoma compared with multidrug resistance-associated protein and P-glycoprotein expression. J Nucl Med 44:1394–1401
96. Gomes CM, Welling M, Que I et al (2007) Functional imaging of multidrug resistance in an orthotopic model of osteosarcoma using 99mTc-sestamibi. Eur J Nucl Med Mol Imaging 34:1793–1803
97. Gorlick R, Liao AC, Antonescu C et al (2001) Lack of correlation of functional scintigraphy with (99m)technetium-methoxyisobutylisonitrile with histological necrosis following induction chemotherapy or measures of P-glycoprotein expression in high-grade osteosarcoma. Clin Cancer Res 7:3065–3070
98. Moretti JL, Hauet N, Caglar M, Rebillard O, Burak Z (2005) To use MIBI or not to use MIBI? That is the question when assessing tumour cells. Eur J Nucl Med Mol Imaging 32:836–842
99. Pusztai L, Wagner P, Ibrahim N et al (2005) Phase II study of tariquidar, a selective P-glycoprotein inhibitor, in patients with chemotherapy-resistant, advanced breast carcinoma. Cancer 104:682–691
100. Fuster D, Vinolas N, Mallafre C, Pavia J, Martin F, Pons F (2003) Tetrofosmin as predictors of tumour response. Q J Nucl Med 47:58–62
101. Gruber A, Arestrom I, Xu D, Liliemark J, Larsson SA, Jacobsson H (1998) Multidrug resistance phenotype in leukaemic cells from patients with acute myelocytic leukaemia can be detected with 99Tc(m)-MIBI. Br J Cancer 77:1732–1736
102. Bates SF, Chen C, Robey R, Kang M, Figg WD, Fojo T (2002) Reversal of multidrug resistance: lessons from clinical oncology. Novartis Found Symp 243:83–96, discussion 102, 80–85
103. Jekerle V, Wang JH, Scollard DA, Reilly RM, Wiese M, Piquette-Miller M (2006) 99mTc-Sestamibi, a sensitive probe for *in vivo* imaging of P-glycoprotein inhibition by modulators and mdr1 antisense oligodeoxynucleotides. Mol Imaging Biol 8:333–339

104. Tatsumi M, Tsuruo T, Nishimura T (2002) Evaluation of MS-209, a novel multidrug-resistance-reversing agent, in tumour-bearing mice by technetium-99m-MIBI imaging. Eur J Nucl Med Mol Imaging 29:288–294
105. Chen CC, Meadows B, Regis J et al (1997) Detection of *in vivo* P-glycoprotein inhibition by PSC 833 using Tc-99m sestamibi. Clin Cancer Res 3:545–552
106. Tunggal JK, Melo T, Ballinger JR, Tannock IF (2000) The influence of expression of P-glycoprotein on the penetration of anticancer drugs through multicellular layers. Int J Cancer 86:101–107
107. Cayre A, Moins N, Finat-Duclos F, Verrelle P, Maublant J (1997) Comparison between technetium-99m-sestamibi and hydrogen-3-daunomycin myocardial cellular retention *in vitro*. J Nucl Med 38:1674–1677
108. Del Vecchio S, Ciarmiello A, Salvatore M (1999) Clinical imaging of multidrug resistance in cancer. Q J Nucl Med 43:125–131

Index

A
Absorbed dose, definition of, 16
ALARA principle, 13
Anger scintillation camera, 8
Attenuation correction, 9

B
Biokinitic model, of ^{99m}Tc MIBI, 13
Bone tumors, 167–168
Brain tumors
    MDR, 181
    hexakis–2-methoxy–2-methylpropyl-
        isontrile technetium–99m, 164–165
Breast cancer, MDR, 179–180

C
Carboxymethylisopropylisonitrile (CPI), 3
Cardiolite™, 4
CPI. *See* Carboxymethylisopropylisonitrile
    (CPI)
CTCA. *See* CT imaging of the Coronary
    Arteries (CTCA)
CT imaging of the Coronary Arteries
    (CTCA), 19
Cumulated activity per injected activity, 17

E
Exercise and pharmacologic stress testing, 68

F
Fatal cancer, induction of, 12, 17
FDG-PET
    lung cancer, 160
    PET-associated incidental positive
        thyroid (PAINs), 144
    thyroid nodule imaging, 143–144

First-pass radionuclide ventriculography
    (FPRNV), 75
Flip-flop-phenomenon, 147

G
Gamma camera, 8
Gamma-ray(s)
    emissions, 10
    release of, 7
    scattering, 10–11
Gastrointestinal tumors, 168

H
Heart-to-organ ratios, 15
Hexakis (2-methoxyisobutyl isonitrile)
        technetium preparation
    ability to drive and use machines, 27
    chemistry and constituents, 25
    interaction with other medicinal
        products and other forms, 27
    organs at risk, 26
    overdosage, 27
    photon energy, 25
    radio-TLC method, 29–30
    special warning and precautions
        for use, 26
    technical aspects
        aseptic procedure, 27–28
        quality control, 28–29
    undesirable effects, 27
Hodgkin's lymphoma, 166
HPLC-chromatogram, of ^{99m}Tc MIBI, 5
Hyperparathyroidism (HPT)
    primary (*see* Primary hyperparathyroidism)
    secondary (*see* Secondary
        hyperparathyroidism)

J. Bucerius et al. (eds.), *^{99m}Tc-Sestamibi*,
DOI 10.1007/978-3-642-04233-1, © Springer-Verlag Berlin Heidelberg 2012

I

Intraoperative parathyroid detection, 41–42
Isonitriles, 4

L

Lung cancers
  FDG-PET, 160
  MDR, 180
  mediastinal lymph node metastases, 161
  non-small cell lung cancers (NSCLC), 159
  small cell lung cancers (SCLC), 159
  SPECT study, 160–162
  types, 159
Lymphomas
  and multiple myeloma, MDR, 181
  hexakis–2-methoxy–2-methylpropyl-
      isontrile technetium–99m, 166–167

M

MDR. *See* Multi-drug resistance (MDR)
2-Methoxy-isobutylisonitrile (^{99m}Tc MIBI)
  and amiodarone-induced thyrotoxicosis,
      145–146
  biokinitic model, 13
  cold/hypofunctioning thyroid nodules
    aim, 135
    benign thyroid nodule, 139
    clinical usage, 141–143
    diagnostic/therapeutic indications, 136
    doses and method of administration, 137
    golden standard, 141
    positive predictive value, 140
    problems with FNAB, 135
    thyroid imaging technique and image
        interpretation, 137–139
    ultrasound, 136
    uptake mechanism, 136
  F–18-FDG-PET
    PET-associated incidental positive
        thyroid (PAINs), 144
    thyroid nodule imaging, 143–144
  imaging medullary thyroid carcinoma,
      150–152
  MPS (*see* Myocardial perfusion scintigra-
      phy (MPS), 99mTc-MIBI)
  and multidrug resistance, 144–145
  radiochemistry and radiopharmacy
    HPLC-chromatogram of, 5
    labelled heart imaging agents, 2–4
    ^{99m}Tc characteristics of, 1–2
    PET/CT-technology, 1
  radiolabelling and quality control, 4–5
  structure of, 4

thyroid, basic anatomy and physiology,
    133–134
  thyroid carcinoma, 146–150
MIBI blood clearance, 13–14
Molybdenum–99 (99Mo), decay of, 7–8
Monte Carlo model, 10
^{99m}Tc
  characteristics of, 1–2
  decay, radiation physics, 7–10
  imaging principles, 7–10
  labelled heart imaging agents, 2–4
  radiation characteristics, 8–9
^{99m}Tc MIBI. *See* 2-Methoxy-isobutylisonitrile
    (^{99m}Tc MIBI)
^{99m}TcN-NOET, structure of, 4
^{99m}Tc-teboroxime, structure of, 4
^{99m}Tc-tetrofosmin, structure of, 4
Multi-drug resistance (MDR)
  -associated protein expression, 39
  brain tumors, 181
  breast cancer, 179–180
  clinical evidences, 178
  computer-aided diagnosis model, 177
  definition, 175
  image acquisition, 177–178
  immunocytochemistry, 176
  lung cancers, 180
  lymphomas and multiple myeloma, 181
  other tumors, 181–182
  P-glycoprotein, 175
  and Tc–99m-MIBI, 144–145
  transporter modulation and regulation, 177
  treatment monitoring/planning, 182–183
Multiple myeloma (MM), 162–163
µ-map, 9–10
Myocardial perfusion imaging
  dose estimates for, 22
  radiation exposure from, 23
Myocardial perfusion scintigraphy (MPS),
      99mTc-MIBI
  acute coronary syndrome, 74–75
  as agent, 67–68
  in assessment, 69–71
  biodistribution, rest and stress, 67
  blood clearance, 66
  ECG-gated SPECT, 75–77
  ejection fraction and regional
      wall motion, 75
  exercise and pharmacologic
      stress testing, 68
  photon energy, 65
  physical and biological half-life, 65
  redistribution, 66

Index 193

risk stratification, coronary artery disease (CAD), 72–74
sensitivity and specificity, 69
stress-only imaging strategy, 68–69
vs. Tl–201 and radiation exposure, 66
uptake, 66
Myoview™, 3

N
Na+/K+ ATPase pump system, 2
Non-Hodgkin's lymphoma, 166
Non-small cell lung cancers (NSCLC), 159

O
Olinda/EXM, 16
Organ dosimetry, 15
Organ residence time, 17

P
Parathyroid imaging
biological factors, 38
concomitant thyroid disease, 40
correlative imaging *vs.* ultrasound, 49
cost-effectiveness, sestamibi, 42
differential diagnosis, thyroid nodules and adenomas, 36
glands, 31
intraoperative parathyroid detection, 41–42
nodular goitre, hyperparathyroidism, 37
pitfalls, 40–41
primary hyperparathyroidism (IIPT)
adenomas, solitary, 43
gamma probe guidance, 44
hypocalcemia rates, 42
minimally invasive parathyroidectomy (MIP) techniques, 43
types of readings, 45
visual inspection, 46
radiation exposure, radiopharmaceuticals, 49, 56
radiochemical purity, 39
recommended injected activity and dosimetry, 36
secondary hyperparathyroidism (HPT)
dual-phase ^{99m}Tc-Sestamibi scintigraphy, 46
high sensitivity and specificity, 48
positive uptake, 47
re-operation, 47
sensitivity and specificity, ^{99m}Tc-Sestamibi, 48–49
sestamibi and histology, 39–40

solid thyroid nodule, 37
SPECT, 36
subtraction and dual-tracer technique, 32–35
Partial volume effect, of SPECT imaging, 11–12
Pertechnetate anion ($[^{99m}$Tc$]$TcO$_4$-), 2
PET-associated incidental positive thyroid (PAINs), 144
PET/CT-technology, 1
P-glycoprotein, 39
Physical and biological half-life, 65
Primary hyperparathyroidism
adenomas, solitary, 43
gamma probe guidance, 44
hypocalcemia rates, 42
minimally invasive parathyroidectomy (MIP) techniques, 43
types of readings, 45
visual inspection, 46

Q
Q12, structure of, 4

R
Radiation dosimetry
for ^{99m}Tc MIBI, 12–13, 16–22
scintimammography, 101–102
Radiation exposure
from myocardial perfusion agents, 23
in tissue, 16
Radiation physics, of ^{99m}Tc, 7–10
Radiochemistry and radiopharmacy, of ^{99m}Tc MIBI
HPLC-chromatogram of, 5
labelled heart imaging agents, 2–4
^{99m}Tc, 1–2
PET/CT-technology, 1
radiolabelling and quality control of, 4–5
Radioiodine-negative metastases, 147–149
Radiolabelling and quality control, of ^{99m}Tc MIBI, 4–5
Radionuclide dosimetry, 16
Radio-TLC method, 29–30
Revised European-American Lymphoma (REAL) classification, 166

S
Scatter correction, 10–11
Scintimammography
axillary lymph node involvement detection, 112–115

chemotherapeutic response, 120
false-positive uptake, 102
female mammary glands characteristics, 87
vs. functional imaging, FDG PET, 103–108
high breast density, 101
histopathological evaluation, 117
hybrid *vs.* planar imaging, 121
image acquisition, 99–100
image-guided percutaneous breast
        biopsy, 91
indications, 93–94
locoregional recurrence, 119
lymph node metastases detection, 118
methods, 96–97
microcalcifications, 118
vs. morphological imaging, 108–112
negative transmembrane potential, 92
number of recurrence, 115–116
occult cancer detection, 117
palliative therapy, 92
physiological distribution, 99
precautions, 97
protective pump, 93
radiation dosimetry, 101–102
receiver operating curve (ROC) analysis,
        120
residual/multifocal disease, 119
response to chemotherapy, 116
risk factors, 103, 107
screening method, 103
screening modality, 91
Society of Nuclear Medicine (SNM) prac-
        tice guide lines, 94–96
sources of error, 101
TNM classification, 88–90
tracer injection, dosage and administration,
        97–99
UICC staging, 88, 90
Secondary hyperparathyroidism
dual-phase ^{99m}Tc-Sestamibi scintigraphy, 46
high sensitivity and specificity, 48
positive uptake, 47
re-operation, 47
Single photon emission gamma camera
        tomography (SPECT)
definition, 8
spatial resolution and and partial volume
        effect, 11–12

Small cell lung cancers (SCLC), 159
SPECT. *See* Single photon emission gamma
        camera tomography (SPECT)
Stannous(II) ions, 2
S-value, 16

T
Tc–99m-hexakis-t-butylisonitrile (Tc–99mT-
        BI), 2
Tc–99m MIBI. *See* 2-Methoxy-isobutyli-
        sonitrile (^{99m}Tc MIBI)
Tc–99mTBI. *See* Tc–99m-hexakis-t-butyli-
        sonitrile (Tc–99mTBI)
TCT. *See* Transmission scans (TCT)
Thallium–201 cation, 2
Thyroid, Tc–99m-MIBI
basic anatomy and physiology, 133–134
carcinoma
        vs. FDG-PET, 149–150
        flip-flop-phenomenon, 147
        radioiodine-negative metastases,
                147–149
        risk factors, 146
nodules
        aim, 135
        benign thyroid nodule, 139
        clinical usage, 141–143
        diagnostic/therapeutic
                indications, 136
        doses and method of administration, 137
        golden standard, 141
        positive predictive value, 140
        prevalence and management, 134
        problems with FNAB, 135
        results of, 139–141
        thyroid imaging technique and image
                interpretation, 137–139
        ultrasound, 136
        uptake mechanism, 136
^{201}Tl myocardial perfusion imaging, 12–13
Transmission scans (TCT), 9

U
Upper-body organ distribution, 14–15

X
X-ray CT imaging, 9